Intelligent Systems Reference Library

Volume 192

The aim of this series is to publish a Reference Library, including novel advances and developments in all aspects of Intelligent Systems in an easily accessible and well structured form. The series includes reference works, handbooks, compendia, textbooks, well-structured monographs, dictionaries, and encyclopedias. It contains well integrated knowledge and current information in the field of Intelligent Systems. The series covers the theory, applications, and design methods of Intelligent Systems. Virtually all disciplines such as engineering, computer science, avionics, business, e-commerce, environment, healthcare, physics and life science are included. The list of topics spans all the areas of modern intelligent systems such as: Ambient intelligence, Computational intelligence, Social intelligence, Computational neuroscience, Artificial life, Virtual society, Cognitive systems, DNA and immunity-based systems, e-Learning and teaching, Human-centred computing and Machine ethics, Intelligent control, Intelligent data analysis, Knowledge-based paradigms, Knowledge management, Intelligent agents, Intelligent decision making, Intelligent network security, Interactive entertainment, Learning paradigms, Recommender systems, Robotics and Mechatronics including human-machine teaming, Self-organizing and adaptive systems, Soft computing including Neural systems, Fuzzy systems, Evolutionary computing and the Fusion of these paradigms, Perception and Vision, Web intelligence and Multimedia.

** Indexing: The books of this series are submitted to ISI Web of Science, SCOPUS, DBLP and Springerlink.

More information about this series at http://www.springer.com/series/8578

Md Atiqur Rahman Ahad · Mosabber Uddin Ahmed
Editors

Signal Processing Techniques for Computational Health Informatics

Springer

Editors
Md Atiqur Rahman Ahad
Department of Electrical
and Electronic Engineering
University of Dhaka
Dhaka, Bangladesh

Department of Media Intelligent
Osaka University
Ibaraki, Osaka, Japan

Mosabber Uddin Ahmed
Department of Electrical
and Electronic Engineering
University of Dhaka
Dhaka, Bangladesh

ISSN 1868-4394 ISSN 1868-4408 (electronic)
Intelligent Systems Reference Library
ISBN 978-3-030-54931-2 ISBN 978-3-030-54932-9 (eBook)
https://doi.org/10.1007/978-3-030-54932-9

This Springer imprint is published by the registered company Springer Nature Switzerland AG
The registered company address is: Gewerbestrasse 11, 6330 Cham, Switzerland

Foreword

I first met Ahad over a decade ago at *IEEE Face and Gesture* where we enjoyed long discussion on computational approaches to human understanding and the importance of including emerging research in Southeast Asia and the Middle East. From those early discussions, we initiated the *1st International Conference on Informatics, Electronics and Vision* (*ICIEV*) in Bangladesh in 2012. The conference series under Ahad's leadership has fostered rich exchange of ideas and collaboration among junior and senior researchers across Asia and the Middle East, Europe, and North America. This edited collection springs from this productive conference series and his passionate efforts to promote computational and signal processing research in biomedicine, mental health, and human behavior more broadly.

Ahad's and Mosabber Uddin Ahmed's comprehensive collection offers a detailed overview of signal processing and healthcare technologies, challenges, applications, and implementations. Chapters come from major research groups and ones newly ascending. The writing is full of knowledge, insight, and spark from international, multi-cultural perspectives. The ideas presented should generate research and new understanding well into the future.

Whether you are graduate student, faculty, or research scientist, you are in for a treat. Enjoy!

Jeffrey F. Cohn
Professor of Psychology
Psychiatry, and Intelligent Systems
University of Pittsburgh
Pittsburgh, PA, USA

Preface

Our edited book titled *Signal Processing Techniques for Computational Health Informatics* is about various signal processing techniques—related to computational health informatics.

Computational health informatics is the interdisciplinary study of the design, development, adoption, and application of information and technology-based innovations, specifically computational techniques that are relevant in health care and often used to describe full range of application and research topics for which biomedical informatics is the pertinent underlying scientific discipline. Given the multitude of techniques and methods used in the field of signal processing, a comprehensive and representative amount of signal processing techniques used in biomedical applications are presented in this book.

These include biosignal origin and dynamics, artifact and noise removal techniques, feature extraction techniques in time, frequency, time–frequency and complexity domain, and image processing techniques in different image modalities like PET, MRI, medical ultrasound, X-ray, computed tomography (CT), etc. Moreover, a comprehensive overview of the security and privacy challenges, opportunities and future directions for computational health informatics in the big data age has been discussed by incorporating recent techniques from the area of artificial intelligence, machine learning and human–computer interaction.

The materials presented in this book are covered in 14 chapters—from basics to methodologies to the challenges ahead. Authors are from 12 countries (Australia, Bangladesh, Canada, China, Denmark, Egypt, France, Hong Kong, Iran, Japan, Sweden, and UK), covering 21 universities/institutes.

Chapter 1 discusses the origin and dynamics of biomedical signals. It initially classifies the biomedical signals based on their origin. Afterward, some representative electrical biomedical signals named ECG, EMG, EEG, etc., along with some nonelectrical biomedical signals are analyzed thoroughly according to their physiological and pathological perspectives.

Chapter 2 provides a detailed overview of different signal artifacts and noises commonly encountered in different biomedical signals and techniques for those artifacts and noise removal. In this chapter, the state-of-the-art signal processing techniques for reliable identification of these offending artifacts, and finally, removing them from the raw recordings without distorting the signal-of-interest are systematically analyzed. Finally, some quantitative and qualitative measures are demonstrated in tables, and the algorithms are assessed in terms of their computational complexity and cost.

Chapter 3 focuses on basic signal processing techniques in time, frequency, and time–frequency domain which are routinely used for feature extraction in health informatics. This chapter provides a tutorial like description of fundamental signal processing techniques such as sampling, windowing, Z-transform, Fourier transform, wavelets, and some advanced data adaptive approaches like empirical mode decomposition, variational mode decomposition, etc. along with some applications.

Chapter 4 introduces the notion of complexity used in health informatics. At first, the definitional controversies for complexity are presented, and signal properties associated with complexity are reviewed. Then, some criteria used to classify complexity measures in the literature are discussed, and finally, some representative complexity measures used in health informatics are described.

Chapter 5 covers the concept of entropy and described some entropy measures that are common in health informatics. Both one-dimensional measures for time series and two-dimensional measures for images are documented in this chapter. For each measure, its theoretical background is detailed and some medical applications are presented.

Chapter 6 reviews the image-processing techniques used in health informatics. As image processing can be executed in 2D, 3D, or even multi-dimensional image domains, it can extract useful information, which can be used for monitoring, diagnosis, and prognosis. In this chapter, both biomedical image enhancement and compression techniques are covered focusing on the three main types of medical images: X-ray/CT, MRI, and ultrasound image. Besides, some representative applications of using the image processing-based techniques in medical imaging system are reported finally.

Chapter 7 provides some more advanced signal processing techniques, which fall under the category of artificial intelligence (AI). The fundamental of AI, machine learning (ML), and machine reasoning (MR) techniques and approaches widely used in health informatics are reviewed first. Afterward, each technique is discussed to show how they can be applied in the development of a decision support system.

Chapter 8 focused on health information retrieval as searching health-related information on the World Wide Web (WWW) has been increasing in the recent past. The methodologies and techniques to access and/or retrieve information related to the health using the process of information retrieval are referred to health information retrieval (HIR). This chapter presents the noticeable challenges in HIR, the most prominent existing methods to solve the problems and future directions. It also includes the details of the datasets, evaluation metrics used, and procedures to validate the performance of any HIR methods.

Health informatics often combines biomedical engineering with information technology to develop modern eHealth system, which needs precise biosignal processing. As most of the biosignal processing units are multichannel systems with extensive datasets, conventional computation techniques often fail to offer real-time data processing. Reconfigurable architecture offers a tangible solution to this problem by utilizing fast parallel computation through hardware acceleration and designing application-specific circuits rather than using the general-purpose processors to do the signal processing. Due to its low cost and fast computation property, reconfigurable architecture is characteristically suitable for health informatics and has become one of the fastest growing research fields of recent years. Chapter 9 summarizes the state-of-the-art research trends in this research field.

Chapter 10 introduces the fundamentals of computational health informatics rigorously. With a view to relate the significance of application domains in health informatics, it represents potential challenges, opportunities, and some recommendations as future directions for health informatics.

Chapter 11 detours to focus toward the available methods of sensing mental health problems through direct and indirect measures. This chapter studies how active and passive sensing by technologies as well as reporting from relevant sources can contribute toward these detection methods. It also reviews available methods of therapeutic treatment available through digital means, and finally, highlights a few key intervention technologies that are being developed by researchers to fight against mental illness issues.

The rest of the three chapters (12–14) actually describe some case studies where different signal processing techniques discussed so far are used in real-life problems. Chapter 12 covers AI, ML, and MR techniques used for advanced Parkinson's disease, stress management, postoperative pain treatment, driver monitoring, and remote health monitoring. In each case, the challenges, current solutions, and limitations are discussed with future directions. Chapter 13 details how the ML is used in risk prediction for Cesarean Section with a view to optimize healthcare operational decisions. Finally, Chap. 14 showcases an application of epileptic seizures classification based on multi-domain feature extraction.

There is no denying the fact that there are numerous aspects of signal processing used in computational health informatics. To cover all aspects in a single monograph is difficult if not impossible. We have tried to cover at least some core aspects of signal processing used in health informatics for that matter. We hope that the systematic analysis of the state-of-the-art techniques covered in this book will help to further our understandings of the physiological processes and increase our capability in medical diagnosis and prognosis.

For any comment, please email. Finally, we would like to thank the authors and reviewers for their valuable time and efforts. Those exchanges facilitate the book to build up and mature different ideas in the line of this book. We are thankful to our former students—Anindya Das Antar (*University of Michigan*); Masud Ahmed (*University of Maryland, Baltimore County*); Kanij Mehtanin Khabir (*Norfolk State University*); and Ferdous Ali Israt (*DigiCon Telecommunication Ltd.*)—as we had a long brain-storming night in December 2018 to outline the concept of the book!

The friendly and amazing personals of Springer made the book realizable, and we would like to thank them specially. Last but not least, we especially thank Prof. Jeffrey F. Cohn for his time to engrave a foreword for this book.

Thank you all!

Osaka, Japan

Md Atiqur Rahman Ahad, Ph.D., SMIEEE
Professor
University of Dhaka

Specially Appointed Associate Professor
Osaka University
atiqahad@du.ac.bd
ahad@am.sanken.osaka-u.ac.jp
http://ahadVisionLab.com

Dhaka, Bangladesh

Mosabber Uddin Ahmed, Ph.D., SMIEEE
Professor
University of Dhaka
mosabber.ahmed@du.ac.bd

Contents

About the Editors

Md Atiqur Rahman Ahad Senior Member, IEEE, is *Professor* of Electrical and Electronic Engineering, University of Dhaka (DU). He is currently working as *specially appointed Associate Professor* at Osaka University, Japan. He works on computer vision, imaging, IoT, health care, etc. He did B.Sc. (Honors) and Masters from the Department of Applied Physics and Electronics, DU; Masters from the School of Computer Science and Engineering, University of New South Wales; and Ph.D. from the Faculty of Engineering, Kyushu Institute of Technology (KIT). He was awarded prestigious UGC Gold Medal 2016 (handed by Honorable President of Bangladesh), JSPS Postdoctoral Fellowship, and 25+ awards/scholarships in different conferences/etc. He was Visiting Researcher at KIT. He published three books as author, two edited books (available in Springer), and a few chapters. He has published 140+ journals/conference papers. Ahad was invited as keynote/invited speakers ~80 times in different conferences/universities in Japan, BD, USA, India, Malaysia, and Indonesia. He has established several international MOU/collaborations (e.g., Clemson University, University of Hyogo, RCCIIT, Fukuoka Women University, and Kyushu University).

He has been involved with some academic and editorial activities, e.g., Editorial Board Member, *Scientific Reports, Nature*; Associate Editor, *Frontiers in ICT*; Editor, *International Journal of Affective Computing*; Associate Technical Editor (former), *IEEE ComSoc Magazine*; Editor-in-Chief: *International Journal of Computer Vision & Signal Processing*http://cennser.org/IJCVSP, General Chair, 2021 *10th International Conference on Informatics, Electronics & Vision, Japan*http://cennter.org/ICIEV; *5th International Conference on Imaging, Vision & Pattern Recognition*http://cennser.org/IVPR; *3rd International Conference on Activity & Behavior Computing*, 2021 https://abc-research.github.io; Workshop Chair, *17th IEEE PiCom*; Publication Chair, *2018 IEEE International Conference on Systems, Man, and Cybernetics* (*SMC*); Vice Publication Co-chair and Vice Award Chair, *Joint 17th World Congress of International Fuzzy Systems Association* (*IFSA*) and *9th International Conference on Soft Computing and Intelligent Systems*; General Chair, *7th International Symposium in Computational Medical and Health Technology*; and several other international conferences.

He served as Guest Editor in *Pattern Recognition Letters*, Elsevier; *Journal of Multimedia User Interface*, Springer; *Journal of Healthcare Engineering*, Hindawi; *International Journal of Innovative Computing, Information and Control*. Ahad is a Member of OSA, ACM, IEEE Computer Society, IAPR, IEEE RAS, IEEE SMC, etc. He is the founder Secretary of *IEEE Computer Society Bangladesh Chapter*, and *Bangladesh Association of Pattern Recognition*, Executive Committee member of *Bangladesh Electronics Society* (BES). He volunteered as a former Executive Committee member of BAPA, the largest environmental group. More: http://ahadVisionLab.com.

Mosabber Uddin Ahmed received B.Sc. (Hons.) and M.Sc. degrees from the Department of Applied Physics and Electronics, University of Dhaka (DU) in 1998 and 1999, respectively. He received a second M.Sc. degree in communications and signal processing and Ph.D. degree in signal processing from the Imperial College London (ICL), UK, in 2006 and 2012, respectively. From 2015 to 2016, he was a postdoctoral fellow at the Department of Electrical and Electronic Engineering at ICL. He is currently a professor at the Department of Electrical and Electronic Engineering, University of Dhaka. Till date, he has authored or co-authored more than 30 research articles that are published in refereed journals, books, and conference proceedings. His research interests include signal processing, brain signal modeling, wind modeling, time–frequency analysis, multivariate time series analysis, complexity analysis, multiscale entropy analysis, embedded system design, network and information security. He has won several fellowships and research grants including the Commonwealth Academic Fellowship, Commonwealth Scholarship, and Charles Wallace Bangladesh Trust (CWBT) grant. He is a senior member of IEEE. He was also a track/area co-chair of the 2nd and 3rd International Conference on Informatics, Electronics and Vision (ICIEV) and a program chair of the International Workshop on Artificial Intelligence and Applications (IWAIA). He has also served in various capacities such as reviewer and editorial board member in different reputed national and international journals.

Chapter 1
Origin and Dynamics of Biomedical Signals

K. M. Talha Nahiyan, A. S. M. Shamsul Arefin, Mamun Rabbani, and Alejandro Lopez Valdes

Abstract The human body is autonomous and self-controlled. It can coordinate and regulate all the activities in the body through various systems. Most of the systems are governed via some inherently generated and propagated stimuli otherwise known as biomedical signals. Biomedical signals can be broadly classified into electrical and non-electrical biomedical signals based on their origin. Major electrical biomedical signals also known as bioelectrical signals include ECG, EMG and EEG. They are extremely important from physiological and pathological perspectives. Most electrical activity in the body arises because of the potential difference created and maintained by the cell membrane. In addition, the generation and propagation of action potential as a result of different internal and external stimuli control various physiological processes. Thus, the origin, characteristics and variability, depending on external impulse and signal acquisition site, of prominent bioelectrical signals require thorough analysis. Apart from the above mentioned ones, there are other bioelectrical signals, originating from various parts and systems of the body, such as the EOG, ECoG and EGG. Furthermore, the dynamic variability of the bioelectrical signals indicates important physiological changes of the body. Also, there are magnetic, thermal, optic, chemical, mechanical and acoustic signals that can be measured from the body which can be broadly termed as non-electrical biomedical signals. These signals are of wide variety and contribute to several monitoring, diagnosis and analysis of human body.

Keywords Biomedical signals · Action potential · Bioelectrical signals · ECG · EMG · EEG · Evoked Potentials

---

K. M. T. Nahiyan (✉) · A. S. M. S. Arefin · M. Rabbani
Department of Biomedical Physics & Technology, University of Dhaka, Dhaka, Bangladesh
e-mail: tnahiyan@du.ac.bd

A. L. Valdes
Cognitive Hearing Sciences, Eriksholm Research Center, Snekkersten, Denmark

M. A. R. Ahad and M. U. Ahmed (eds.), *Signal Processing Techniques for Computational Health Informatics*, Intelligent Systems Reference Library 192,
https://doi.org/10.1007/978-3-030-54932-9_1

1.1 Introduction

Knowledge of the biomedical signals is essential in better understanding of the physiological systems. Any variation in biomedical signal characteristics is indicative of change in the part of the body or system from where it originates. Thus, the origin of biomedical signals allows understanding the physiological systems more precisely. This facilitates better diagnosis and monitoring of health conditions by leading to development of novel methods. In this chapter, biomedical signals which are of most interest in signal processing techniques have been given focus. The chapter provides classification of biomedical signals based on different aspects. Then the attention moves to bioelectrical signals. The role of cell membrane is discussed in generation of action potential which is the basic building unit of most bioelectrical signals. In the discussion of major bioelectrical signals; ECG, EMG and EEG, the dynamic and evoked responses of these signals are also addressed apart from their origin and basic characteristics. Some other bioelectrical signals such as EOG, ECoG and EGG are also explained briefly. Finally, the chapter presents an overview of some non-electrical biomedical signals.

1.2 Biomedical Signal Classification

The variation in nature of biomedical signals makes them difficult ones to categorize them under any general classifications. However, an approach of classifying them based on three generic criteria can be demonstrated in Fig. 1.1.

1.2.1 Based on Signal Origin

Biomedical signals initially can be classified based on their origins as illustrated in Fig. 1.1. Electric and magnetic biomedical signals originate from electromagnetic sources inside the body. Optic biomedical signals can be measured to interpret the optical properties of the biologic system. Chemical biomedical signals represent the composition and temporal changes in living tissues in terms of chemical properties. Moreover, thermal biomedical signals reflect the losses and absorptions of heat in the body by virtue of various mechanisms. Apart from these, mechanic biomedical signals reflect the mechanical functionalities of the biologic system, like motion, displacement, vibration, pressure, tension and flow signals etc. Lastly, acoustic biomedical signals represent sounds and noises in diverse frequency bands produced by different human body parts and systems.

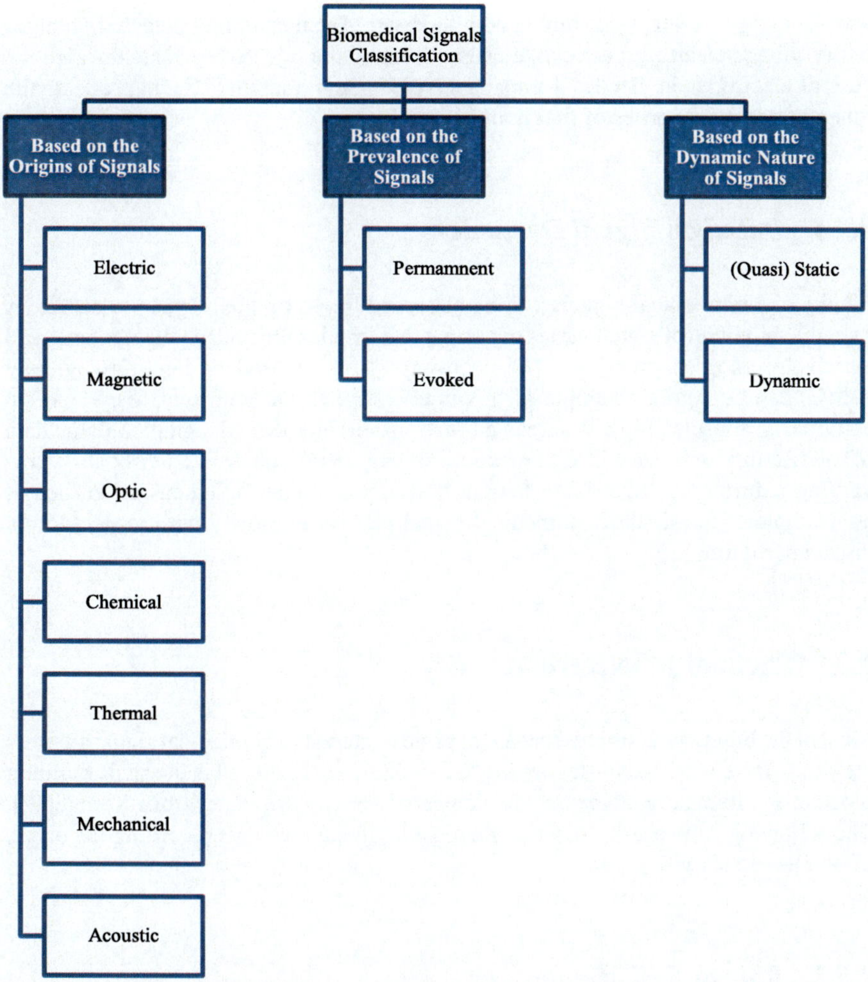

Fig. 1.1 A classification approach of biomedical signals

1.2.2 Based on Signal Prevalence

Biomedical signals can be further classified based on the prevalence of the signals. On one hand, the biomedical signals that are continuously or periodically available without any external stimulus are known as permanent biomedical signals. These signals originate from the sources that are within the human body, like electrocardiograms available via electrocardiography (ECG) represent the heart muscle activities that depict the functionality of the heart [43].

On the other hand, evoked biomedical signals express themselves in the presence of external excitation or trigger and depending on the underlying biologic properties usually end just after the stimulus is withdrawn. As an example, detected voltages in the voltage electrodes are evoked signals due to the injected currents through the current electrodes in electrical impedance plethysmography (IPG) that reflects the inherent tissue properties of that body region [46].

1.2.3 Based on Signal Dynamics

Finally, the biomedical signals can be classified based on their dynamic nature. A dynamic biomedical signal varies over time that implies the underlying dynamic and varied physiological processes. The electromyogram acquired via electromyography (EMG) can be a good example of this type of signal that represents the electrical activities in muscles [43]. Whereas a (quasi) static biomedical signal contains data of interest in a stationary level, i.e., does not vary over time or in a reasonably slow varying nature over time. Core human body temperature, as discussed earlier, is an example of quasi-static biomedical signal that varies slowly with respect to the circadian rhythm [30].

1.3 Origin of Bioelectric Activity

Most of the biomedical signals that are of utmost interest in biomedical signal analysis are due to the electric activities arising at cellular levels. The cell is the basic building block of any living organism and the bioelectric activity originates from the cell [12]. The following sub-sections discuss the most pertinent concepts regarding the origin of bioelectric activities.

1.3.1 Role of Cell Membrane

Human cell membrane is a very thin (7.5–10 nm) semi permeable membrane that encapsulates the human body cell [39]. The base of the membrane is made by phospholipid bilayer in which various types of proteins are embedded. This mosaic structure is dynamic in nature and is held together by the hydrophobic interactions among the phospholipid molecules. Due to the hydrophilic and hydrophobic orientations of the phospholipid molecules, non-polar molecules can enter into the cell, however, ions and polar molecules, like water cannot access through the membrane [12].

The primary role of the cell membrane is to regulate the exchange of chemical substances. Phospholipids grant access to non-polar hydrophobic molecules, such as hydrocarbons as discussed earlier. On the other hand, transfer of ions and polar molecules require special assistance from integral proteins. A kind of integral proteins are known as *ion channels* as they facilitate the transfer of particular polar molecules or ions. These channels help the diffusion of ions from a higher concentration to a lower concentration according to the specific ion concentration gradient and thus are passive in nature [6]. On the contrary, a different group of proteins are known as *ion pumps*. These pumps utilize energy to transport ions across membrane against a potential and/or concentration gradient. The activities of these pumps and channels thus maintain ion concentrations differences in intracellular and extracellular mediums and determine the electrical properties of a cell. Hence, there exists a potential difference across the cell membrane in the resting state unless it is disturbed. This phenomenon is the primary factor behind the origin of the biosignals [39].

1.3.2 Resting Membrane Potential

Ions diffusing through the ion channels and ion pumps as discussed earlier tend to accumulate across the cell membrane and thus develop an electric field within the membrane. This electric field acts opposite to the concentration gradient and impedes further diffusion of ions. The more diffusion occurs, the more electric field increases. Consequently, these two forces, electric-field force and diffusional force balance each other and an equilibrium is attained for all permeable ions. The potential across the cell membrane at this point is known as the resting or equilibrium membrane potential. The typical amplitude range of the potential is −40 to −90 mV with respect to extracellular matrix [48].

The variations in concentrations of Na, K, Cl and other relevant ions between intracellular and extracellular mediums induce the resting membrane potential. Nernst Equation can be utilized to measure this potential. However, the equilibrium potential due to multiple ions can be approximated using the Goldmann-Hodgkin-Katz Equation [19] as in Eq. 1.1.

$$V_m = \frac{kT}{q}\ln\left(\frac{P_K[K^+]_o + P_{Na}[Na^+]_o + P_{Cl}[Cl^-]_i}{P_K[K^+]_i + P_{Na}[Na^+]_i + P_{Cl}[Cl^-]_o}\right) \tag{1.1}$$

where, V_m is the resting membrane potential, P_x is the permeability coefficient for a particular ion X, k is the Boltzmann's constant, T is the absolute temperature in degrees Kelvin, $[X]_o$ and $[X]_i$ are concentrations of ions in extracellular and intracellular mediums respectively and q is the amount of the electric charge.

1.3.3 Action Potential

Due to an external or internal stimulation, excitable cells, like neurons in the body can alter the resting potential. This results in a sudden change of permeability of ions like K^+ and Na^+. This alteration of membrane permeability from resting state to excited state and then back again triggers an electric phenomenon that is known as *action potential* [6]. The cell thus behaves as an electrical source generating a current that propagates through the human body volume conductor.

Action potential emerges due to the abrupt incoming of Na^+ ions via the Na channels due to an adequate stimulus that is sufficient to overcome the threshold potential to initiate an action potential. The influx of Na^+ initiates a reduction of the magnitude of the polarized resting potential to an extent up to +30 to +40 mV which is known as *depolarization* [56]. The K channels get opened at this point and the cell tends to repolarize to its equilibrium potential due to the efflux of more positive K^+ ions. Due to a relatively extended period of K channels opening, sometimes there is an increase in the magnitude of polarized resting potential which is called *hyper-polarization* [59]. A typical nerve action potential is exhibited in Fig. 1.2 indicating the various phases.

A cell's ability to react to any other stimuli to generate another action potential just after it has produced one is limited by a certain time interval. This period is generally known as the *refractory period* of an excitable cell and has two sub-classes. The *absolute refractory period* is a time interval during the initial portion of the action potential where irrespective to the intensity of the stimulus, it is completely impossible for another action potential to be activated. Following that the *relative refractory period* is the time interval where another action potential can be activated by a stimulus greater than the normal threshold value crossing stimulus [19]. Refractory periods are demonstrated in Fig. 1.2 as well.

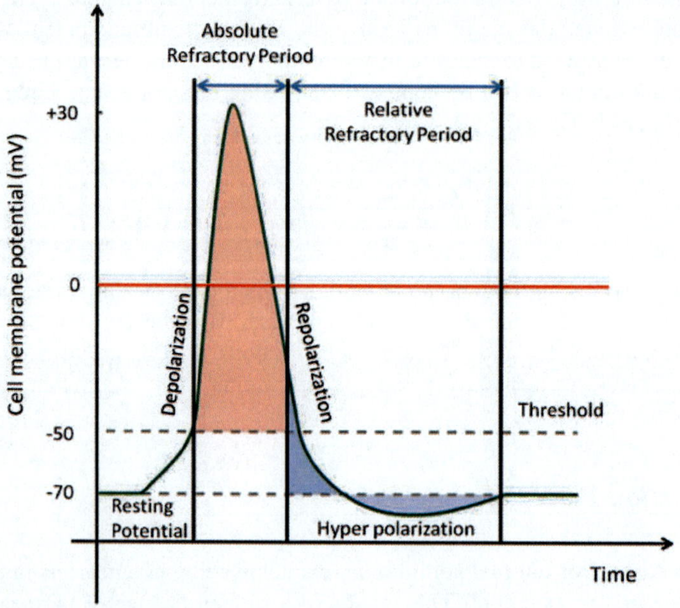

Fig. 1.2 A typical nerve action potential schematic of a neuron

An initial depolarization in a membrane patch of a particular neuron initiates depolarization in the adjacent membrane patch provided that the initial depolarization acts as an adequate stimulus as discussed earlier. Depolarization thus propagates through the length of the cell membrane indicating a wave like propagation. Consequently, the depolarization reaches the far end of the neuron from the soma and the axon terminals of the initial neuron provide stimuli to other neurons to initiate action potentials in succession.

In the following sections the most prominent bioelectrical signals are discussed.

1.4 ECG

The Electrocardiogram or ECG records the electrical activity of the heart. ECG is essential in monitoring and diagnosis of heart diseases. It can be captured through electrodes from the body surface, the body being a volume conductor. An ECG commonly comprises of P wave, QRS complex and T wave (Fig. 1.3), along with PR interval and ST segment. The origin of these waves is in the cardiac muscle cells or myocytes. All myocytes together create a global electrical excitation in the heart and the resultant signal is the ECG.

1.4.1 Cardiac Action Potential

The mechanism of cardiac action potential is very similar to generation of action potential in excitable cells. Each individual myocyte is capable of generating action

Fig. 1.3 An ECG signal

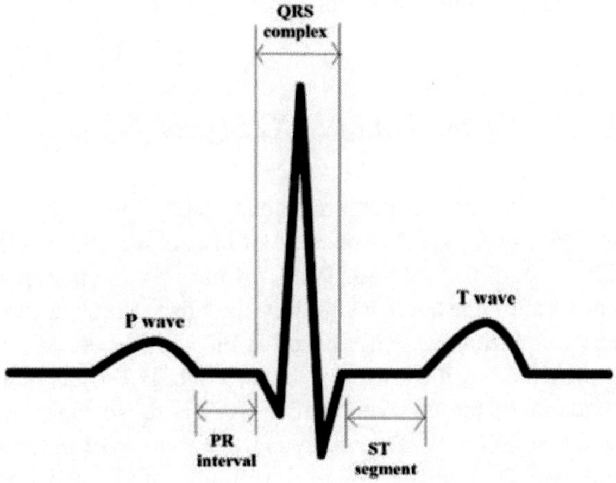

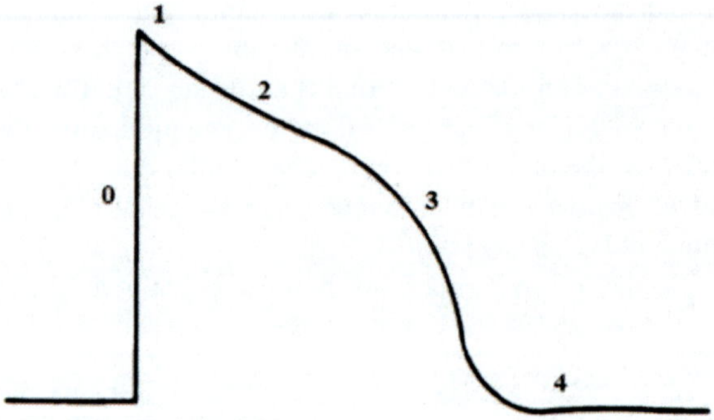

Fig. 1.4 Phases of cardiac action potential in atrial and ventricular cells

potential upon receiving threshold stimulus. The factors that control the depolarization and repolarization are activation-inactivation of the voltage-gated Na^+, Ca^{2+} and K^+ channels. As illustrated in Fig. 1.4, the cardiac action potential cycle consists of five phases.

Phase 0 is the *rapid depolarization* state. Whenever the excitation threshold is exceeded a rapid depolarization takes place. It is initiated by activation of voltage-gated Na^+ and Ca^{2+} channels with subsequent inward flow of Na^+ and Ca^{2+} currents. The Na^+ channel quickly inactivates and the K^+ channel is activated. It results in outward flow of K^+ currents and the membrane potential decreases rapidly to initiate repolarization. This is called *early rapid repolarization* and indicates phase 1. Phase 2 is also called a *plateau*, a slow repolarization phase. This is a distinct configuration of the cardiac action potential. The outward K^+ currents are counterbalanced by inward current of slower Ca^{2+} channels which is the reason for a slow repolarization. Phase 3 is the *final rapid repolarization* which starts when the Ca^{2+} channels close and the cell is rapidly repolarized by outward K^+ currents. In phase 4, repolarization takes the membrane potential to the resting state and this is the value of membrane potential during diastole of heart [52, 61].

1.4.2 Formation of ECG Signal

The cardiac action potential generated in one myocyte propagates to neighboring myocytes very quickly because of low resistance of cellular gaps between myocytes. The sinoatrial (SA) node is the primary pacemaker of the heart. An action potential generated at the SA node quickly spreads to the atria and initiates contraction by depolarization. Subsequently blood is ejected into both ventricles. This phenomenon is represented by the *P wave* in ECG. There is a slight delay in the propagation of action potential at the atrioventricular (AV) node so that the ventricles can be filled with blood completely. This delay is the *PR interval* in the ECG. Then the action potential spreads readily through the Bundle of His and Purkinje fibers depolarizing the ventricles. The *QRS complex* in ECG represents this phase of ventricular excitation which results in contraction of ventricles and ejection of blood into arteries. The *ST segment* denotes the interval between ventricular depolarization and repolarization. Finally the *T wave* is reminiscent of ventricular repolarization [30, 39].

1.4.3 12-Lead ECG

The volume conductor effect allows recording of ECG from various sites on the body surface. But the shape and size of the signal is different due to distance from the signal source (the heart). These variations have significant importance in diagnosis from ECG.

Mostly 12 lead ECG is required in clinical practice. Figure 1.5a shows an Einthoven triangle for placement of electrodes for measuring 3 frontal plane leads; Lead I, Lead II and Lead III. The electrodes are attached at three points; wrist of right arm, wrist of left arm and ankle of left leg. A reference electrode is also required to be attached in lower part of the torso, most commonly at the ankle of right leg. There are also three augmented frontal leads; aVR, aVL and aVF, which can be calculated as:

$$
\begin{aligned}
\text{aVR} &= -(\text{Lead I} + \text{Lead II})/2 \\
\text{aVL} &= (\text{Lead I} - \text{Lead III})/2 \\
\text{aVF} &= (\text{Lead II} + \text{Lead III})/2
\end{aligned}
$$

The transverse plane chest leads placements are shown in Fig. 1.5b. Leads V1 and V2 are placed just right and left of the sternum in the fourth intercostal space. V4 is placed directly below the left mid-clavicular line in the fifth intercostal space. V3 is placed halfway between V2 and V4. V5 and V6 are placed on the same horizontal line with V4. V5 is placed directly below anterior axillary line and V6 directly below the mid-axillary line. The typical variation of 12 lead ECG signal shape and size is shown in Fig. 1.6 [40].

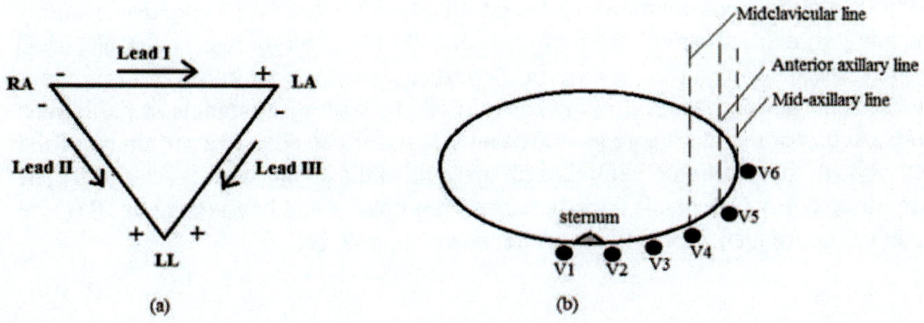

Fig. 1.5 **a** Einthoven triangle for 3-lead ECG, **b** ECG Chest leads

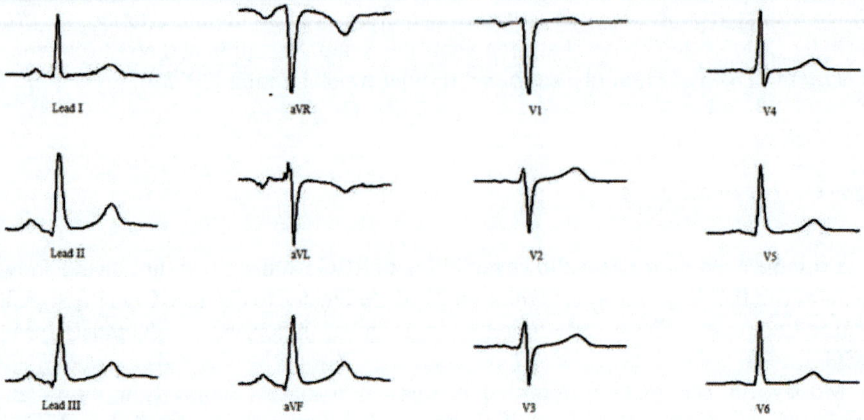

Fig. 1.6 Signal variation in 12 lead ECG

1.4.4 Heart Rate Variability

The RR interval between two consecutive heartbeats is never the same and represents a dynamic nature. Heart rate variability (HRV) is the oscillation in the RR interval between consecutive heartbeats. HRV analysis is based on RR interval time series which is an event series. The variations can be analyzed by a number of methods. Most common are time domain methods and frequency domain methods. The HRV have correlation with various cardiological and non-cardiological diseases such as myocardial infarction, congestive heart failure, diabetic neuropathy, obstructive sleep apnea, Parkinson's disease, epilepsy etc. [33, 55].

1.5 EMG

Electromyogram (EMG) is one of the basic biosignals to be observed in the human body. The word electromyogram originates from the Greek work 'electros' roughly meaning signal and 'myo' meaning muscle. So electromyogram is the electrical signal generated from the muscles in the human body. As we know from previous discussions, action potential is the basis of all the biological signals in the human body. Action potentials are generated in muscle tissue cells due to a certain muscular activity. All these action potentials sum up to form the signal we treat as EMG. The amplitude of EMG depends upon the observing muscle and has a range of 50 μV to 30 mV. The frequency component is between 7 and 20 Hz.

1.5.1 Generation and Propagation of EMG

A great deal of external and internal demands and constraints are dealt by a motor unit in humans which include movements, locomotion, gestures and postures. A motor unit is considered as the functional unit. It is made up of motor neurons from the nervous system and skeletal muscle fibers. The muscle fibers are connected with the neurons through the axonal terminals [11]. The primary signaling of the motor unit takes place in the premotor cortex and other areas of the cortex. Signals from these areas unite at the primary motor cortex, generating or inhibiting the primary cortex neurons. Each motor unit consists of a α-motoneuron which is situated in the spinal cord. It is considered as the addition point for all the reflex and motor signals. Whcn thc nct mcmbranc currcnt rcachcs thc α-motoncuron, it crcatcs a ccrtain firing pattern for the different synaptic innervation sites in the motor unit. When the signal reaches the neuromuscular junction, it originates an emission of acetylcholine (ACh), a neurotransmitter, in the gap between the muscle fiber membrane and axonal terminal of the nerve. The release of ACh stimulates the muscle fiber membrane in producing a membrane potential. This membrane potential is propagated into various muscle fibers. The summation of the output of all the motor units establishes EMG. The number of motor units may vary in humans and may range from 100 to 1000 depending on the size of the muscle [26]. The force generating capacity also varies from motor unit to motor unit [23, 53].

1.5.2 Detection Montages of EMG

EMG can be detected using surface electrodes which are mounted on the skin and intramuscular electrodes which are inserted in the muscle tissue. Intramuscular electrodes are useful in detecting electric potentials very close to the source. Such detection minimizes the effect of current propagation in volume conductor on the acquired signal. Signals from various motor units have a reasonably separation in the time domain when acquired through this montage. The prominent drawback of this method is that the electrodes are invasive in nature and requires the involvement of specialized personnel. Surface electrode montage is more preferred in detection of EMG. The most commonly used method of detection in this montage is the bipolar montage where two electrodes are used at a small distance of 1–3 cm of the muscle fiber to detect the EMG signal. Monopolar electrodes are also used in some cases where the reference electrode is situated is a far-away site on the body. Although the surface electrode method is non-invasive, it possesses some complexities [21]. The position of electrode placement is an important issue here as the distance between the point of source and detection plays a significant role. The power line interference and spatial low-pass filtering effect of the tissues between the source and electrodes are the common mode components which should be removed during detection. In comparison, intramuscular electrode montage gives a better outcome than surface electrode montage [47].

1.5.3 Evoked EMG

Evoked EMG is the result of external stimulation applied to the motor nervous system. Non-invasive stimulation of the motor cortex through the scalp is known as motor evoked potential (MEP). Electric pulses of 1000–1500 V and 50–100 μs durations are typically applied in the motor cortex to generate MEP and were first reported by Merton and Morton [41]. Transient magnetic fields with variable flow and having intensity of 1.5–2.5 T were proposed by Barker et al. which are used to generate MEP [5]. The magnetic stimulation is preferred over the electric method due to the minimal attenuation faced by magnetic signals than that by electric signals.

Several parameters are considered in evaluating motor evoked potentials. The lowest intensity of stimulation capable of producing a MEP which causes muscle relaxation or contraction is known as the threshold of stimulation. It refers to the excitability of the corticospinal connections. The time taken by impulses to reach the intended muscle is known as latency of the signal. Latencies vary as a function of muscle length. The peak to peak amplitude of the signal is another parameter of MEP which is expressed as a percentage of the maximum amplitude of response recorded in the same muscle.

The MEPs provide valuable information for diagnosis. On analyzing the evoked potential waves, various segments are noted and observed. A direct stimulation of the motor nerve records the M-wave. This is also known as Compound Muscle Action Potential (CMAP). A generic wave shape of the M-wave is shown in Fig. 2.7. The M-wave is generated when stimulus is applied at a muscle site which is proximal to the motor nerve. This stimulation activates the motor neurons directly. A stimulation which is capable of stimulating all the motor neurons in a bundle is known as supramaximal stimulation. The amplitude of M-wave is maximum during supramaximal stimulation.

The parameters for analysis of M-wave are peak to peak amplitude and M-wave area. Although M-wave latency is considered as a measuring parameter by many [37], it is found to be rather constant and less sensitive to changes. M-wave area is

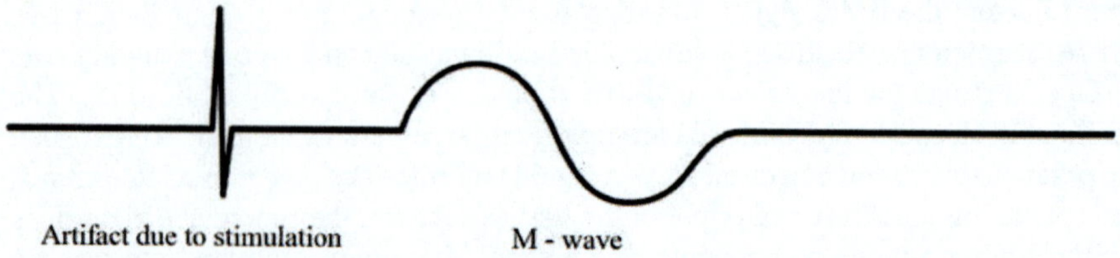

Fig. 1.7 M-wave generated due to stimulation

considered more reliable compared to M-wave amplitude as M-wave area is found to be uninterrupted in repeated measurements [2]. The stimulation rate should be kept at three stimuli per second in measuring these parameters.

One of the other waves observed during evoked EMG is the Hoffmann reflex or the H-reflex or simply H-wave. H-wave is evoked by a submaximal stimulus to the peripheral nerve. H-wave analysis is important is measuring the excitability of the motoneurons. A stimulus in the peripheral nerve activates the afferent fibers which in turn activates the motoneurons and initiates the H-wave. Such stimulation bypasses the muscle spindle. Another wave observed in the evoked EMG is the V-wave. When a supramaximal stimulation is applied, the subject experiences a maximal isometric contraction. This records a response which is termed as V-wave [58]. In general, the V-wave can be contemplated as the amount of central drive to the motoneurons in a state of maximal contraction. The F-wave is another response recorded from the muscle in an event of evoked stimulation. F-wave is generated due to the antidromic reactivation or simply put as 'backfiring' of motoneurons. After stimulation, a motoneuron action potential travels to the spinal cord antidromically and then is reflected back to the muscle along the motoneuron pathway. The difference between F-wave and H-wave is that F-wave is not generated by afferent fibers, rather by the backfiring of the motoneurons.

1.6 EEG

The Electroencephalogram (*electro—electrical, encephalo—brain, gram—writing*) represents the summated cortical potentials that are generated by the synchronous pyramidal neurons in the brain due to internal or external triggering [45]. The ionic currents, flowing across the cell membranes of active neurons and glia cells due to action potentials, induce the cortical electrical potentials. The summated cortical potentials can be recorded by surface electrodes from the human scalp [10]. German psychiatrist Hans Berger is the first man to scientifically report the recording of EEG [9]. Several electrodes are placed above the brain scalp according to some standard nomenclature, e.g., the international 10-20 rule [27]. Typically, a passive reference electrode which is to record minimum of activity is also added in general. The differential potential between individual active electrodes and the reference is amplified and processed for visualization and further analysis. A display of the complex fluctuations of these potentials as a function of time due to various physiological control processes, memory processes, thought processes and external triggering is known as EEG [8, 29].

1.6.1 Basic EEG Characteristics

The amplitude of EEG ranges from 0.001 to 0.01 mV. The frequency bandwidth has a range of 0.5–40 Hz. Sometimes, greater than 40 Hz oscillations are observed in EEG signals as well [56]. EEG signals are prone to artifacts as signals of small amplitude face interference passing through the scalp. EEG artifacts can be primarily categorized into physiological, electronic and environmental noise sources [3]. Physiological noises arise from ECG, chewing, respiration, EMG, eye blinking, etc. [18]. Furthermore, environmental noises emanate due to the interference of external electromagnetic (EM) waves and power line EM radiations. Moreover, EEG signals are contaminated with electronic noises that are byproducts of poorly tuned electronic circuitry [50]. Last but not the least, EEG signal artifact may arise from the recording electrodes as well due to impedance mismatch and/or improper contacts in the form of *electrode pop* [3, 18].

1.6.2 EEG Waves

EEG continues to be one of the leading non-invasive brain imaging technique to understand the neurophysiology, to monitor neural mechanisms due to different physiological and psychological activities for the diagnosis of neural disorders like epilepsy, and for brain–computer interfacing, feedback and control [45, 50]. However, EEG signals are intricate to realize as they are the accumulated representation of activities performed by numerous neurons that are spread in the brain in a complex nature via multiple mediums like brain tissues, fluids, and scalp [3]. Some of the features can be detected via direct observation, like interictal spikes in epilepsy, transients and other oscillations associated with nervous system disorders [44]. On the other hand, some of the EEG signals represent different waves with distinct bandwidths that are commonly known as *brainwaves*. Utilizing minimal signal processing techniques like Discrete Fourier Transform (DFT) or Power Spectra, these brainwaves can be easily detected in the brain [43]. The prevalence and/or disappearance of these rhythms are of utmost clinical importance as they indicate vital underlying physiological functionalities [7]. The general characteristic of these brainwaves can be found in Table 1.1 [3, 8, 18, 39].

1.6.3 Evoked Potentials in EEG

Evoked potentials (EPs) are the induced EEG signals that are the resultant electrical responses from the brain or brain stem due to various external stimuli. As the name suggests, an EP is a transient waveform that generally appears following a time interval that is associated with the period of production of the stimulus. On the

Table 1.1 Typical features of common EEG brainwaves

EEG waves	**Bandwidth (Hz)**	**Features**
Delta (δ)	0.5–4	Typically appear in infants and at deep-sleep stages for adults
Theta (θ)	4–8	Generally obtained from children and at the beginning stages of sleep for adults
Alpha (α)	8–13	Predominant resting oscillation of the brain, commonly available in the occipital region in resting adults when eyes are closed
Beta (β)	13–30	Flight-and-fight response rhythms that are usually obtained over the frontal and parietal lobes
Gamma (γ)	30–80	Induced oscillations due to external stimuli, sensory processing requiring attention, memory processing etc.

contrary, EEG activities are always present and the changes in oscillations are usually random in nature. EPs can be obtained with the scalp electrodes in the similar EEG recording configuration. They are generally in the range of 0.1–10 μV in amplitude, hence, buried under the background EEG signals that are in the range of 10–100 μV in amplitude [54]. These non-invasively recorded EPs can objectively provide information on abnormalities in visual, sensory and auditory nervous system pathways and disorders related to vision, speech and sensing etc. [14, 60]. Depending on the nature of stimuli, most commonly used clinical EP modalities are visual evoked potential (VEP), auditory evoked potential (AEP) and somatosensory evoked potential (SEP). Latencies and amplitudes are computed from the averaged EPs in all modalities and comparative analyses are performed to distinguish healthy subjects from subjects with abnormalities to detect the underlying abnormalities [17].

VEP analysis is one of the most common clinical routines in investigating optic nerve disorders, retinopathy, maculopathy and demyelinating diseases [49, 60]. In VEP clinical setup, the subject under test is presented with a visual stimulus for a number of times. Generally two types of stimuli are presented, pattern reversal or chequer-board and flashing, to one eye keeping the other one covered for neurologic purposes. The resultant VEPs are then recorded for analysis [14]. Clinically pertinent information from VEPs in the occipital regions is usually available from 75 ms onwards [16].

AEP analysis is one of the most valuable techniques for the assessment of hearing, brainstem disease diagnosis, intraoperative monitoring of nerve integrity of the auditory pathways during neurosurgery and monitor the prognosis of coma patients in intensive care unit (ICU). AEPs are elicited due to transient external acoustic stimuli. Simultaneously, EEG signals are recorded according to the frequency of the stimuli being played. Recorded AEPs represent the neural information that managed to propagate through the auditory pathways with latencies ranging from 2 to 500 ms [15, 35, 60].

SEP analysis is a great clinical aid in investigating neuro disorders due to demyelination and myoclonus, intraoperative monitoring of nerve integrity of the sensory pathways during neurosurgery and coma patient monitoring in ICU as discussed earlier for AEP [4, 60]. SEPs are generated with latencies ranging from 30 to 60 ms in the central nervous system (CNS) due to electrical stimulations on a particular nerve from the upper or lower limbs [54]. The stimuli are carried by the nerves from the stimulation point to the cerebral cortex via the spinal cord. The resultant responses to these stimuli in the brain, i.e., SEPs are then recorded, measured and analyzed for clinical assessments [43].

1.6.4 Event Related Potentials in EEG

EPs discussed in the earlier section generate exogenous or stimulus-based signals that are devoid of a subject's attention or interest as we have seen in the cases of AEP and SEP that are being used for coma patient's prognosis monitoring. On the contrary, some endogenous or event-based potentials can be recorded due to certain external stimuli otherwise known as events [24]. These events require attention or higher order processing from a subject in distinguishing a particular stimulus (target stimulus) from a train of stimuli (baseline stimulus). The generated potentials due to the events can be obtained with the scalp electrodes in the similar EEG recording configuration. When a number of these EEG epochs are averaged, brain activity related to the specific stimulus or event becomes measurable. This time-locked average waveform is known as Event Related Potential (ERP) [51].

Due to the averaging of the random EEG epochs, the signal-to-noise ratio (SNR) gets improved proportionately to the square root of the average of number of epochs [32]. Pre-stimulus epoch provides reference line electrical activity which remains relatively constant if sufficiently averaged and post-stimulus-onset contains the ERP waveform with components which are basically the peaks and troughs that represent the responses depending on the stimulus modalities. These components are usually characterized in terms of amplitude, polarity, scalp distribution and latency from the onset of the stimulus [38].

ERP analyses with the distinct features like non-invasiveness, high temporal resolution and relatively lower cost have broadened the horizon of in vivo human brain research [57]. Furthermore, ERP analyses are getting popular day by day in clinical routines to investigate cognitive disorders, depression and disorders affecting memory and attention [24, 38].

Last but not the least, there exists a whole lot of other EEG analysis techniques like frequency domain analysis, forward and inverse modelling, component analysis etc. But a detailed discussion is beyond the scope of this chapter.

1.7 Other Bioelectric Signals

The most common bioelectrical signals have been discussed extensively already. In this section some other bioelectrical signals with clinical significance are discussed briefly.

1.7.1 Electrooculogram (EOG)

The Electrooculogram is the potential generated due to the movement of the eye. Thc human cyc can bc considcrcd as a dipolc whcrc thc cornca is takcn as positivc potential compared to the retina. Hence there is a potential difference between the cornea and the retina. This corneo-retinal potential ranges from 0.4–1.0 mV and varies with the movement of the eyes. When electrodes are placed at the vicinity of the eyes, they record the corneo-retinal potential. The electrode which is closer to the cornea after movement registers a positive potential while the one which is closer to the retina registers a negative potential. A potential difference is found in comparing the two electrodes and this potential depends on the movement of eye. This potential measurement can be analyzed as EOG [13, 28].

The corneo-retinal potential changes with the intensity of incident light on the eyes, hence constant illumination should be maintained during recording of EOG. Moreover EOG can be affected by the artifacts from EEG, EMG, etc. EOG has the advantage of being non-invasive and easy to assemble. It creates minimal patient discomfort and is effective than other methods of ocular detection. It can detect eye movement with closed eyelids and head movement which adds to the versatility. For being low-cost and easily applicable, EOG is the most practical method of recording eye movements [25].

1.7.2 Electrocorticogram (ECoG)

The Electrocorticogram is a semi-invasive technique to determine the electrical signals generated from the brain. While EEG measures the brain signals from the cortex, ECoG measures the generated signals from the exposed surface of the cerebral cortex. Electrodes are implanted on the cerebral cortex by craniotomy. These electrodes may reach the epidural or subdural regions. In some cases a grid electrode is used which consist of 4–256 electrodes covering a large area of the cerebral cortex [42]. Compared to EEG, ECoG has a high spatial resolution for the fact that the generated signal does not need to travel to the scalp. The spatial resolution of ECoG is in the tenth of millimeter range while EEG has a nearly 100 fold lower resolution. As the brain signal faces less attenuation on reaching the electrode, ECoG has amplitude of 50–100 μV which is higher than the typical amplitude of EEG.

ECoG has a lower clinical risk than other invasive techniques as the electrode does not need to penetrate the cortex. Moreover, artifacts from EMG and EOG have less impact on ECoG and the electrodes are less affected by environmental noise. For the advantages over EEG, ECoG is one of the preferred techniques in Brain Computer Interfacing (BCI) [36].

1.7.3 Electroglottogram (EGG)

The measurement of the extent of contact between the two vibrating vocal folds during the production of sound is known as Electroglottogram. This method is non-invasive where a pair of electrodes is placed on the surface of the neck and a current of low amplitude and high frequency is applied through the electrodes. This records the changes in transverse electrical impedance of the larynx and nearby tissues during voice production [22, 34]. The EGG signal consists of two components. A high frequency component due to the vibrating vocal cords during production of sound and a low frequency component due to the movement of larynx while swallowing. The amplitude of the EGG signal is highly dependent on the position of electrodes. EGG signals are widely used in many applications like stroboscope synchronization, tracking the fundamental frequency of voice, tracking the movements of vocal fold abduction, studying of singing voice, determining the quality of voice, assessing the range of speaking voice, voice therapy, etc. [31].

1.8 Non-electrical Biomedical Signals

Other than the electrical biomedical signals there are varied categories of biomedical signals which originate from the body. As introduced already in Sect. 1.2, there are magnetic, thermal, optic, chemical, mechanical and acoustic signals that can be measured from the body. An example of magnetic biomedical signal is Magnetoencephalography (MEG) which reflects the magnetic field due to neuronal activities inside the brain. Core human body temperature can be termed as a thermal signal which is a vital parameter of human body. It is usually high in day times and relatively low in night times [30]. Photoplethysmogram (PPG) obtained via non-invasive optical measurement method, can help calculate the arterial oxygen saturation (SpO_2) in the blood [1]. Partial pressure of Oxygen (pO_2) in the lungs or blood, cortisol levels in the blood are examples chemical signals [20]. A type of mechanical signal is a vibromyogram (VMG) which is a vibration signal. It is usually acquired with the help of contact microphones or accelerometers that manifests the mechanical contraction of a skeletal muscle. Different systems and movements in the human body produce sounds which can be categorized as acoustic signals. Breathing, tracheal, lung and chest sounds, snoring sounds, gastrointestinal or bowel sounds are some example of acoustic signals [50].

1.9 Conclusions

In this chapter, origin of several biomedical signals has been explained extensively along with other necessary aspects which change the signal characteristics such as dynamic variability and evoked responses. With emergence of novel signal processing techniques and machine learning, there is endless possibility that biomedical signals can aid in disease diagnosis and health monitoring. Also with better analysis tools and enhanced computational ability, it is possible to disseminate biomedical signals through simulation which are otherwise unfavorable to perform in clinical practice.

References

1. Abay, T.Y., Kyriacou, P.A.: Photoplethysmography for blood volumes and oxygenation changes during intermittent vascular occlusions. J. Clin. Monit. Comput. **32**(3), 447–455 (2018). https://doi.org/10.1007/s10877-017-0030-2
2. Aiello, I., Sau, G.F., Bissakou, M., Patraskakis, S., Traccis, S.: Standardization of changes in M-wave area to repetitive nerve stimulation. Electromyogr. Clin. Neurophysiol. **26**, 529–532 (1986)
3. Aminoff, J.M.: Electroencephalography: General Principles and Clinical Applications. In: Aminoff, J.M. (ed.) Electrodiagnosis in Clinical Neurology, 5th edn, pp. 37–84. Elsevier Inc., Philadelphia, PA (2005). ISBN 0-443-06647-7
4. Aminoff, J.M., Eisen, A.: Somatosensory Evoked Potentials. In: Aminoff, J.M. (ed.) Electrodiagnosis in Clinical Neurology, 5th edn, pp. 553–576. Elsevier Inc., Philadelphia, PA (2005). ISBN 0-443-06647-7
5. Barker, A.J., Jalinous, R., Freeston, I.L.: Non-invasive stimulation of human motor cortex. Lancet **2**, 1106–1107 (1985)
6. Barr. R.C.: Basic electrophysiology. In: Bronzino, J.D. (ed.) The Biomedical Engineering Handbook, 2nd edn. CRC Press, Boca Raton, FL (2000). ISBN 978-0849385940
7. Başar, E.R., Schürmann, M.A., Demiralp, T.A., Başar-Eroglu, C.A., Ademoglu, A.H.: Event-related oscillations are 'real brain responses'—wavelet analysis and new strategies. Int. J. Psychophysiol. **39**, 91–127 (2001)
8. Bentin, S.: Electrophysiological studies of visual word perception, lexical organization, and semantic processing: a tutorial review. Lang. Speech **32**, 205–220 (1989)
9. Berger, H.: Über das Elektrenkephalogramm des Menschen. Archiv für Psychiatrie und Nervenkrankheiten **87**(1), 527–570 (1929)
10. Bronzino, J.D.: Principles of electroencephalography. In: Bronzino, J.D. (ed.) The Biomedical Engineering Handbook, 2nd edn. CRC Press, Boca Raton, FL (2000). ISBN 978-0849385940
11. Buchtal, F., Schmalbruch, H.: Motor unit of mammalian muscle. Physiol. Rev. **60**(1), 90–142 (1980)
12. Campbell, N.A., Reece, J.B.: Biology, 8th edn. Pearson, San Francisco (2008). ISBN 9780805368444
13. Carpenter, R.H.S.: Movements of the Eyes, 2nd edn, pp. 405–426. Pion, London (1988)
14. Celesia, G.G.: Visual evoked potentials in clinical neurology. In: Aminoff, J.M. (ed.) Electrodiagnosis in Clinical Neurology, 5th edn, pp. 453–471. Elsevier Inc., Philadelphia, PA (2005). ISBN 0-443-06647-7
15. Celesia, G.G., Brigell, M.G.: Auditory evoked potentials. In: Niedermeyer, E., da Silva, F.L. (eds.) Electroencephalography: Basic principles, clinical applications and related fields, pp. 994–1013. Williams & Wilkins, Baltimore, MD (1999)

16. Celesia, G.G., Peachey, N.S.: Visual evoked potentials and electroretinograms. In: Niedermeyer, E., da Silva, F.L. (eds.) Electroencephalography: Basic principles, clinical applications and related fields, pp. 968–993. Williams & Wilkins, Baltimore, MD (1999)
17. Chabot, R.J., John, E.R.: Normative evoked potential data. In: da Silva, F.L., van Leeuwen, W.S., Remond, A. (eds.) Handbook of Electroencephalography and Clinical Electrophysiology: Clinical Applications of Computer Analysis of EEG and Other Neurophysiological Signals, pp. 263–309. Elsevier, New York (1986)
18. Chong, D.J., Sahlem, G.L., Bazil, C.W.: Introduction to electroencephalography. In: Barkoukis, T.J., Avidan, A.Y.: (eds) Review of Sleep Medicine, 2nd edn., pp. 105–141. Butterworth-Heinemann (2007). https://doi.org/10.1016/b978-075067563-5.10008-2
19. Clark J.W.: The origin of biopotentials. In: Webster, J.G. (ed.) Medical Instrumentation: Application and Design, 4th edn. Wiley, Hoboken, NJ (2011). ISBN 978471676003
20. Cohen, A.: Biomedical signals: origin and dynamic characteristics; frequency-domain analysis. In: Bronzino, J.D. (ed.) The Biomedical Engineering Handbook—Medical Devices and Systems, 3rd edn., pp. 1–1 to 1–22. CRC Press, Boca Raton, FL (2006)
21. Farina, D., Stegeman, D.F., Merletti, R.: Biophysics of the generation of EMG signals. In: Farina, D., Merletti, R. (eds.) Surface Electromyography: Physiology, Engineering, and Applications, pp 30–53. IEEE (2016)
22. Fourcin, A.J., Abberton, E.: First applications of a new laryngograph. Med. Biol. Illus. **21**, 172–182 (1971)
23. Garnett, R.A.F., O'Donovan, M.J., Stephens, J.A., Taylar, A.: Motor unit organization of human medial gastrocnemius. J. Physiol. London **287**, 33–43 (1979)
24. Goodin, D.S.: Event-related potentials. In: Aminoff, J.M. (ed.) Electrodiagnosis in Clinical Neurology, 5th edn, pp. 609–626. Elsevier Inc., Philadelphia, PA (2005). ISBN 0-443-06647-7
25. Heide, W., Koenig, E., Trillenberg, P., Koempf, D., Zee, D.S.: Electrooculography: technical standards and applications. In: Deuschl, G., Eisen, A. (eds.) Recommendations for the Practice of Clinical Neurophysiology: Guidelines of the International Federation of Clinical Physiology. International Federation of Clinical Neurophysiology, Elsevier (1999)
26. Henneman, E., Mendell, L.M.: Functional organization of the motoneuron pool and its inputs. In: Brooks VB (ed.) Handbook of Physiology: The Nervous System, pp. 423–507. American Physiological Society, Bethesda (1988)
27. IFSECN—International Federation of Societies for Electroencephalography and Clinical Neurophysiology: The ten twenty electrode system. Am. J. EEG Technol. **1**(1), 13–19 (1961). https://doi.org/10.1080/00029238.1961.11080571
28. Jung, R., Kornhuber, H.H.: Results of electronystagmography in man: the value of optokinetic, vestibular, and spontaneous nystagmus for neurologic diagnosis and research. In: Bender, M.B. (ed.) The Oculomotor System, pp. 428–488. Harper and Row, New York (1964)
29. Kaiser, D.: Basic principles of quantitative EEG. J. Adult Dev. **12**, 99–104 (2005)
30. Kaniusas, E.: Biomedical Signals and Sensors I: Linking Physiological Phenomena and Biosignals. Springer, Berlin, Heidelberg (2012). https://doi.org/10.1007/978-3-642-24843-6
31. Kitzing, P.: Clinical applications of electroglottography. J. Voice **4**(3), 238–249 (1990)
32. Kropotov, J.D.: Event-related potentials. In: Kropotov, J.D. (ed.) Functional Neuromarkers for Psychiatry, pp. 59–78. Academic Press (2016). https://doi.org/10.1016/b978-0-12-410513-3.00006-1
33. Kuusela, T.: Methodological aspects of heart rate variability analysis. In: Kamath, M.V., Watanabe, M.A., Upton, A.R.M. (eds.) Heart Rate Variability (HRV) Signal Analysis, pp. 10–42. CRC Press
34. Lecluse, F.L.E., Brocaar, M.P., Verschurre, J.: The electoglottography and its relation to glottal activity. Fol. Phoniatr. **27**, 215–224 (1975). https://doi.org/10.1159/000263988
35. Legat, A.D.: Brainstem auditory evoked potentials: methodology, interpretation, and clinical application. In: Aminoff, J.M. (ed.) Electrodiagnosis in clinical neurology, 5th edn, pp. 489–524. Elsevier, Philadelphia, PA (2005). ISBN 0-443-06647-7
36. Leuthardt, E.C., Schalk, G., Wolpaw, J.R., Ojemann, J.G., Moran, D.W.: A brain–computer interface using electrocorticographic signals in humans. J. Neural Eng. **1**(2), 63–71 (2004)

37. Linnamo, V., Strojnik, V., Komi, P.V.: EMG power spectrum and maximal M-wave during eccentric and concentric actions at different force levels. Acta Physiologica Pharmacologica Bulgarica **26**, 33–36 (2001)
38. Luck, S.J. An introduction to the event-related potentials and their neural origins. In: An Introduction to the Event-Related Potential Technique, pp. 1–50. MIT Press (2005). ISBN 978-0262122771
39. Malmivuo, J., Plonsey, R.: Bioelectromagnetism: Principles and Applications of Bioelectric and Biomagnetic Fields. Oxford University Press, New York. (1995). https://doi.org/10.1093/acprof:oso/9780195058239.001.0001
40. Mcfarlane, P,W.: Lead systems. In: Macfarlane, P.W., van Oosterom, A., Pahlm OKligfield, P., Janse, M., Camm, J. (eds.) Comprehensive Electrocardiology, pp. 377–425. Springer (2011)
41. Merton, P.A., Hill, D.K., Morton, H.B., Marsden, C.D.: Scope of a technique for electrical stimulation of human brain, spinal cord, and muscle. Lancet **2**, 597–600 (1982)
42. Mesgarani, N., Chang, E.F.: Selective cortical representation of attended speaker in multi-talker speech perception. Nature **485**(7397), 233–236 (2012). https://doi.org/10.1038/nature11020
43. Najarian, K., Splinter, R.: Biomedical Signal and Image Processing, 2nd edn. CRC Press, Boca Raton, FL (2012). ISBN 978-1-4398-7034-1
44. Niedermeyer, E.: Depth electroencephalography. In: Niedermeyer, E., da Silva, F.L. (eds.) Electroencephalography: Basic principles, clinical applications and related fields. Williams & Wilkins, Baltimore, MD (1999)
45. Nunez, P.L., Srinivasan, R.: Electric Fields of the Brain: The Neurophysics of EEG, 2nd edn. Oxford University Press, New York (2006)
46. Nyboer, J., Kreider, M.M., Hannapel, L.: Electrical impedance plethysmography: a physical and physiologic approach to peripheral vascular study. Circulation **2**(6), 811–821 (1950). https://doi.org/10.1161/01.CIR.2.6.811
47. Perry, J., Easterday, C.S., Antonelli, D.J.: Surface versus intramuscular electrodes for electromyography of superficial and deep muscles. Phys. Ther. **61**(1), 7–15 (1981). https://doi.org/10.1093/ptj/61.1.7
48. Plonsey, R., Barr, R.C.: Bioelectricity: A Quantitative Approach, 3rd edn. Springer, New York (2007). ISBN 978-0-387-48865-3
49. Porciatti, V., Sartucci, F.: Retinal and cortical evoked responses to chromatic contrast stimuli: specific losses in both eyes of patients with multiple sclerosis and unilateral optic neuritis. Brain **119**, 723 (1996)
50. Rangayyan, R.M.: Biomedical signal analysis, 2nd edn. Wiley—IEEE Press, Hoboken, New Jersey (2015). ISBN 978-1-119-06793-1
51. Rugg, M.D.: Event-related potentials (ERPs). In: Squire, L.R. (ed.) Encyclopedia of Neuroscience, pp. 7–12. Academic Press (2009). https://doi.org/10.1016/b978-008045046-9.00752-x
52. Shih, H.T.: Anatomy of the action potential in the heart. Tex. Heart Inst. J. **21**(1), 30–41 (1994)
53. Stephens, J.A., Usherwood, T.P.: The mechanical properties of human motor units with special reference to their fatigability and recruitment threshold. Brain Res. **125**, 91–97 (1977)
54. Sörnmo, L., Laguna, P.: Evoked potentials. In: Sörnmo, L., Laguna, P. (eds.) Biomedical Engineering, Bioelectrical Signal Processing in Cardiac and Neurological Applications, pp. 181–336. Academic Press (2005). https://doi.org/10.1016/b978-012437552-9/50004-0
55. TFESCNASP—Task Force of the European Society of Cardiology the North American Society of Pacing Electrophysiology: Heart rate variability. Circulation **93**(5), 1043–1065 (1996)
56. Thakor, N.V.: Biopotentials and Electrophysiology Measurement. In: Webster, J.G. (ed.) Measurement, Instrumentation, and Sensors Handbook, CRC—IEEE Press, Boca Raton IL (1999). ISSN 1523-3014
57. Thingpen, N.N., Keil, A.: Event-Related Potentials. Reference Module in Neuroscience and Biobehavioral Psychology. Elsevier (2017). https://doi.org/10.1016/b978-0-12-809324-5.02456-1
58. Upton, A.R., McComas, A.J., Sica, R.E.: Potentiation of "late" responses evoked in muscles during effort. J. Neurol. Neurosurg. Psychiatry **34**, 699–711 (1971)

59. Varghese, A.: Membrane models. In: Bronzino, J.D. (ed.) The Biomedical Engineering Handbook, 2nd edn. CRC Press, Boca Raton, FL (2000). ISBN 978-0849385940
60. Walsh, P., Kane, N., Butler, S.: The clinical role of evoked potentials. J. Neurol. Neurosurg. Psychiat. **76**(Suppl II), ii16–ii22 (2005). https://doi.org/10.1136/jnnp.2005.068130
61. Zaza, A., Wilders, R., Opthof, T.: Cellular electrophysiology. In: Macfarlane, P.W., van Oosterom, A., Pahlm OKligfield, P., Janse, M., Camm, J.: (eds.) Comprehensive Electrocardiology, pp. 107–144. Springer (2011)

Chapter 2
Signal Artifacts and Techniques for Artifacts and Noise Removal

Md. Kafiul Islam, Amir Rastegarnia, and Saeid Sanei

Abstract Biosignals have quite low signal-to-noise ratio and are often corrupted by different types of artifacts and noises originated from both external and internal sources. The presence of such artifacts and noises poses a great challenge in proper analysis of the recorded signals and thus useful information extraction or classification in the subsequent stages becomes erroneous. This eventually results either in a wrong diagnosis of the diseases or misleading the feedback associated with such biosignal-based systems. Brain-Computer Interfaces (BCIs) and neural prostheses are among the popular ones. There have been many signal processing-based algorithms proposed in the literature for reliable identification and removal of such artifacts from the biosignal recordings. The purpose of this chapter is to introduce different sources of artifacts and noises present in biosignal recordings, such as EEG, ECG, and EMG, describe how the artifact characteristics are different from signal-of-interest, and systematically analyze the state-of-the-art signal processing techniques for reliable identification of these offending artifacts and finally removing them from the raw recordings without distorting the signal-of-interest. The analysis of the biosignal recordings in time, frequency and tensor domains is of major interest. In addition, the impact of artifact and noise removal is examined for BCI and clinical diagnostic applications. Since most biosignals are recorded in low sampling rate, the noise removal algorithms can be often applied in real time. In the case of tensor domain systems, more care has to be taken to comply with real time applications. Therefore, in the final part of this chapter, both quantitative and qualitative measures

Md. K. Islam (✉)
Department of Electrical and Electronic Engineering, Independent University, Bangladesh, Dhaka, Bangladesh
e-mail: kafiul_islam@iub.edu.bd

A. Rastegarnia
Department of Electrical Engineering, Malayer University, Malayer 65719-95863, Iran
e-mail: rastegarnia@malayeru.ac.ir

S. Sanei
School of Science and Technology, Nottingham Trent University, Nottingham NG11 8NS, UK
e-mail: saeid.sanei@ntu.ac.uk

M. A. R. Ahad and M. U. Ahmed (eds.), *Signal Processing Techniques for Computational Health Informatics*, Intelligent Systems Reference Library 192,
https://doi.org/10.1007/978-3-030-54932-9_2

are demonstrated in tables and the algorithms are assessed in terms of their computational complexity and cost. It is also shown that availability of some a priori clinical or statistical information can boost the algorithm performance in many cases.

Keywords Artifact · Biosignal · ECG · EEG · Neural signal · Noise, etc.

2.1 Introduction

2.1.1 Background and Motivation

Human body is composed of several complex systems including nervous, cardiovascular and musculoskeletal systems. Each system has a particular structure and carries its own physiological, functional and pathological processes. These complex biological systems are dependent on each other and the processes involved are often considered as non-linear, nonstationary, and stochastic process. The resultant biosignals generated from these complex biological processes can be recorded in both invasive and non-invasive ways. The signals recorded by non-invasive electrodes often have extremely low amplitudes (ranging from μV to mV) due to the attenuation by various body tissues. In addition, due to the non-invasive nature, the recordings are more prone to many external noise sources such as artifacts and interferences resulting in low signal-to-noise ratios (SNRs). Thus, the acquired biosignals and their associated important clinical/biological events are often submerged under noise and required to be processed properly by removing such artifacts and interferences before any further analysis and decision can be made. However, often traditional signal processing techniques, e.g., digital filtering, are not suitable enough to effectively remove such artifacts. Therefore, advanced signal processing techniques have been proposed in the literature for this purpose. Figure 2.1 illustrates the general steps involved in a typical biosignal processing system from signal acquisition until classification.

2.1.2 Objectives

The objectives of this chapter are as follows:

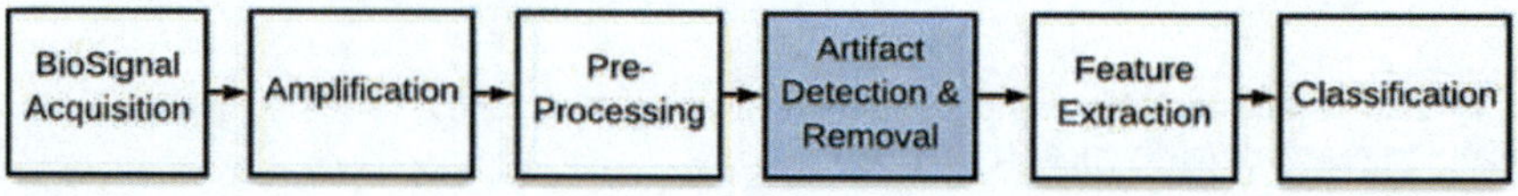

Fig. 2.1 Typical process flow of a biosignal processing system. Only artifact detection and removal is covered in this chapter

- Identify biosignal characteristics and their applications,
- Identify artifact sources and their characteristics,
- Compare and identify suitable signal analysis and processing techniques for artifact detection and removal,
- Demonstrate the influence of reliable artifact detection and removal on the later-stage detection or classification of clinically significant biological events.

2.2 Biosignals and Artifact/Noise Modeling and Characterization

2.2.1 Different Types of Biosignals

Four major types of biosignals including their properties is shown in Fig. 2.2.

2.2.1.1 Biosignals Generated by Cardiac Activity

Electrocardiography

Electrocardiography (ECG aka EKG), shows the electrical activity of heart over a period of time. ECG is recorded via the electrodes that are placed on the chest. Small changes in electrical potentials are picked up by these electrodes due to the cardiac muscle's electrophysiological pattern of depolarizing and repolarizing during each heartbeat. It generally is composed of QRS complexes, P waves and T waves. Figure 2.3 shows an ECG signal of a heart in normal sinus or regular rhythm, at a heart rate of 60–100 beats per minutes.

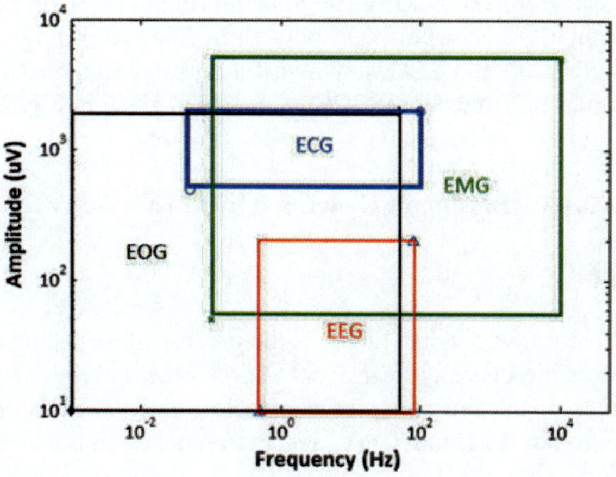

Fig. 2.2 Typical characteristics of some commonly used biosignals in terms of amplitude and frequency range

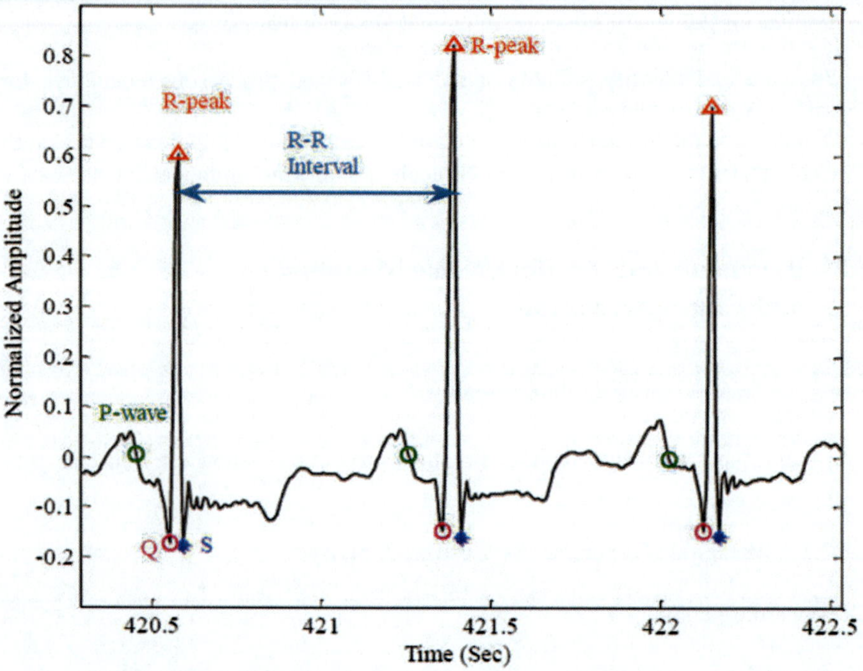

Fig. 2.3 A sample ECG recording with its characteristics points (P-wave, QRS complex) during a cardiac cycle of a normal sinus rhythm

Seismocardiography

Seismocardiography (SCG) is the non-intrusive estimation of cardiovascular vibrations transmitted to the chest divider by the heart and usually recorded by an accelerometer. SCG can provide information of all the activities during cardiac cycle which may not be found only from ECG recordings. Simultaneous recordings of both ECG and SCG may reveal a lot more diagnostic information related to heart diseases. An example SCG recording is given in Fig. 2.4.

2.2.1.2 Biosignals Generated by Muscle Activity

EMG

Electromyography (EMG) is the process of recording electrical potential generated from muscle cells during contraction. Electromyogram is the combined action potentials of the muscle cells of muscle tissue. The amplitude of an EMG signal lies between 0.01 and 1 mV, and its frequency range is 20–1000 Hz. If this signal is

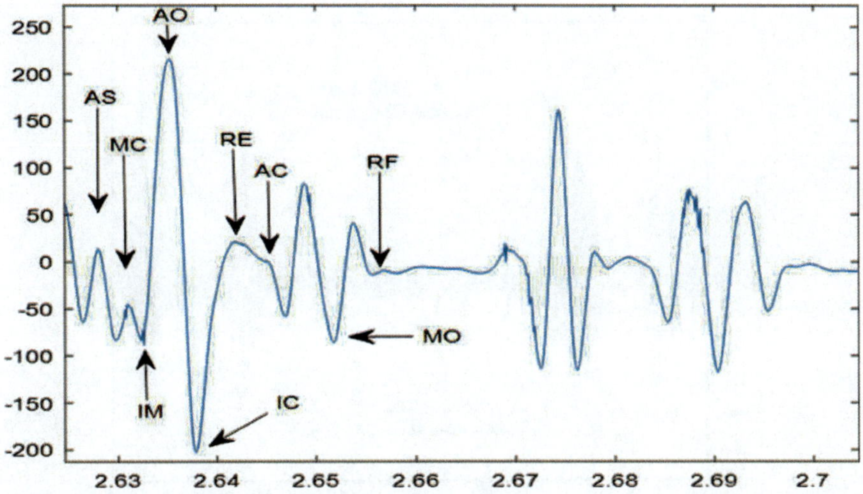

Fig. 2.4 An example of SCG recording during one complete cardiac cycle with annotation proposed by Salerno [1]. Where AS, MC, IM, AO, IC, RE, AC, MO, RF refer to atrial systole, mitral value closure, isovolumic movement, aortic valve opening, isovolumic contraction, rapid systolic ejection, aortic valve closure, mitral valve opening and rapid diastolic filling respectively. X-axis and Y-axis referring to the signal amplitude (in mV) and time (in second) respectively

detected from the surface of the skin, it will be the superposition of messages from all the muscles underneath. A sample raw EMG recording is given in Fig. 2.5.

2.2.1.3 Biosignals Generated by Ocular Activity

Electrooculography

Electrooculogram (EOG) signal is generated due to the potential difference between retina and cornea of the eye which is modeled as an electrical dipole that moves with eyeball movement. The dynamic range of EOG signal is typically 0.05–3.5 mV (peak to peak). The bandwidth of EOG is between 0 and 1000 Hz; however, maximum usable energy of EOG signal lies between 0.1 and 40 Hz [2]. A sample raw EOG recording consisting of both horizontal and vertical eye movements is illustrated in Fig. 2.6.

Eye Blinks

Eye blinks are common ocular artifacts that are found in EEG signals which is due to the blinking of eyes (both voluntary and involuntary). During eye blinks, movement

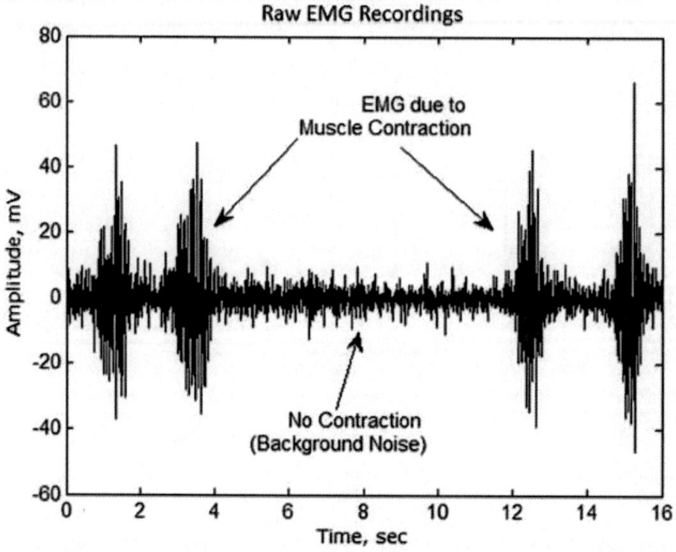

Fig. 2.5 Sample raw EMG signal recorded from arm (after analog amplification) using Ag-AgCl disposable electrodes

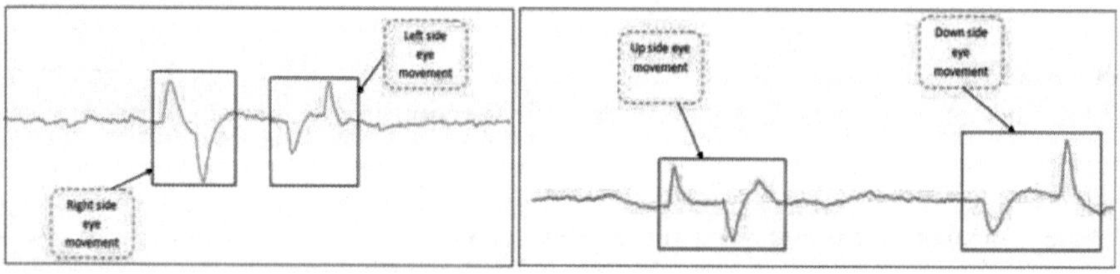

Fig. 2.6 Sample EOG signal recording with disposable electrodes during horizontal (left plot) and vertical (right plot) movement of the eyeball [2]. X-axis and Y-axis referring to the normalized signal amplitude and time (in second) respectively

of eyelid muscles generates such potentials which are counted as artifacts to the neural signal recordings, such as EEG.

2.2.1.4 Biosignals Generated by the Brain

Different biosignals generated due to neural activities in the brain are mainly classified based on their location of recording (i.e. placement of recording electrodes) which is shown in Fig. 2.7 while their characteristics in terms of amplitude and frequency is shown in the Table 2.1.

Table 2.1 Different types of neural signals and their characteristics

Signal type	Frequency range (Hz)	Amplitude range (mV_{pp})
EEG	0.05–128	0.02–0.4
ECoG	0.1–64	0.02–0.1
LFP	0.1–100	0.1–1
EAP	100–10 k	0.04–0.2
IAP	100–10 k	~100

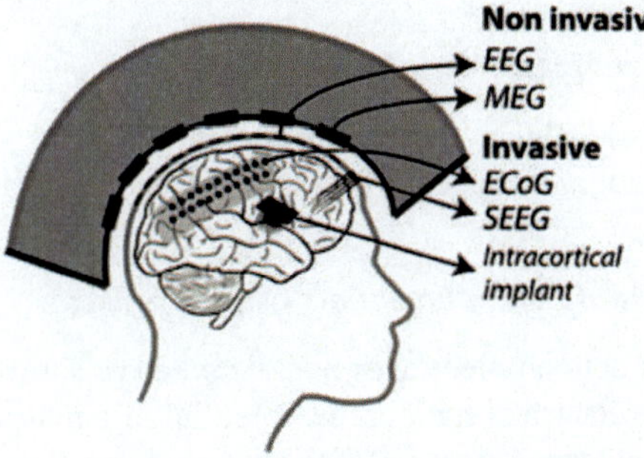

Fig. 2.7 Different types of brain recordings based on the placement of electrodes/sensors. *Courtesy* http://www.frontiersin.org/files/Articles/103134/fnsys-08-00144-HTML/image_t/fnsys-08-00144-g003.gif

Non-invasive Brain Recordings

The most popular non-invasive brain recording technique is Electroencephalography (EEG) that measures the integrated electrical activities produced by billions of neurons in the brain by placing electrodes on the scalp. It is the most commonly used brain recording technique for diagnosis of different neurological disorders along with other applications such as brain-computer interface and basic neuroscience research. The EEG recordings are described in terms of rhythms and transients while the rhythmic activity of EEG is composed of non-overlapping bands of frequency. The most common EEG rhythms are Delta (0–4 Hz), Theta (4–8 Hz), Alpha (8–12 Hz) and Beta (12–30 Hz) waves. Recently a relatively high frequency Gamma wave (>30 Hz) is also considered. On the other hand, artifacts are transient events, although epilepsy seizure events can also be transient but they are more oscillatory than artifacts [3].

To provide a model for recorded raw EEG data, let's denote the clean EEG background activity/rhythm as E_c with weight w_c; Artifact event as A_{T_n} with weight w_{T_n} and time delay τ_{T_n}; where $n = 0, 1, \ldots, N$ denotes the type of artifact. E.g. if it is a Type-1 artifact [4], then denoted by A_{T_1} with weight w_{T_1} and time delay τ_{T_1}. Now the recorded raw EEG signal is usually modeled as the linear combination of these two signal components.

$$E_R(t) = w_c E_c(t) + \sum_{n=1}^{N} w_{T_n} A_{T_n}\left(t - \tau_{T_n}\right) \tag{2.1}$$

Semi-invasive Brain Recordings

Electro-cortiography (ECoG) or intracranial EEG (iEEG) refers to measuring brain signals from the surface of the brain after opening the skull. The temporal resolution of ECoG is better than scalp-EEG but as it requires brain surgery to open up the skull, often it is discouraged in human subject.

Fully Invasive Brain Recordings

Local Field Potentials

Extracellular local field potentials (LFP) are produced by the collective and simultaneous activity of many nearby neurons by synaptic transmission.

Neural Action Potentials (Neural Spikes)

An action potential or neural spike is a short-lasting event (usually 2–3 ms) in which the electrical membrane potential of a neuron rapidly rises (i.e. depolarization) and falls (repolarization), following a consistent trajectory. Such activity gives rise to a specific waveform shape known as action potential. The extracellular action potentials are typically about 100 μV–1 mV), smaller than an intracellular action potential. Microelectrodes (with a tip size of approx. 1 μm) are usually implanted into the brain of a living animal to detect such electrical activity generated by the nearby neurons which is known as 'single-unit' recording. Such recordings of single neurons in living animals can be used to understand the process of information the brain.

2.2.2 *Different Sources of Artifacts and Noises*

Artifacts can originate from both external and internal sources. Internal sources of artifacts are due to different body activities (both voluntary and involuntary activities). On the other hand, external artifacts arise from coupling due to unwanted external interferences. In addition to that, artifacts in broad sense can be categorized into two classes: 'local' and 'global'. Local artifacts are confined in space, i.e. appear only in a single recording channel while global artifacts are found across multiple channels at the same temporal window. An example of global artifacts found in all recording channels of two different neural recordings is shown in Fig. 2.8.

On the other hand, sometimes an artifact is found once in the whole recording sequence (high entropy) while sometimes can have regular/periodic pattern due to any periodic activities/motions of the subject. An example of such artifacts is shown in Fig. 2.9. Table 2.2 summarizes the artifact classification from different perspectives.

Other noise sources are described below:

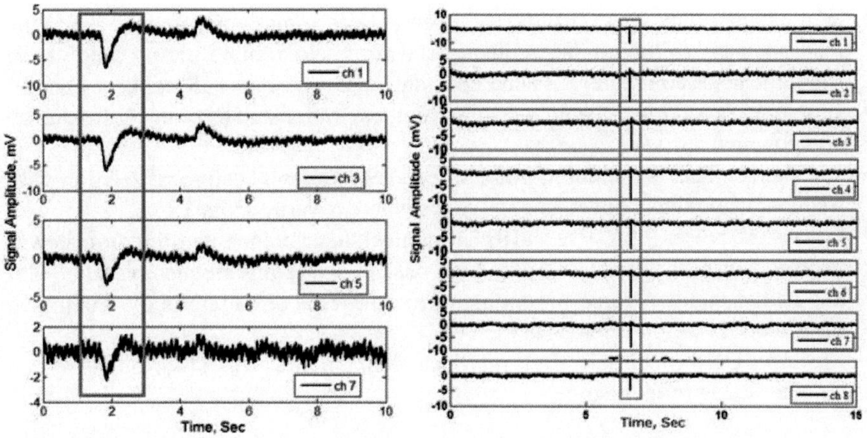

Fig. 2.8 Example of global artifacts from two different datasets of invasive neural signals

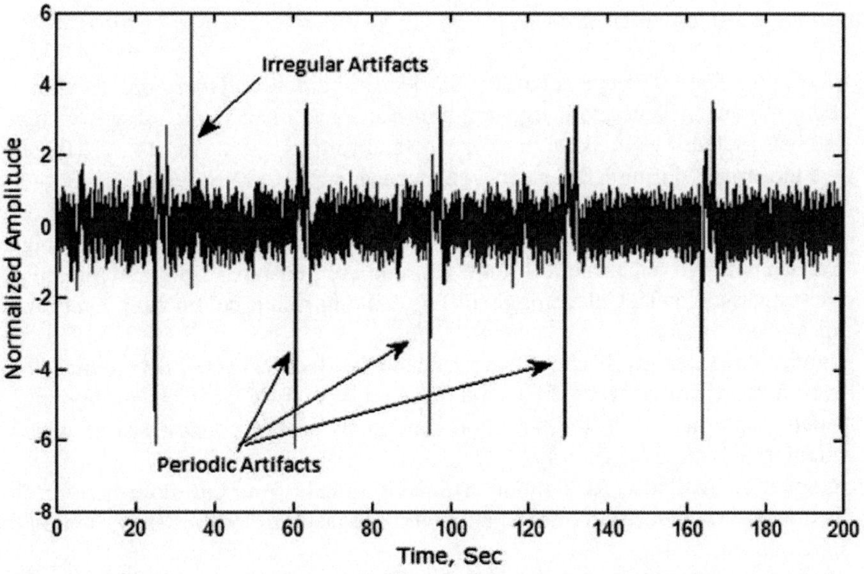

Fig. 2.9 An example of irregular artifact due to electrode pop (left) and periodic artifact due to periodic motion activity of the subject (right) found in invasive neural recordings

Table 2.2 Summary of artifact classification from different perspectives

Perspective	Artifact category	
Repeatability	Irregular/No	Periodic/Regular/Yes
Origin	Internal	External
Appearance	Local	Global

- White Noise: This noise results from thermal electronics noise mainly due to thc resistance and follows a flat frequency spectrum. No digital filtering can remove the white noise completely as it has constant noise power over all frequency bands.
- Baseline Wandering: It usually results from respiration and has sub-Hz frequency components.
- $1/f$ Noise: This is a colored noise whose PSD follows reciprocal relation with frequency and thus known as $1/f^{\alpha}$ noise where α varies from 1 to 3.
- Power-line noises (50/60 Hz and its harmonics): Interference resulting from power sources which usually have a very high peak at power line frequency (50/60 Hz) and its harmonics. Proper grounding of electrodes is often required to minimize the effect of such interference.
- Electrode Offset: Skin-electrode interface often is modeled as a DC voltage source known as electrode offset.

2.2.2.1 Different Artifacts in Neural Signals (EEG, ECOG)

Physiological/Internal Artifacts

- Ocular Artifacts: The eyeball acts as an electrical dipole and therefore any movement in eyeball generates large-amplitude artifacts in EEG recordings. Ocular artifacts include eye blink, both horizontal and vertical eye movement, eye flatter, eye movement during REM sleep, eye saccade, etc.
- Muscle Artifacts: One of the most prominent physiological artifacts comes from muscle activity of the subject (EMG). Usually muscle artifacts are of high frequency range (e.g. from 20 to 40 Hz) and are generated from activities like chewing, swallowing, clenching, sniffing, talking, scalp contraction, eyebrows raising, etc.
- Cardiac Artifacts: Cardiac artifacts are due to the electrical activities produced by heart and are of two types: ECG and pulse artifacts. ECG artifacts are rhythmic regular activities while the pulsation sometimes can cause slow waves which might mimic the EEG activity.
- Respiration Artifacts: Respiration artifacts originate from the movement of an electrode with inhalation or exhalation and can take the form of slow, rhythmic EEG activity.
- Sweat Artifacts: Electrodermal or sweat artifacts originate from changes in electrolyte concentration of electrode due to sweat secretion on the scalp and take the shape of a long, slow baseline drift in the spectral band of 0.25–0.5 Hz [5].

Extra-Physiological/External Artifacts

- Motion Artifact: Movement of patient especially in an ambulatory EEG monitoring system [6–8], generates a lot of motion artifacts. This artifact often has

Table 2.3 Different types of artifacts and their sources found in EEG signals

Physiological or internal				Extra-physiological or external		
Ocular	Cardiac	Muscle	Others	Instrumental	Interference	Movement
Eye blink artifacts, eye movement artifacts (both vertical and horizontal EOG), eye flatter, etc.	ECG artifacts; pulse artifacts	Swallowing, chewing, sniffing, clenching, talking, scalp contraction, etc.	Glossokinetic, respiration, skin, etc.	Electrode pop-up or displacement, cable motion, No/poor grounding, etc.	Electrical, sound, optical, magnetic, etc.	Tremor, movements of head, body, and limbs

extremely high amplitude such that it can saturate the recordings. Head movement, body movement, limbs movement, tremor, walking, running, browsing PC, and many other movements in daily activities are responsible for this type of artifact.

- Environmental Artifact
  - Loose electrode: Loose contact between electrode and scalp leads to change of impedance on the tissue-electrode interface and results in prolonged EEG spike-like artifact.
  - Electrode Pop and Movement: Another common source of artifact is due to electrode pop which produces sudden change in impedance in the electrode-tissue interface and results in high amplitude sharp waveform-shaped artifacts. Electrode movement occurs when it moves with respect to the scalp and produces high-amplitude deflection in EEG generally in the low frequency range of 1–10 Hz.
  - EM Interferences: This type of artifacts is due to the interferences coming from the surrounding electrical/electronic devices/machines that produce EM waves. Also any sound or optical interference may also be picked up by the EEG electrodes as artifacts. In addition, one of most common source of artifacts in any biomedical signal acquisition is the 50/60 Hz main voltage and its harmonics. A summary of different artifact types and their sources is provided in Table 2.3.

2.2.2.2 Properties of Artifacts in Neural Recordings

Usually the artifacts have very large magnitude and/or sharper transitions/edges compared to the biosignals of interest. The frequency range for artifacts may vary from very low (e.g. motion artifact) to high frequency (e.g. artifacts due to residue charge on electrodes) range suggesting artifact spectra overlap with biosignal of interest.

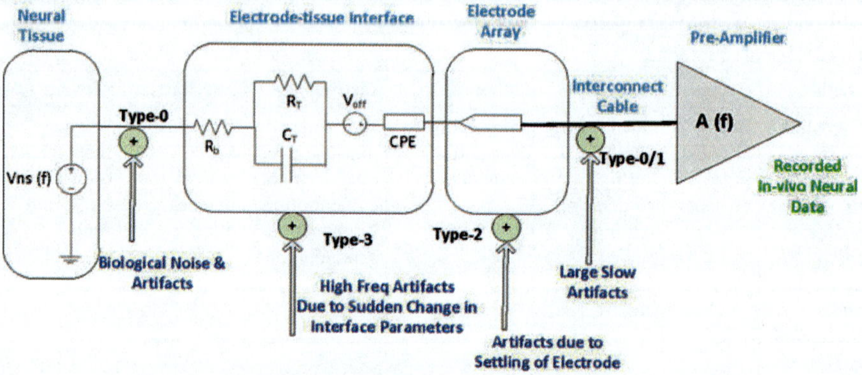

Fig. 2.10 Illustration of origins of different artifact during invasive neural recordings

In order to characterize the spectrum statistics of artifacts as described in [9], different artifact segments have been manually identified and then three artifact templates (Type-1, 2, and 3) were extracted as shown in Fig. 2.11 (a, b, c). Later, artifact spectrum is estimated using windowed Fourier Transform. The results are summarized in Fig. 2.11 (d, e), where it is clearly seen that artifacts tend to display varied spectrum shape and span over broad frequency band of $0 - 6\,\text{kHz}$. Type-1 and type-2 artifacts are dominating at low frequency range while type-3 has higher

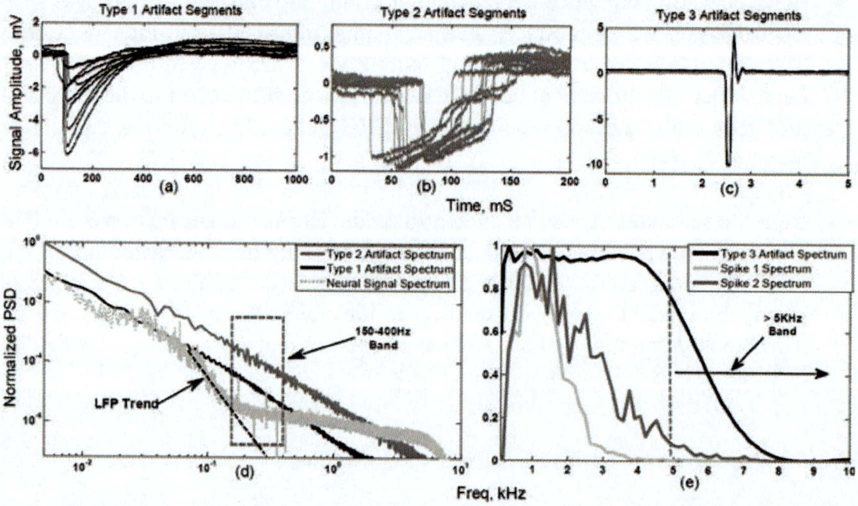

Fig. 2.11 An example of varied artifact characteristics compared with neural signal of interest. **a, b,** and **c**: Three different types of artifact templates: type-1, type-2, and type-3, collected from invasive neural recordings. **d**, averaged PSD of type-1 and type-2 artifacts in comparison with LFP. **e**, type-3 artifact spectrum and neural spike (action potentials) spectrum. Spikes are randomly selected from two different templates

frequency bandwidth. Figure 2.10 shows different artifacts' origin during invasive neural recordings.

To estimate power spectrum density of LFP only, data recorded from rat's superficial layer cortex have been analyzed and spectrum are averaged over 8-channels. Figure 2.11d shows that PSD drops to the level of noise floor at frequency over 150 Hz.

To estimate neural spike spectrum, larger grouped spikes are smoothed and averaged to extract different spike templates. As an example, only two spike templates are used to estimate PSD as plotted in Fig. 2.11e, and found that PSD of spikes drops to noise floor at frequency beyond 5 KHz.

2.3 Signal Analysis and Processing Techniques for Handling Artifacts and Noises

Artifact detection and reduction/removal is one of the most faced challenges for EEG and other bio-signal processing applications and is an open research problem. Most of the biosignal recordings are prone to artifacts and interferences. The variety of artifacts and their overlapping with signal of interest in both spectral and temporal domain, even sometimes in spatial domain, makes it difficult for simple signal preprocessing technique such as typical digital filtering or amplitude thresholding to identify them from desired biosignals. Therefore the use of traditional filters often results in poor performance both in terms of signal distortion and artifact removal. Many attempts have been made to develop suitable methods for artifact detection and removal with the help of recent advancement in signal processing techniques/algorithms in the past decade and a half. However, there is no universal complete solution yet and hence still an active area of research. After careful reviewing almost all the major artifact detection and removal techniques found in the literature, in this section we present a comparative analysis among these SPTs considering their brief theoretical background, pros and cons based on their suitability and performance and finally challenges in implementing them in different biosignal applications.

2.3.1 Pre-processing

2.3.1.1 Epoch-by-Epoch Analysis/Segmentation

The recorded sequence of biosignals is often divided to small duration segments known as epoch. The duration of epoch is such that it contains at least one cycle of biological event of interest or such that the signal within the epoch duration can be considered as stationary since most of the biosignals exhibit non-stationary characteristics. The size of epoch also plays role in determining the computational complexity of the signal processing algorithm in later stage which can be critical in real-time application. The epoch duration is a trade-off between accuracy and real-time computational ability of the SPTs. For EEG, the epoch duration is often decided as one second since within this one second, it can be considered non-stationary whereas EEG is typically a non-stationary signal.

2.3.1.2 Re-Referencing

For multi-channel EEG recordings, re-referencing is often used. Any potential recorded at a particular electrode is with respect to a reference electrode (e.g. in EEG recordings, the mastoid is often chosen as a reference electrode since it is closest to the other electrodes as well as least chance to be influenced by neural potentials). However, still the typical reference electrode may contain some neural information as it also closer to the brain. Therefore, for high density EEG recordings, average activities of all the electrodes may be chosen as reference. This re-referencing can be done offline after the recordings are imported on a software toolbox such as EEGLAB [10].

2.3.1.3 DC Offset Removal

Usually DC signal remains in the biosignal recordings due to electrode-skin interface offset voltage which can be reduced by subtracting the average/mean value of the biosignal from the biosignal itself. If $X(t)$ is a raw biosignal recording and if the mean of $X(t)$ is μ, then the signal after removing DC offset would be $X'(t)$ such that

$$X'(t) = X(t) - \mu \tag{2.2}$$

2.3.1.4 Digital Filtering

Digital filtering, which is nothing but a discrete-time LTI system, is a common part of preprocessing the recorded biosignals to attenuate out-of-band noises and artifacts. Both FIR and IIR filters have been found to be used in such preprocessing stage depending on the application and given specification. The trade-off between FIR and IIR filter is filter-order and stability, respectively. The transfer function of a digital filter can be written as

$$H(z) = \frac{\sum_{l=0}^{M} b_{ml} z^{-l}}{1 + \sum_{k=1}^{N} a_k z^{-k}} \tag{2.3}$$

where $H(z)$ is the z-transform of the impulse response of the LTI system, $h(n)$ knows as system/transfer function while a_k and b_m are the co-efficients of outputs, y(n − k) and inputs, $x(n-l)$ of a Discrete-time LTI system respectively. The difference equation based on which the present output, $y(n)$ is related with the present input, $x(n)$, past inputs, $x(n-l)$ and past outputs, $y(n-k)$ is as follows:

$$y(n) = b_m x(n-l) + a_k y(n-k) \tag{2.4}$$

Low-Pass Filtering

Depending on different biosignals, if desired bandwidth of the recorded signals is known, then a typical FIR low-pass filter is used to cancel out high frequency out-of-band noises and artifacts from the raw recordings. This can be done either in analog domain or in digital domain.

High-Pass Filtering

Sometimes a very steep-slop (IIR or higher order if FIR) high-pass filter with cut-off frequency as low as 0.05–0.1 Hz is used to cancel out electrode (DC) offset including slow-wave artifacts (e.g. motion artifacts).

Notch Filtering

In most of the literatures, a 50 or 60-Hz 3rd or 4th order IIR notch filter is used to remove the 50/60 Hz power line interference (PLI) and its harmonics. Since most of the biosignals have maximum frequency up to 100 Hz (except EMG or invasive neural signals), therefore, often it is good enough to remove the fundamental frequency of the power line interference and removal of higher harmonics (2nd or 3rd harmonic) are not required. However, the problem with notch filtering is that it not only removes the PLI at the fundamental frequency but also removes signal component at that notch frequency. In addition to that, the notch frequency has to be determined in advance to design the notch filter, but in reality, there might be some fluctuations in the notch frequency (e.g. it can be 49.8 or 50.1 Hz instead of exactly 50 Hz). In such cases, the PLI doesn't get removed properly and instead the desired signal component (e.g. Gamma rhythm in EEG recordings) may be removed. In some literatures, researchers proposed the use of adaptive filtering (given that the reference channel can record the power line noise) to remove the PLI without attenuating the signal of interest in that particular (i.e. 50 or 60 Hz) frequency. In [11], a regression approach was proposed to predict the PLI and its harmonics through a mathematical model which doesn't require an extra reference channel and which also doesn't bring any distortion to the signal of interest. An example of application of notch filtering on ECG recordings is illustrated in Fig. 2.12 to remove 50-Hz PLI and its harmonics.

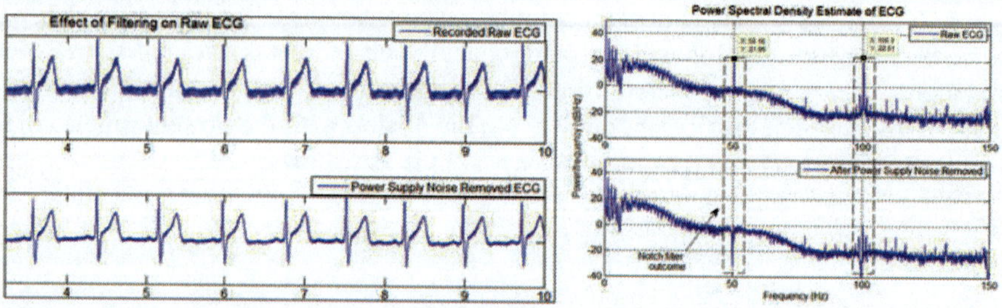

Fig. 2.12 Effect of notch filtering on ECG signals (time domain on left and frequency domain in right) to remove 50-Hz power supply noise and its harmonics

2.3.2 Artifact Avoidance

This is a preventive technique to avoid artifacts or minimize the effect of artifacts by ensuring proper recording environment and protocol such as asking the subject to have least amount of movements or eye-blinks, proper grounding of the recording devices, using enough gel for better connectivity of the wet electrodes, etc. However, artifact avoidance is not the ultimate way of getting rid of artifacts completely, in some applications such as continuous ambulatory monitoring or BCI/HCI applications, subject's movement is inevitable. Moreover, some of the internal or physiological artifacts are involuntary and not possible to avoid, e.g. pulse and eye blink artifacts found in EEG recordings. In addition, the subject may not limit the movement for more than a specific period of time, especially if it is a child. Therefore, these unavoidable artifacts should be removed in the later stage, i.e. digital signal processing (DSP) domain.

2.3.3 Artifact Detection

Reliable identification of artifact contaminated segments of biosignal recording is the most important step for handling artifacts. If any application requires to separate or detect artifacts in real-time, therefore having prior knowledge of characteristics or properties of either the artifact or the signal of interest is really necessary in order to detect them faster. Artifact detection may refer to detection of a specific epoch or an independent component (IC) as artifactual. The detection domain (time or frequency or wavelet) is influenced by the type of artifacts and/or applications. The detection method also varies depending on whether a reference artifact source is available or not, whether the no. of channels is enough, whether artifact removal is required after detection and so on.

2.3.3.1 Simple Amplitude Threshold

Often simple amplitude threshold based approach is taken to detect certain types of artifact or artifactual epoch from artifact-free epoch in time domain. Usually the signal amplitude higher than the set threshold is detected as artifact(s) and lower than the threshold is assumed to be clean epoch. However, due to the non-stationary nature of most biosignals as well as due to variety of artifact types, a pre-defined threshold is not reliable to detect artifact. The following type of threshold value is often seen to be used in the literature for a time series signal, x:

$$Thr = 3 * rms(x) \tag{2.5}$$

2.3.3.2 Machine Learning

Recently machine learning based methods are being used (mostly supervised learning) for artifact separation from useful biosignal of interest by extracting important dominating features. Identified artifactual epochs are either marked as annotator of artifacts for clinicians to make decision (e.g. epileptic onset detection) or rejected before sending for examination to clinician or before sending to automated system [12]. Machine learning techniques are mainly categorized as: supervised (labeled training samples) and unsupervised learning (unlabeled samples). Artificial Neural Network (ANN) [13–17] and Support Vector Machine (SVM) [12, 18–21] are two widely used classifiers among supervised algorithms for separation between artifact and brain signals. While popular unsupervised learning algorithms are k-means clustering and outlier detection in artifact detection applications [12]. A typical process of classifying artifacts from EEG using machine learning is illustrated in Fig. 2.13.

Deep Learning

Deep learning is an advanced version of artificial neural network with representation learning which uses multiple deep layers of neurons to progressively extract higher level features from the raw input and recently has been very popular for separation or identification of artifactual epochs/artifacts from artifact-free epochs [22, 23].

2.3.4 Artifact Rejection

A simple approach to remove the influence of artifacts after detection is to reject/cancel the artifact contaminated epoch or segment. This process not only removes artifact but also removes signal of interest since both overlaps in temporal domain which eventually results in the loss of critical information. This used to

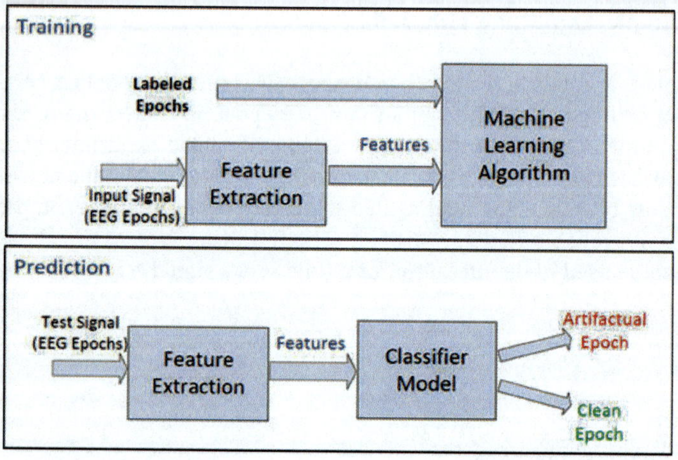

Fig. 2.13 Machine learning approach for classifying artifactual epochs from clean epochs

be traditional way of handling artifacts, but recently with advancement of signal processing techniques, the priority is towards removal or correction of artifactual segments without distorting signal of interest instead of completely rejecting the epoch. However, in some applications, this approach may still be useful, such as offline analysis or training of machine learning classifiers. Artifact rejection can be of following two types:

(a) Full sequence/channel rejection: Bad channels are completely rejected from analysis if found too noisy or artifactual.
(b) Particular Epoch(s) rejection: Only the bad/noisy epochs are rejected from further analysis instead of full channel rejection.

2.3.5 *Artifact Removal*

Artifact removal refers to cancelling or correcting the artifacts without distorting the underlying biomedical signal of interest. This is mainly performed in two means: (i) by filtering or regression and (ii) by separating or decomposing the biosignal recording to other domains.

2.3.5.1 Regression

In this approach, a multi-modal linear model is assumed between observed artifact-contaminated EEG channel and a reference channel containing artifact source. Then, the samples that do not fit with the model are considered as outliers. Physiological artifacts e.g. ocular and ECG artifacts may be removed using such technique from

EEG recordings. However, if no reference channel is available, then such regression will be able to function. In addition, most biomedical signals originate from non-linear and non-stationary process, which makes the linear regression method not useful for artifact removal from such biosignals.

Single-Variate Autoregressive

In an autoregressive model the current sample of the signal is estimated from its previous samples using a set of prediction coefficients optimally calculated using Yule-Walker equations. Denoting the single biosignal as

$$x(t) = \sum_{i=1}^{p} a_i x(t-i) + e(t) \tag{2.6}$$

where p denotes the prediction order, i.e., the number of previous samples used in prediction of the current sample, and $e(t)$ is the residual signal and needs to be minimized and temporally during the prediction coefficient, a_i, estimation. Smaller values of p result in a smoother estimation of the signal by rejecting more redundancy in the signal considering it as noise. On the other hand, larger p will include more redundancy or noise within the estimated signal. Akaike Criterion [24] was one of the first methods in estimating an acceptable value for p. This criterion however, was improved by the approach proposed by Bengtsson [25] for a more accurate estimation of p.

Multi-variate Autoregressive

This is an extension of single variate (univariate) autoregressive. assuming the main multichannel EEGs are both time and space (channel) correlated, then prediction of one sample from one channel from not only the same channel but samples of other channels, which exploits the correlations between channels, can lead to rejecting noise. This has application in brain connectivity, more robust spectrum estimation, and most importantly denoising.

Variational Bayes

Variational Bayesian methods are some useful techniques to solve the problem of estimating an original signal from degraded observations [26–29]. Unlike the Bayesian methods (such as the Bayesian estimation methods based on Markov Chain Monte Carlo (MCMC) algorithms, in VBA methods the intractable true posterior distribution is approximated using a tractable one from which the posterior mean can be easily calculated. In addition, VBA methods usefully have a lower computational complexity compared with the sampling-based methods.

2.3.5.2 Blind Source Separation/Subspace Signal Separation

Blind Source Separation (BSS) is known as useful technique for artifact detection from biosignals. Here, the measured biosignals, X are considered as linear mixture of the sources, S along with AWGN vector, N in multi-channel recordings

$$X = AS + N \tag{2.7}$$

In BSS methods, the ultimate goal is to develop an iterative algorithm which estimates the linear mixture matrix, A. Then, the estimated matrix (denoted by W) is used to estimate the source signals, S' by following formula:

$$S' = WX \tag{2.8}$$

In order to use BSS, it is required that the number of sources must be equal or less than the number of observed channels. In addition, the sources should be maximally uncorrelated (for CCA) or independent (for ICA) from each other. A basic BSS based artifact removal technique is illustrated in Fig. 2.14.

Independent Component Analysis

In general, the Independent Component Analysis (ICA) based algorithms require that the source signals are linearly independent and non-Gaussian distributed. In order to apply these algorithms artifact detection and removal, it is also may require manual intervention to reject independent source components (known as ICs) with visually identified artifacts. It may be made automated by combining ICA with another complementary method such as Empirical Mode Decomposition (EMD) or Wavelet Transform (WT). It also may be used with machine learning classifiers such as SVM or even with a help of a reference channel [30]. However, artifactual ICs may also contain few residual neural or biosignals. Therefore, if the artifactual IC is

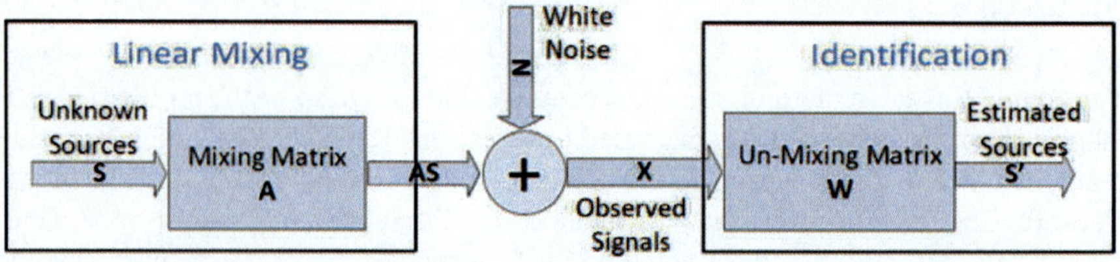

Fig. 2.14 Illustration of a basic blind source separation technique

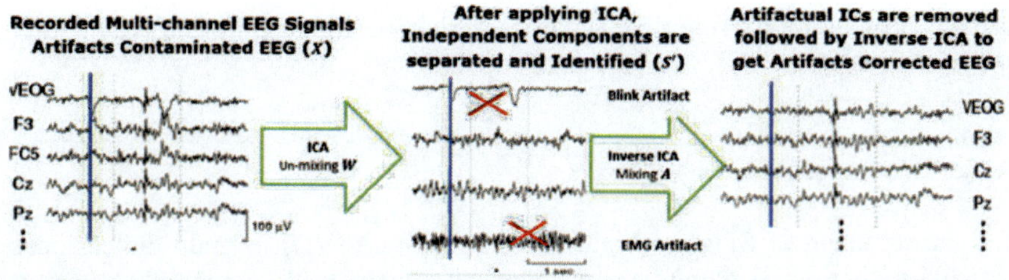

Fig. 2.15 A typical example of application of ICA to identify and remove artifacts (ocular and muscle) that can be separated as an independent sources from multi-channel EEG recordings. Adopted from [40, 41]

completely rejected then distortion to the background neural (or bio) signals occurs. In addition, ICA requires multi-channel recordings to operate which suggests that it cannot be applicable for single (or few channels) recordings. Another challenge that restricts the suitability of ICA for artifact removal (especially in real-time applications) is its high computational complexity. This is because ICA based algorithm usually requires multiple iterations to converge. Considering these factors, ICA may be a suitable choice to remove global artifacts, i.e. ocular artifacts [15, 31–34] or sometimes other physiological artifacts, but not external artifacts. The following works used modified ICA [35] or constrained ICA [36–39] for making it automated artifact detection and removal. An example of ICA based ocular and muscle artifact detection and removal is illustrated in Fig. 2.15.

Canonical Correlation Analysis

A different BSS technique for separating mixed signals is Canonical Correlation Analysis (CCA). In this method, second-order statistics (SOS) is used in order to generate components based on their uncorrelated properties. Considering the uncorrelated components, CCA has weaker criteria than statistical independence used by ICA. CCA addresses temporal correlation unlike ICA, therefore, CCA has maximum temporal or spatial correlation within each component [42].

Morphological Component Analysis

The idea behind the Morphological Component Analysis (MCA) is to decompose the recorded signals into components which have different morphological characteristics and each component is sparsely represented in an over-complete dictionary [43]. It is only applicable to certain artifact types whose waveform shape or morphological characteristics are known in advance and stored in a database. MCA-based method's performance largely depends on the availability of the artifact-template database. An example use of MCA is found in [44] for removing ocular artifacts and few EMG artifacts originating from muscle activities during swallowing, jaw clenching, and eye-brow raising.

Tensor Decomposition

It is an extension of Singular Value Decomposition (SVD) to multi-dimensional space where in the case of multichannel medical signals can decompose the data into its constituent components in a multi-dimensional (time, frequency, space- which is the channel domain-, trial, subject, and even subject groups) or multi-way space. This method separates the disjoint signals, including noise, and localizes the sources. Tensor decomposition best exploits the diversity in the data and its variation in any possible domain. Therefore, generally it is more effective than any other fusion or decomposition technique such as PCA, ICA, or time-frequency method for detecting and localizing events [45, 46].

Time-Frequency Representation

Time-frequency analysis is often performed for biomedical signals as suitable for non-stationary time-series data such as EEG signals. Time and frequency domain analysis are performed simultaneously since non-stationary biosignals have varied statistical and spectral properties with time. Therefore, any change in the instantaneous frequency of each signal component [e.g. either artifact or seizure [47, 48] can be detected in a particular temporal window. An excellent example of the use of such analysis is found in [49] where it is observed that frequencies up to 181 Hz can be present in a subject's EOG signal for certain tasks after simultaneous time-frequency representation was performed for the recorded ocular artifacts (OA) including saccades and blinks. This result suggests that if EOG recording is used as a reference channel for removing ocular artifact from EEG recordings, then sampling rate of EOG recording must be at least 362 Hz (2×181) to avoid aliasing.

The short-time Fourier Transform (STFT) is a widely used time-frequency representation. In this method a uniform time-frequency resolution is used for all signal spectrum (frequency values). The spectrum of most biomedical signals is around 0.5–100 Hz and the spectrum of most artifacts appear in frequency region (< 10 Hz). This means that having high frequency resolution in the lower frequency region is required. But, clearly due to uniform frequency resolution, STFT cannot satisfy such requirement. A nice solution of this issue is to use wavelet transform since it provides a decent time-frequency resolution for most biosignals.

Short-Time Fourier Transform

Short-Time Fourier transform (STFT) is one of the common time-frequency representation techniques which is obtained by segmenting the whole recording sequence

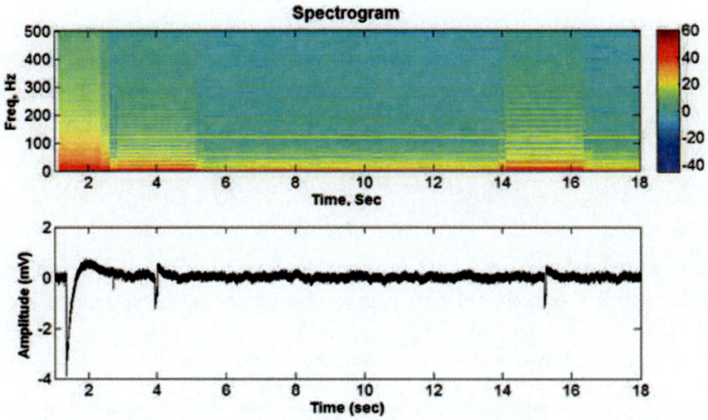

Fig. 2.16 Real neural signal contaminated with both type-1 and type-2 artifacts (bottom) and its Spectrogram (top) shows relatively high frequency components at the temporal locations of these artifacts

into many short-duration epochs by applying window function and then, its frequency representation is calculated by FFT for each of this epochs:

$$F_x(t, f; h) = \int_{-\infty}^{+\infty} x(u) * h(u - t)e^{-i2\pi uf} du \tag{2.9}$$

Here, $h(t)$ denotes the STFT sliding window. For a finite energy window it can be represented as:

$$x(t) = E_h \int_{-\infty}^{+\infty} \int_{-\infty}^{+\infty} F_x(u, f; h)h(t - u)e^{i2\pi tf} dudf \tag{2.10}$$

where $E_h = \int_{-\infty}^{+\infty} |h(t)|^2 dt$. Consequently, STFT is used to determine the energy distribution of any time-series signal (e.g. biosignals) in simultaneous time-frequency domain. Figure 2.16 shows how STFT-based spectrogram can be useful in identifying artifacts by plotting the biosignal energy in both temporal and spectral domain simultaneously.

Wavelet Transform

Wavelets are localized in both temporal and spectral domains compared to the typical Fourier transform which is localized in only frequency. Although STFT offers time-frequency representation, but wavelets provide a better signal representation in terms of higher frequency resolution in lower frequency region and thus more suitable for biosignal time series analysis as most biosignals have dominant frequency components in the low frequency region. The wavelet transform decomposes original signal f(t) into dilated and translated versions of a basis function ψ(t) known as mother wavelet [50]. Any Wavelet is generated from a mother wavelet via:

$$\psi_{j,k}(t) = 2^{j/2}\psi\left(2^{j/2}t - k\right) \tag{2.11}$$

where k is the translation in time with scaling factor of 2 and j indicates the resolution level. Wavelet decomposition follows linear expansion expressed as follows:

$$f(t) = \sum_{k=-\infty}^{+\infty} [c_k\varphi(t-k)] + \sum_{k=-\infty}^{+\infty}\sum_{j=0}^{\infty} d_{j,k}\psi\left(2^j t - k\right) \tag{2.12}$$

where $\varphi(t)$ is known as the scaling function or father wavelet and c_k and d_j, k are the coarse and detail level expansion coefficients, respectively. Theoretically, the expansion coefficients c_k and $d_{j,k}$ are calculated from the inner product of $f(t)$ with $\varphi(t)$ and $\psi(t)$, respectively. A function may serve as mother wavelet by satisfying the following condition:

$$\int_{-\infty}^{+\infty} \psi(t)dt = 0 \tag{2.13}$$

There are various types of wavelet methods such as wavelet approximation and decomposition, wavelet packet decomposition (WPD), discrete and continuous wavelet transform (CWT), stationary wavelet transform (SWT), and so forth. Among them, Discrete Wavelet Transform (DWT) is the most commonly used technique. The relation between input and output of DWT can be expressed as:

$$x_{a,L}[n] = \sum_{k=1}^{N} x_{a-1,L}[2n-k]g[k] \tag{2.14}$$

$$x_{a,H}[n] = \sum_{k=1}^{N} x_{a-1,L}[2n-k]h[k] \tag{2.15}$$

where $g[n]$ is a low-pass filter mimicking scaling function and $h[n]$ is a high-pass filter similar to mother wavelet. Briefly, discrete wavelet transform decomposing a signal into its low frequency component and high frequency components through these two filters known as approximate and detailed coefficients. The wavelet filter decomposition structure is shown in Fig. 2.17.

Once the signal is decomposed, thresholding is applied to denoise the signal from artifacts. At that point the new sets of detailed and approximate coefficients are

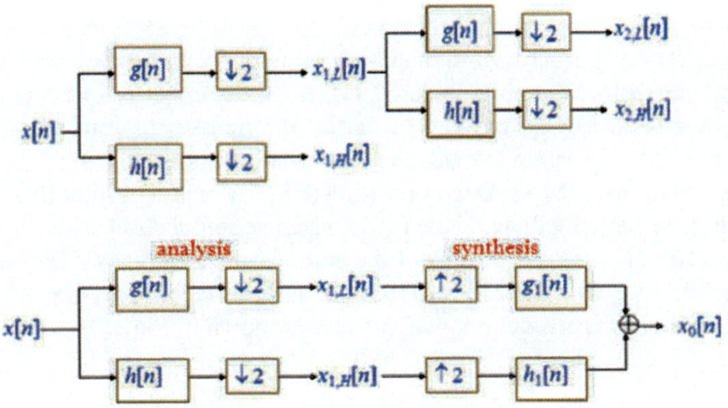

Fig. 2.17 The decomposition (analysis) and reconstruction (synthesis) structures of wavelet filters

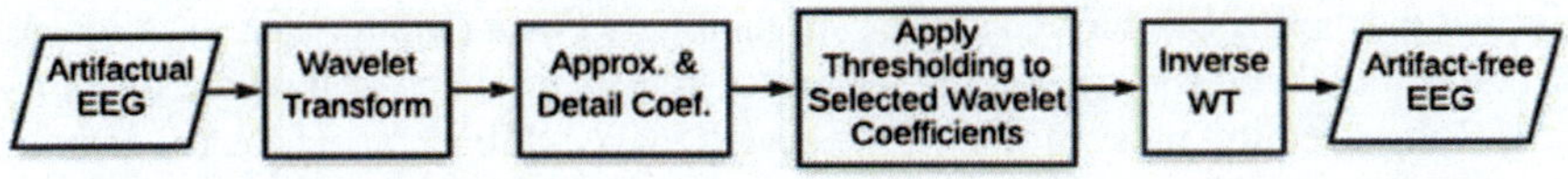

Fig. 2.18 Typical process flow of wavelet-based denoising technique

added up to reconstruct back the artifact-free signal. A typical wavelet denoising based artifact removal from EEG signal as an example is illustrated in Fig. 2.18.

In recent years, wavelet transform based denoising (e.g. DWT) have gained special attention in EEG signal processing due to their suitability in non-linear and non-stationary signal processing [51]. Wavelet transform can be used to separate the energy of the EEG recording into different frequency bands. When it is applied to artifactual EEG signal, it yields the wavelet coefficients representing correlation between the noisy EEG and the wavelet function. Based on the selection of mother wavelet, larger coefficients correspond to the artifactual segment, while smaller coefficients correspond to the actual EEG. It is important to note that suitable mother wavelet and thresholds are required to ensure the effective separation of the artifact coefficients and the EEG signal coefficients. The problem remains how to select the proper mother wavelet and how to choose the parameters for achieving best performance in an automatic fashion.

Empirical Mode Decomposition

Empirical mode decomposition (EMD) is an empirical and data-driven technique applicable for non-stationary, non-linear, stochastic processes, such as EEG signals. However, the computational burden of EMD is higher doubting its ability to perform in online applications. EMD algorithm decomposes the original signal, $s(n)$ into a sum of the band limited functions, $d_m(n)$ known as intrinsic mode functions (IMF) with well-defined instantaneous frequencies [52–54]. An IMF should satisfy the following criteria: (i) at any point, the mean value of the two envelopes defined by local maxima and local minima is zero [54], (ii) the number of extrema has to be equal (or at the most differ by one) to that of the number of zero crossings. The flowchart of EMD algorithm to calculate IMF is shown in Fig. 2.19.

Enhanced Empirical Mode Decomposition (EEM is modified from EMD to make it robust to noise which will avoid the mode mixing complication arises in EMD. To achieve this EEMD uses mean value of the number of ensembles (IMFs) as optimal IMFs allowing it to offer a noise-assisted data analysis technique [42]. An example of simple EMD-based artifact removal process is shown in Fig. 2.20.

Wiener Filtering

Unlike adaptive filters, in Wiener filter a reference signal is not required. However, it assumes that both the signal and artifact are stationary linear random processes, where their spectral characteristics are known and also the signal and artifact are uncorrelated. But in reality, most of the biomedical signals exhibit non-stationary characteristics and are believed to be originated from a complicated non-linear stochastic process. Again, although the spectral characteristics of most biomedical signals are known, due to the uncertainty of different types of artifact sources, the spectral characteristics of artifacts cannot be determined accurately. In addition, the wiener filter is unable to be implemented in real-time, thus may not be suitable for applications where real-time processing is requires such as closed-loop Human-machine interfacing (HMI) through which external devices/machines (e.g. wheelchair, computer, prosthetic limbs) are controlled by biomedical signals (e.g. EEG, EMG, EOG, etc.).

Adaptive Filtering

Adaptive filters have been manifested to prove useful in great deal of biomedical applications. For example, most biosignals, such as ECG or EEG signal acquisition, the information-bearing signals may be contaminated by noise and disturbances caused by the 50/60 Hz power-line, high frequency interference and random body voltages. In such problems, both required signal and noise occur in an identical frequency band and so the noise cannot be discriminately filtered out by removing any specific frequency band. In such cases, filters that can adjust to the changing noise are required. Adaptive filters, systems with variable as an alternative to fixed filter coefficients, can overcome these difficulties. This is achieved by employing adaptive filters such as least-mean-square (LMS) algorithm, recursive-least-square (RLS) algorithm, and Kalman filter-type algorithms, as the analytical implementation of Bayesian filtering recursions for linear Normal state-space models. Adaptive filters are preferably designed as FIR filters, as shown in Fig. 2.21, known for their good stability properties and ease of implementation.

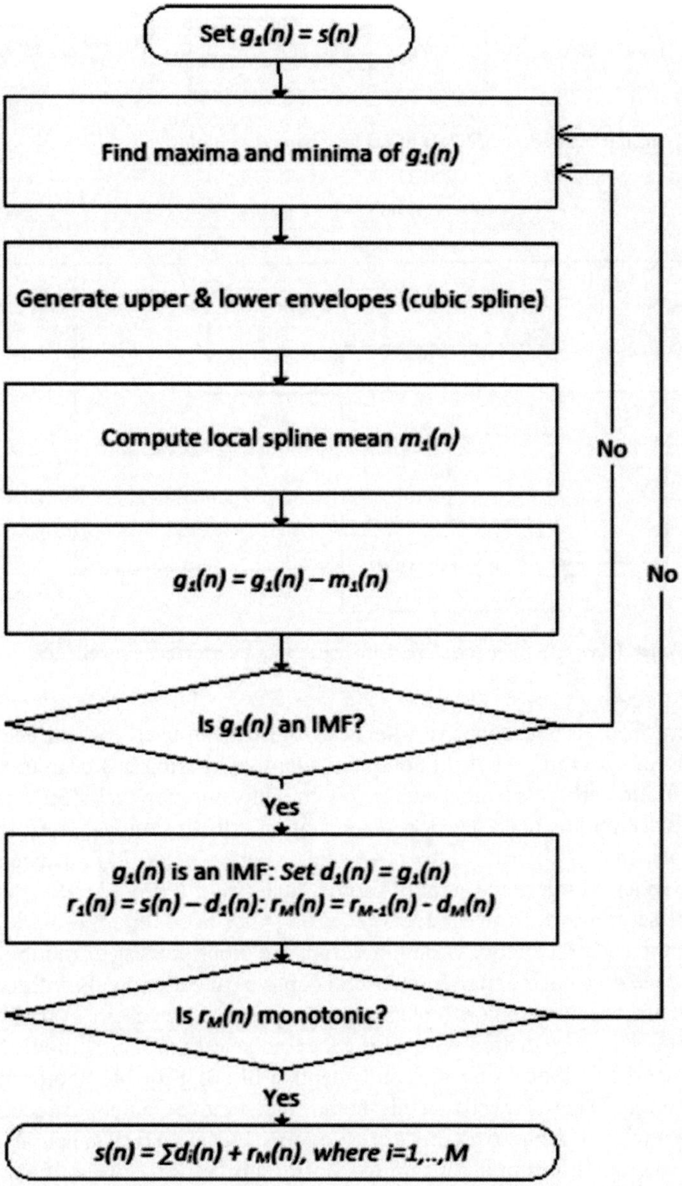

Fig. 2.19 The general process flow of EMD algorithm to generate IMFs

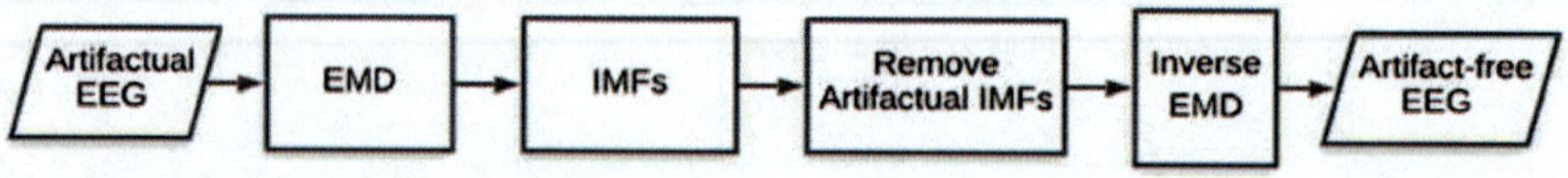

Fig. 2.20 Typical process flow of EMD-based denoising technique

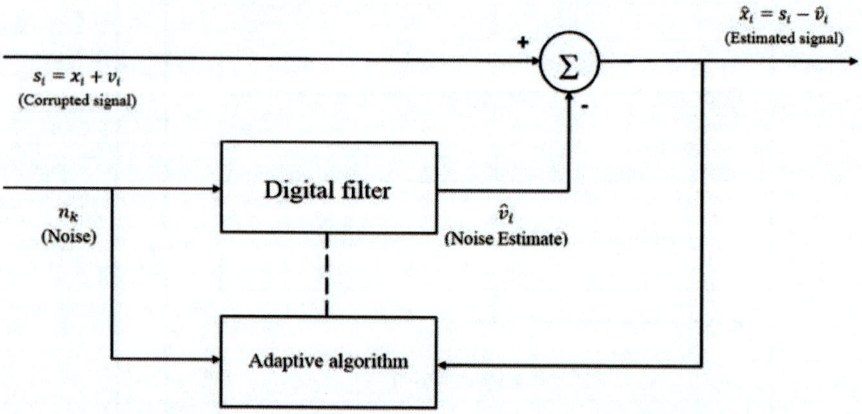

Fig. 2.21 General adaptive filter structure, with concept of interference cancellation

As mentioned earlier, adaptive filters have also been used for artifact removal from biosignals. In [55], a hybrid nonlinear adaptive filtering has been reported for removing motion artifacts from wearable photoplethysmography. In [56] an adaptive filtering algorithm has been developed for motion artifact removal from capacitive ECG signals. In this algorithm, the power-line interference (PLI) has been used to extract the required reference signal. Another adaptive filtering based algorithm for motion artifact removal from the ECG recordings has been reported in [57]. In this algorithm, the spectral energy variation during the input process of motion artifacts is used to develop a cosine transform LMS adaptive cancellation algorithm. In [58], a motion artifact removal algorithm has been proposed which uses a cascade of LMS adaptive filters, in conjunction with a reference noise estimation method. Kim et al. [59] developed a method using ICA and adaptive filtering for MI (motor imagery)-BCI applications. They showed that this method can remove Ocular Artifacts from the EEG signals without measuring Electrooculogram (EOG). In [60], a neural network-enhanced adaptive filtering algorithm has been reported for EEG artifact removal. In order to remove EOG artifacts from EEG recording, it is usually required to have multi-channel EEG recording or an additional EOG recording in real-time. In [61] a new method has been developed which uses a cascade of RLS adaptive filters and sparse autoencoder (SAE) to remove EOG artifacts from EEG recordings. A novel time-domain linear filtering algorithm to remove ocular artifacts from EEG signals has been introduced in [62], where the eye-blink signal is obtained by a small

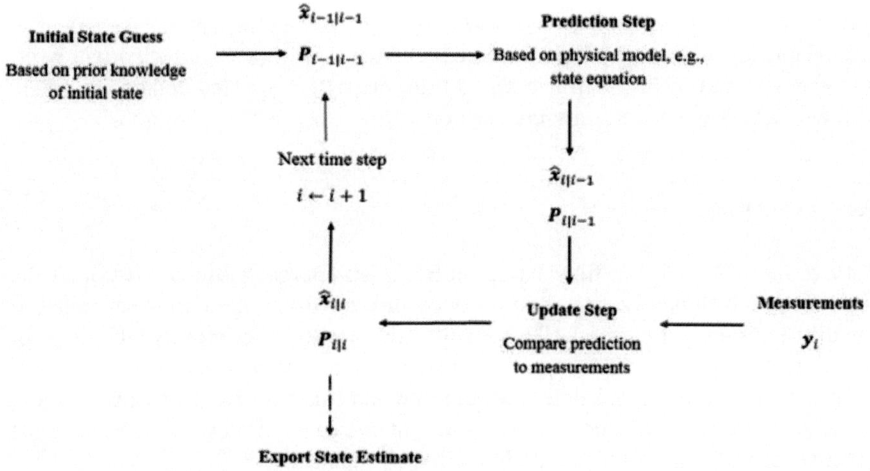

Fig. 2.22 A schematic of the Kalman filter structure

number of frontal electrodes (instead of directly estimating the artifact-free signal) and applying a multichannel Wiener filter (MWF).

Kalman Filtering

Kalman Filter is an estimator based on Minimum Mean Square Error (MMSE) which is often used to extract or smooth physiological signals. Moreover, Kalman filtering may be used to denoise, separate signals or fuse sensor data, all three in a single architecture. The main advantage of Kalman filter, compared to other filtering or signal separation techniques, is its lower systemic delays in real-time computations.

In order to apply the Kalman Filter, the observations should follow a state-space model. In this model an equation shows the evolution of the state model, and the other equation describes the relation of the parameters with the observations:

$$\boldsymbol{x}_i = \boldsymbol{A}\boldsymbol{x}_{i-1} + \boldsymbol{w}_i \tag{2.16}$$

$$\boldsymbol{y}_i = \boldsymbol{B}z_i + \boldsymbol{v}_i \tag{2.17}$$

In the above model $\boldsymbol{x}_i$ are represents the state of model at time i, $\boldsymbol{y}_i$ are the noisy measurements (observations), $\boldsymbol{w}_i$ is the state noise, $\boldsymbol{v}_i$ is the observation, $\boldsymbol{B}$ is the observation matrix and $\boldsymbol{A}$ is the state transition matrix. A schematic diagram of the Kalman Filter is demonstrated in Fig. 2.22.

The Kalman filter consists of two prediction and update steps, which are sequentially executed through time. In the prediction step, the available the data up to time $i+1$ is used to estimate $\boldsymbol{x}_i$. The forecast is denoted as $\hat{\boldsymbol{x}}_{i|i-1}$ and subject to uncertainty quantified by the prediction error covariance $\boldsymbol{P}_{i|i-1}$. When the new measurement $\boldsymbol{y}_i$ is available, the update step is performed. In this step, $\boldsymbol{y}_i$ is leveraged to correct $\hat{\boldsymbol{x}}_{i|i-1}$ and generate an updated estimate $\hat{\boldsymbol{x}}_{i|i}$. At this step $\boldsymbol{P}_{i|i-1}$ is also updated to obtain $\boldsymbol{P}_{i|i}$ to quantify the uncertainty imposed on $\hat{\boldsymbol{x}}_{i|i}$.

Particle Filtering

Particle filter is a kind of filter based on Bayesian approach which overcomes the limitation of Kalman filter as it does not require the data follow a linear model or the distribution to be unimodal. But it still needs a priori user input which may not be available always in EEG-based applications. And there is very little work has been done by far to use particle filter to remove artifacts in EEG signals. Hence it is not guaranteed to be a successful choice, but one can definitely try to observe the outcome of such filter implementation in removing artifacts.

Spatial Filtering

Principal Component Analysis (PCA) is one kind of spatial filtering that typically transforms the original dataset from temporal domain to a new domain by rotating the axes in an N-dimensional space (N is the no. recording channels) where each dimension in the resultant space having minimum variance as well as axes are being orthogonal to each other [63]. It reduces dimensionality of the dataset and highlights dominant features of data that are usually hard to detect in the original domain. In [64] a robust PCA is used after wavelet-based denoising is done as preprocessing while in [65], a comparison is made between PCA and ICA for artifact removal and it is found that ICA outperforms PCA. Since both these articles evaluated the performance qualitatively; therefore, it is difficult to assess the efficacy of the use of PCA in artifact removal. One significant drawback of PCA is that it cannot be used to identify artifacts when signal and artifact amplitudes are comparable to each other (e.g. ocular artifacts from EEG) as it relies on the higher order statistics of the data [36].

Hybrid Methods

In recent years, many works are reported that have utilized the advantages of different SPTs by combining two or more techniques in multiple stages into a single technique for detecting and removing artifacts from biosignals. Some of such hybrid methods are described as follows:

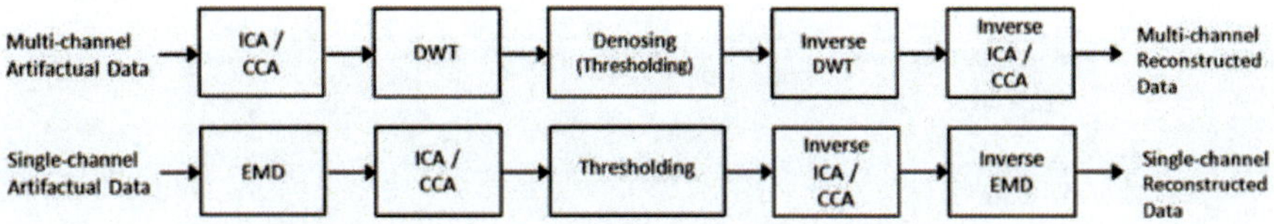

Fig. 2.23 General process flow of wavelet-BSS and EMD-BSS methods

Wavelet-BSS

Wavelet-BSS is formed by combining two commonly used methods: wavelet transform in the first stage followed by blind source separation in the later stage. It is mainly inspired since BSS based separation of artifactual independent components (i.e. ICs) is often flawed as the separated IC may also contain residual biosignals which eventually results in significant distortion in reconstructed signals. To overcome this issue, multi-channel biosignal recordings are converted to ICs or CCs by applying BSS and then potential artifactual component is further decomposed by wavelet decomposition into detail and approximate coefficients of different frequency bands. After that, wavelet denoising is applied which eventually preserves the residual bio signals of low amplitude after thresholding is used to remove the higher amplitude artifactual segments. The reference articles are [66–68] for wavelet-ICA, [69, 70] for wavelet-CCA. On the other hand, for single-channel recording, reversing the order of wavelet transform and BSS i.e. BSS-Wavelet may be used. E.g. [71, 72] reported artifact removal by first decomposing signal into wavelet coefficients; after that BSS is applied on the artifactual coefficients to separate artifacts from background neural/bio signal. However, the former method is more popular to the research community which is known as wavelet enhanced ICA (wICA) or wavelet enhanced CCA (wCCA).

EMD-BSS

It includes BSS with EMD technique. The initial stage of EMD-BSS is to decompose the signal into IMFs by applying EMD or EEMD and then BSS (either ICA or CCA) is applied on the IMFs to identify artifactual components and finally rejecting the artifactual ICs or CCs. (E)EMD-BSS are reported in [42, 73, 74]. Figure 2.23 illustrates typical steps involved in both wavelet-BSS and EMD-BSS based methods.

BSS-SVM

A hybrid BSS-SVM was reported in [20] for removing eye blink and ECG artifacts from EEG recordings where features extraction is performed from separated source components (after BSS is applied) to feed the SVM classifier to separate artifact components followed by removal of the artifact components. Finally in order to

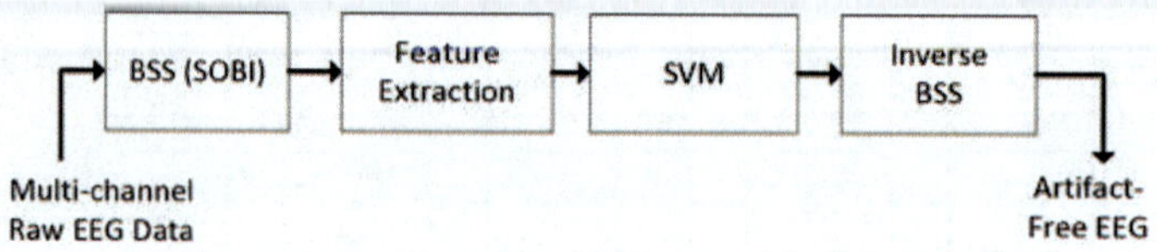

Fig. 2.24 Typical process flow of BSS-SVM method for artifact removal

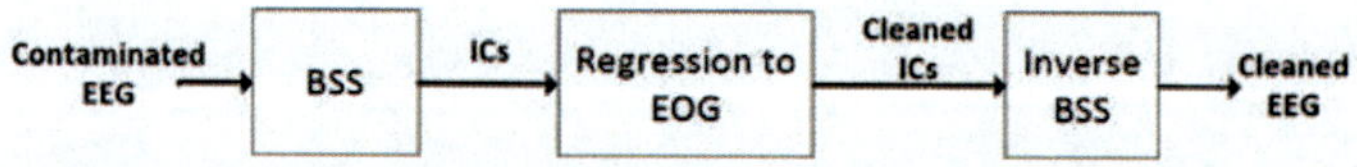

Fig. 2.25 Process flow of REG-BSS hybrid method for artifact removal

reconstruct artifact-free EEG, the remaining source components are re-projected. The whole process is illustrated in Fig. 2.24.

REG-BSS

In [31] a hybrid methodology was reported by combining BSS and regression for removal of ocular artifacts where both vertical EOG and horizontal EOG were used as reference channels as shown in Fig. 2.25. Similar approach has been proposed by Guerrero-Mosquera [26] to remove ocular artifacts by involving ICA and adaptive filtering. Another work [75] proposed to combine ICA and Auto-Regressive eXogenous (ARX) to implement a robust ocular artifact removal where ARX reduced the negative effect induced due to ICA.

Other Approaches

Nguyen et al. [76] reports removing EOG artifacts from EEG using the combination of Wavelet decomposition and Artificial Neural Network, i.e. WNN where EOG reference channel is only required during training of ANN classifier. Another work [77] proposed a hybrid method combining DWT and ANC (Adaptive noise canceller) to remove EOG artifacts (the reference signal is estimated from DWT coefficients required for the adaptive filter). On the other hand, [78] proposed the use of both EMD and adaptive filter (using RLS algorithm) to remove cardiac artifacts from EEG recordings. The authors in [16] reported a new hybrid method to remove EOG and EMG artifacts from EEG recordings by combining functional link neural network (FLNN) and adaptive neural fuzzy inference system (ANFIS).

2.3.5.3 Statistical Features

Statistical features are also used in machine learning in feature extraction stage or during calculation of threshold value used in different SPTs (wavelet, EMD, ICA, etc.) for identifying artifacts from biosignal of interest. Some of the commonly used features are discussed below:

Time Domain Features

Among time domain features, most commonly used features are: Entropy, Kurtosis, Line Length, NEO, Maximum, Minimum, Variance, Mean, etc. [51].

Frequency Domain Features

Among spectral domain features, most commonly used features are mean, maximum, minimum and variance of the absolute value of FFT or PSD. E.g. EEG rhythms are non-overlapping frequency bands and therefore, spectral features may be useful to separate artifacts from a targeted EEG rhythm in consideration for a specific application.

Spatial Features

Spatial distribution of the recordings can be known from spatial features which allows to identify the origin of brain signals as well as some artifact types (e.g. ocular artifacts are mostly found in frontal electrodes as closest to the origin of that artifact). In addition, global artifacts (e.g. eye blinks) can be differentiated from local artifacts based on spatial mapping. Therefore spatial features of data with both temporal and spectral contents can be useful to separate artifacts from EEG signals [14, 79].

Auto-Regressive Features

Refer to Sect. 3.5.1.1, the AR model parameters, α_i can be considered as features for classification.

2.3.6 Summary and Comparison Between SPTs

See Table 2.4.

Table 2.4 Comparison of different SPTs used in artifact removal from different biosignals

Main methods used	References	Type of bio signal	Type of artifacts/noise	Applications	Remarks
Adaptive filtering/ANC	[55–61]	PPG, ECG, EEG	Motion/Ocular/EMG + ECG + EOG/	Cardiac diagnosis	Extra channel (EOG, ECG, Accelerometer, Gyroscope, Eye tracker, motion captured camera, contact impedance measurement, etc. required to record reference signal
Kalman Filtering	[80–82]	ECG	Gaussian/Non-Gaussian/muscle artifact/PLI	Cardiac diagnosis	Automated and real-time processing, no a-priori info required, not suitable for non-linear and non-stationary process like EEG

(continued)

Table 2.4 (continued)

Main methods used	References	Type of bio signal	Type of artifacts/noise	Applications	Remarks
Wiener Filtering	[62]	EEG	Eye Blink	General	Proposed for multi-channel EEG recording. Also can work on single-channel data. A-priori user input required and cannot operate online in general
(c)ICA	[31–35, 37, 39, 83]	EEG	Mostly ocular, few motion and other Physiological artifacts	Epilepsy diagnosis, BCI, general purpose	Most of them are semi-automated, few require additional sensor(s) while
CCA	[84, 85]	EEG	Muscle/ocular	Ictal EEG source imaging, Epilepsy monitoring	Not online/real-time processing, requires multi-channel recordings
PCA	[35, 57, 64]	EEG	General	SSVEP for emotion detection	Robust PCA

(continued)

Table 2.4 (continued)

Main methods used	References	Type of bio signal	Type of artifacts/noise	Applications	Remarks
Wavelet transform	[51]	EEG	All types: ocular, muscle	Epileptic seizure detection	Can work for both single and multi-channel recordings, no extra reference channel required
Tensor decomposition	[46, 86]	EEG	Ocular	Epileptic Seizure detection and localization, diagnosis in Preterm babies and many other EEG related applications	Tensor decomposition may involve wavelet transform, ICA, etc.
(E)EMD	[42, 54]	EEG	EOG	General	Extra reference of Fractional Gaussian Noise required and can work for single channel recordings
Hybrid methods					

(continued)

Table 2.4 (continued)

Main methods used	References	Type of bio signal	Type of artifacts/noise	Applications	Remarks
Wavelet-BSS (W-ICA/W-CCA)	[66–69, 71]	EEG	Ocular + muscle + electrical shift	General	Mostly applicable for multi-channel recordings
(E)EMD-BSS (ICA/CCA)	[42, 73, 74]	EEG	Muscle, motion, EOG	Ambulatory single-channel applications, ictal EEG, diagnosis	Can work for single channel and mostly automated
BSS-SVM	[20]	EEG	Eye blink	General; e.g. ERP analysis	Applicable only for multi-channel recordings
REG-BSS	[31, 87, 88]	EEG	Ocular	General	vEOG and hEOG reference channel required
Others (WNN/DWT-ANC/EMD-ANC/ICA-ANC/FLNN-ANFIS)	[16, 76–78]	EEG	EOG, ECG, EMG	General, diagnosis, portable applications	Reference channels are required for ANC related methods

2.3.7 *Currently Available Software Plug-Ins*

Different biosignal processing and analysis toolboxes are listed in the following table where it is shown what are the SPTs used for these toolboxes along with type of biosignal and artifact types handled.

2.4 Discussion

2.4.1 *Limitations and Suitability of the SPTs*

2.4.1.1 Real-Time/Online Implementation

There are some applications that require real-time or online processing of biosignals such as HMI or real-time seizure detection (i.e. BCI, neural prosthetics, EOG-controlled wheelchair, etc.). Therefore, choice of artifact removal technique for such application would be such that it has the required low computational complexity to be compatible with real-time/online processing. In that case, trade-off between computational complexity and performance of the artifact removal algorithm is to be made. On the other hand, there are applications such as diagnosis of neurological disorders/diseases that may allow offline processing. In such case, one can only focus on achieving highest performance without much considering about computational time.

2.4.1.2 Single or Multi-channel

As seen from both Tables 2.4 and 2.5 that some SPTs are suitable for both single and multi-channel biosignal recordings while few of them (such as BSS based techniques) require multi-channel recordings to be applied. On the other hand, wavelet or EMD based techniques can be applied for a single-channel recording. So it is critical to select SPT for appropriate application considering the no. of channels in mind.

2.4.1.3 Reference Channel

Refer to Table 2.5, some of the available SPTs require an additional dedicated reference channel to record artifact source for functional. Example of such reference channels: EOG, ECG, Motion Sensors, and Contact Impedance Measurement channels to remove ocular artifact, cardiac/pulse artifact, motion artifacts, artifacts due to electrode popup or movement, respectively. However, having an extra reference channel is not always feasible in some applications such as portable and continuous monitoring if the reference sensor is not integrated with the original biosignal

Table 2.5 Existing software toolboxes for handling different types of artifacts from biosignals

Name of toolbox	References	Main methods used	Type of bio-signal	Type of artifacts/noises	Extra features or specs	Platform/compatibility	Free/open source?
EEGLAB	[10]	ICA, Time-frequency Analysis, standard averaging	EEG, MEG, ECoG	Almost all types of Artifacts except motion artifacts	Supports importing of multi-format database, high-density recordings scrolling, artifact removal (semi-automated), EVENT and channel location handling, forward and inverse head or source modeling, over 100 advanced plug-ins/extensions	MATLAB	Y
BCILAB	[89]	Similar to EEGLAB	EEG	Almost all types of artifacts except motion artifacts	BCI Applications and classification	EEGLAB/MATLAB	Y
Bio-SP	[90]	Signal-specific algorithms Mainly IIR digital filtering (Elliptic, Gaussian, or Butterworth)	Peripheral Physiological Signals (ECG, EDA, EMG, BP, or ICG)	General types of artifacts and noises including PLI	Feature extraction and critical events or parameters detection	MATLAB (Any version) Windows, macOS, Linux	Y

(continued)

Table 2.5 (continued)

Name of toolbox	References	Main methods used	Type of bio-signal	Type of artifacts/noises	Extra features or specs	Platform/compatibility	Free/open source?
BioSig	[91]	Linear regression for EOG artifacts removal from EEG, and time/frequency domain features such as slope, amplitude or spectral edge frequency for EMG artifacts detection from EEG	EEG, ECoG, ECG, EOG, EMG, and Respiration signals	Removal EOG artifacts and only detection of EMG artifacts from EEG	Real-time BCI system implemented in MATLAB and Simulink	MATLAB or octave and python	Y
ANSLAB	[92]	Threshold-based, digital filtering	ECG, EDA, EMG, eye blinks, respiration signals	General types	Analysis of long-term recordings from ambulatory settings	MATLAB	Open ANSLAB—Y ANSLAB Professional—Partly
Clean rawdata	[93]	ASR and digital filtering	EEG	Low-frequency drifts, flat line, eye blinks, muscle activity, sensor motion	default EEGLAB method for removing artifacts from EEG	EEGLAB/MATLAB	Y
BioSigKit	[94]	RLS adaptive Filter, variable leaky ALE filter	ECG, EMG and EEG	Motion artifacts	Fetal-ECG extraction from both single and multi-channel maternal ECG	MATLAB	Y

(continued)

Table 2.5 (continued)

Name of toolbox	References	Main methods used	Type of bio-signal	Type of artifacts/noises	Extra features or specs	Platform/compatibility	Free/open source?
biosppy	[95]	Digital filtering	BVP, ECG, EDA, EEG, EMG, Respiration	Out of band noise and DC offset	Support for various biosignal processing, detection of events and clustering	Python	Y
WFDB	[96]	Not found	ECG, EEG, EMG, fetal ECG, PLETH (PPG), ABP, respiration, etc.	Not mentioned	Allows reading, writing, and processing of physiological signals and time series signals from PhysioBank databases	MATLAB/Octave	Y
BSP	[97]	Non-linear filtering (Rank Filters, Median Filters)	ECG, ABP, ICP, and SpO2	Movement artifact and quantization noise	Nonlinear filtering, detection algorithms, spectral analysis, multi-signal analysis, non-stationary signal visualization.	MATLAB	Y
EMGLAB	[98]	Digital filtering	EMG	Low frequency artifacts, DC offset, out of band noises	Decomposing EMG into MUAP trains and averaging MUAP waveforms	MATLAB	Y

(continued)

Table 2.5 (continued)

Name of toolbox	References	Main methods used	Type of bio-signal	Type of artifacts/noises	Extra features or specs	Platform/compatibility	Free/open source?
SASICA	[99]	Reject/select independent components based various features/properties	EEG	Muscle artifacts	Semi-automated guided selection of artifactual ICs	EEGLAB/MATLAB	Y
FASTER	[100]	ICA	EEG	EOG, EMG artifacts, linear trend and white noise	Fully automated and unsupervised; supports high-density EEG recordings	EEGLAB/MATLAB	Y
OSET	[101]	Semi BSS and digital filtering	Any Bioelectric signals	Cardiac and EOG artifacts	Biological signal generation, modeling, processing, and filtering	MATLAB and C ++	Y
AAR	[102]	Regression/adaptive algorithms (LMS, RLS), BSS and Spatial Filters + ICA	EEG	Ocular and muscular artifact	Automated algorithm (ICA-based)	EEGLAB/MATLAB	Y
ADJUST	[14]	ICA	EEG	Ocular (blinks, eye movements)	Automated; no MATLAB toolbox is needed to run	EEGLAB/MATLAB	Y
FOOBI	[103]	Underdetermined blind source separation	EEG	Ocular	Automated, no extra channel required	–	–

(continued)

Table 2.5 (continued)

Name of toolbox	References	Main methods used	Type of bio-signal	Type of artifacts/noises	Extra features or specs	Platform/compatibility	Free/open source?
LAMIC	[104]	Temporal extension of ICA (TDSEP) followed by clustering based on AMI	EEG	Ocular, EMG and ECG	Automatic clustering algorithm	–	–
FORCe	[83]	Combination of WT, ICA and thresholding	EEG	Eye blink, EOG and EMG artifacts	Fully online and automated artifact Removal for BCI applications	MATLAB Wavelet Toolbox/EEGLAB	Y
PRANA	[105]	Digital filtering + BSS	EMG, ECG, EEG, EOG, EDA, pulse oxymetry, respiration, blood pressure, temperature, sound, light intensity activity, etc.	Not mentioned (mainly ocular artifacts)	GUI for different Biosignals processing and time series analysis	MATLAB	Y
PFEIFER	[106]	Digital filtering	ECG	Signal noise, drift, etc.	Computationally efficient GUI	MATLAB	Y

(continued)

Table 2.5 (continued)

Name of toolbox	References	Main methods used	Type of bio-signal	Type of artifacts/noises	Extra features or specs	Platform/compatibility	Free/open source?
Brainstorm	[107]	Signal Space Projections, ICA, Digital filtering	MEG, EEG, fNIRS, ECoG, invasive neural recordings	Eye blinks, ECG	Supports wide verities of data file formats and brain recording modalities with automated detection of artifacts, 2D/3D visualization, time-series analysis, head and source modeling, functional connectivity, decoding and pattern analysis	MATLAB (executable, OS platform independent, doesn't require to own a License)	Y
FieldTrip	[49]	Digital filtering and ICA	MEG, EEG, iEEG and NIRS	EOG, ECG, EMG artifacts and line noise	Both manual and automatic artifact rejection. Allows time-frequency analysis, dipoles-based source reconstruction, and non-parametric statistical testing	MATLAB	Y

(continued)

Table 2.5 (continued)

Name of toolbox	References	Main methods used	Type of bio-signal	Type of artifacts/noises	Extra features or specs	Platform/compatibility	Free/open source?
REST	[108]	Online RLS Whitening, Online ICA	EEG	General noise	Real-time source localization	MATLAB/EEGLAB	Y
BERGEN	[109]	Digital IIR filters (band-pass) and Moving average correction based on artifact templates	simultaneous EEG-fMRI	Gradient artifacts from fMRI	Head movements are taken into account for better removal of gradient artifacts	EEGLAB/MATLAB	Y
CIAC	[110]	ICA (semi-automated)	EEG	Electrical artifacts originating from cochlear implants	Allows to identify and cluster artifactual ICs across subjects	EEGLAB/MATLAB (Statistics toolbox)	Y
CORRMAP	[111]	Template based identification (Semi-automatic) and clustering of independent components	EEG	Ocular and heartbeat artifacts	Allows to identify and cluster artifactual ICs across subjects	EEGLAB/MATLAB (Statistics toolbox)	Y
FMRIB	[75]	FASTR: FMRI artifact slice template removal	EEG-fMRI	fMRI-environment artifacts: e.g. gradient artifacts, BCG artifacts and scanner-related artifacts from EEG	GUI software	EEGLAB/MATLAB	Y

(continued)

Table 2.5 (continued)

Name of toolbox	References	Main methods used	Type of bio-signal	Type of artifacts/noises	Extra features or specs	Platform/compatibility	Free/open source?
MARA	[112, 113]	Linear classifier to classify independent components as 'accept' or 'reject'	EEG	Ocular artifacts, muscular artifacts and loose electrodes	Not limited to a specific artifact type; uses supervised machine learning algorithm	EEGLAB/MATLAB (toolboxes required: Statistics, Optimization and Signal Processing)	Y
REGICA	[31]	Regression performed on ICA components	EEG	EOG artifacts	Semi-automated	EEGLAB/MATLAB	Y
CleanLine	[114]	ICA + Regression technique (frequency-domain)	EEG	50/60 Hz line noise + harmonics	Both manual and automatic artifact rejection, supports computationally efficient GUI	EEGLAB/MATLAB	Y

recorder. In addition, these reference channels must synchronize (e.g. in terms of sampling rate or dynamic range), with relevant biosignal recordings to be able to apply regression or adaptive filtering technique.

2.4.1.4 Robustness

Robustness is another important issue to decide on the selection of any artifact removal technique since diverse types of artifacts contaminate and/or affect different biosignals differently for different recording protocols and for different environments. In order to evaluate a particular SPT on its ability to detect and remove artifacts from a specific biosignal, it is very critical to prove its robustness under different experimental setups (or different applications or environments) and different set of subjects.

2.4.2 Future Challenges and Opportunities

With the advancement of technology (e.g. improved sensors, flexible and wearable electronics, analog front-ends, wireless data transfer, cloud computing, AI and machine learning), biomedical signals are going to be recorded and processed real-time in an ambulatory settings where the subjects can move freely and able to perform daily activities. The purpose of such continuous ambulatory recording is not only to monitor patient's condition or to diagnose diseases, but also to predict future health condition and utilize continuous biomedical signals for preventive healthcare. In addition to that, such recording will be used in the area of games and sports and evaluation of one's overall fitness. This potential future scope will come up with new challenges such as handling extreme motion artifacts due to subject's movements in daily activities. Another challenge will be the processing of huge amount of data samples for such continuous recording which will require advanced SPTs to be able to operate in real-time. In addition to that, transferring the samples wirelessly and eventually to store this big data for future reference is another potential challenge to address. In such case, before transferring the samples wirelessly, instead of transferring raw data, extracted and selected features along with compression may be important which again requires new improved SPTs to be proposed and tested.

2.4.3 Recommendations

2.4.3.1 Application Specific Models

The choice of SPT should be application specific. Often it is not required to remove each and every artifact type for a particular application, instead the preference should be given only on those artifacts that affect the application most. For example, in Motor Imagery based BCI, the frequency bandwidth of EEG signal of interest is 8 − 32 Hz (i.e. Alpha and Beta rhythms) which means artifacts present in that frequency range must be handled carefully and removed without distorting targeted signal of interest. Artifacts due to muscle activities (EMG) lie in that frequency range while EOG/ECG or motion artifacts belong to less than 8 Hz frequency bandwidth. This implies that one should not bother about removing EOG/ECG/motion artifacts that much for MI based BCI applications, rather concentrate on only removing EMG artifacts as it affect both the Alpha and Beta rhythms most. Therefore, to choose the right SPT for removing artifacts, one should consider the particular application and required specifications to be met given a certain computational resources and recording protocol available. Only those artifacts should be removed which affect the later stage decision making. If an extra reference channel is available to record artifact source (e.g. EOG, ECG, motion sensors, etc.), then SPTs such as regression or adaptive filtering technique may be applied. In case of ambulatory and continuous monitoring applications, no. of channels is lower and reference channel is not available, then it is recommended to use computationally efficient methods that are capable of functioning without reference channel and with single or few channels. Examples of such SPTs are wavelet based methods. In some applications, if prior knowledge about artifacts is available and some training samples are available, and finally if the it only requires to identify artifacts without removing them, at that time machine learning may be a realistic choice. If the biosignals have high-density channels, then PCA can be applied to reduce the dimensionality of the data before applying SPTs for artifact removal (e.g. BSS involved techniques). If the application does not require real-time computation (i.e. involves offline analysis), then computationally expensive techniques with high performance such as cICA or EEMD may be applicable. An example of different application-specific models is as follows:

- Biosignal Specific: EEG, iEEG/ECoG, ECG, EMG, etc.
- Diagnostic/Clinical Application Specific:
- Artifact Specific: Ocular, Muscle, or Motion artifacts.

2.4.3.2 Standard Performance Evaluation

Lack of standard performance evaluation metrics/criteria for the SPTs is a big concern. Most works proposing SPTs for artifact removal found in the literature mentioned some qualitative plots in either time or frequency domain to visually assess the performance (e.g. assessment by clinical experts). (K. T. Sweeney et al. [52] proposed a recording protocol for correct assessment and comparison between different SPTs for physiological signals which may be suitable for some applications that allow intervention to the recording protocol and an extra artifact reference channel is available. However, applications such as portable EEG recordings for ambulatory monitoring may not be compatible with this proposed method. Although it is highly encouraged to evaluate a particular SPT by the domain experts, however, such qualitative assessment varies from one expert to another and therefore difficult to compare between SPTs for different recording protocols or different biosignals. Therefore, it is high time to develop few standard evaluation criteria for the SPTs which may consist of both qualitative and quantitative metrics to make it more realistic and have a fair comparison.

2.4.3.3 Ground Truth Data

The unavailability of ground truth data (i.e. clean reference biosignals) is another reason for not being able to evaluate performance of a SPT quantitatively. Thus it is also essential to develop a public database with clean biosignal of all types, especially EEG. This is because EEG is the most prone to noise and artifacts among all other non-invasive biosignal recordings and there is no ground truth data of EEG found to the best of our knowledge. So to record ground truth biosignals, recording protocols and experiment should be designed carefully. In addition to that an acceptable mathematical model to generate/simulate basic biosignals may also be developed for quantitative evaluation of any existing or future SPTs. Finally, more research is required to identify and characterize artifacts as many as possible. Therefore, it will be feasible to label both ground truth biosignals as well as artifact templates.

2.5 Conclusions

The chapter summarizes different sources of artifacts and their characteristics found in different biomedical signals and discusses the advances in signal processing techniques and their suitability for handling these artifacts from different perspectives in a variety of biosignal based applications starting from patient monitoring to disease diagnosis, basic physiology/neuroscience research to brain-machine interfacing, evaluating therapeutic intervention to preventive healthcare, etc. The motivation of deciding to use a particular SPT to remove artifacts must be followed by enhancing the overall detection or classification performance, e.g. it in terms of reduction of false alarms for epileptic seizure detection or increasing accuracy for BCI studies. If it does not add any significant value to the later-stage performance, then it is better not to use that SPT for removing artifacts or noises since only improving SNR will not make any sense then. Finally, this chapter discusses the current limitation of the available SPTs, possible future challenges, and potential recommendations to overcome those challenges. More research will be required in developing new SPTs such that they can handle extreme motion artifacts during ambulatory recordings, enabling online/real-time processing, allowing on-chip implementation (if applicable), being compatible with cloud-computing, storing and utilizing the recorded Big data for appropriate decision making and more importantly customizable for different applications and/or different biosignal types.

Appendix

Abbreviation	Definition	Abbreviation	Definition
AAR	Automatic Artifact Removal	LAMIC	Lagged Auto-Mutual Information Clustering
ABP	Arterial Blood Pressure	LFP	Local Field Potential
ADJUST	Automatic EEG artifact detector based on the joint use of spatial and temporal features	LMS	Least Mean Square
ALE	Adaptve Line Enhancer	LTI	Linear Time Invariant
ANC	Adaptive Noise Canceller	MARA	Multiple artifact rejection algorithm
ANFIS	Adaptive Neural Fuzzy Inference System	MCA	Morphological Component Analysis
ANN	Artificial Neural Network	MCMC	Markov Chain Monte Carlo
ARX	Auto-Regressive Exogenous	MEG	Magnetoencephalography
ASR	Artifact Subspace Reconstruction	MI	Motor Imagery
AWGN	Additive White Gaussian Noise	MMSE	Minimum Mean Square Error
BCG	Ballistocardiography	MUAP	Muscle Unit Action Potential
BCI	Brain-Computer-Interface	MWF	multichannel Wiener filter
BioSigKit	BioSignal Analysis Kit	NB	Naïve Bayes
Bio-SP	Biosignal-Specific Processing (A toolbox)	NEO	Non-linear Energy Operator
Biosppy	Biosignal Processing in Python (toolbox)	OSET	Open-source electrophysiological toolbox
BSP	biomedical signal processing toolbox	PCA	Principal Component Analysis
BSS	Blind Source Separation	PCG	Phonocardiogram
CCA	Canonical Correlation Analysis	PFEIFER	Preprocessing Framework of Electrograms Intermittently Fiducialized from Experimental Recordings
CWT	Continuous Wavelet Transform	PLI	Power Line Interference
DWT	Discrete Wavelet Transform	PPG	Photoplethysmogram
EAP	Extracellular Action Potential	PRANA	Polygraphic Recording Analyzer
ECG/EKG	Electrocardiography	PSD	Power Spectral Density
ecg-kit	A Matlab toolbox for cardiovascular (ECG, EKG, ABP, PPG) signal processing	REM	Rapid Eye Movement
ECoG	Electrocorticography	RLS	Recursive Least Square

(continued)

(continued)

Abbreviation	Definition	Abbreviation	Definition
ECoG	Electrocorticography	RMS	Root Mean Squares
EEG	Electroencephalography	SAE	Sparse Autoencoders
EEMD	Ensemble Empirical Mode Decomposition	SCG	Seismocardiography
EMD	Empirical Mode Decomposition	SNR	Signal to Noise Ratio
EMG	Electromyography	SOS	Second-Order Statistics
EOG	Electrooculography	SPT	Signal Processing Techniques
ERP	Event Related Potential	SSS	Subspace Signal Separation
FASTER	Fully Automated Statistical Thresholding for EEG Artifact Rejection	SSVEP	Steady State Visual Evoked Potential
FFT	Fast Fourier Transform	STFT	Short Time Fourier Transform
FIR	Finite Impulse Response	SVD	Singular Value Decomposition
FLNN	Functional Link Neural Network	SVM	Support Vector Machine
FOOBI	Fourth-order Tensor method	SWT	Stationary Wavelet Transform
FORCe	Fully online and automated artifact removal for BCI	TDSEP	Temporal De-correlation source SEParation
HCI	Human-Computer Interfacing	VBA	Variational Bayes Approximation
HMI	Human-Machine Interfacing	W-CCA	Wavelet Enhanced CCA
IAP	Intracellular Action Potential	WFDB	WaveForm DataBase
ICA	Independent Component Analysis	W-ICA	Wavelet Enhanced ICA
iEEG	intracranial electroencephalography	WNN	Wavelet Neural Network
IIR	Infinite Impulse Response	WPD	Wavelet Packet Decomposition
k-NN	K- Nearest Neighbor	WT	Wavelet Transform

References

1. Salerno, D.M., Zanetti, J.M., Poliac, L.C., Crow, R.S., Hannan, P.J., Wang, K., Goldenberg, I.F., Tassel, R.A.V.: Exercise seismocardiography for detection of coronary artery disease. Am. J. Noninvasive Cardiol. **6**(5), 321–330 (1992)
2. Kabir, A.U., Bin Shahin, F., Islam, M.K.: Design and implementation of an EOG-based mouse cursor control for application in human-computer interaction. In: 4th International Conference on Data Processing and Robotics (ICDPR 2020). Singapore (2020)
3. Islam, M.K., Rastegarnia, A., Yang, Z.: Methods for artifact detection and removal from scalp EEG: a review. Neurophysiol. Clin. Clin. Neurophys. **46**(4–5), 287–305 (2016)

4. Islam, M.K., Rastegarnia, A., Nguyen, A.T., Yang, Z.: Artifact characterization and removal for in vivo neural recording. J. Neurosci. Methods **15**(226), 110–123 (2014)
5. Sweeney, K.: Motion artifact processing techniques for physiological signals. Ph.D. Thesis, National University of Ireland Maynooth (2013)
6. Chang, B.S.: Atlas of Ambulatory EEG. Elsevier (2005)
7. Holmes, G.L., Jones, H.R., Moshé, S.L.: Clinical Neurophysiology of Infancy, Childhood, and Adolescence. Elsevier, Amsterdam (2006)
8. Shahrokhi, Farzaneh, Abdelhalim, Karim, Serletis, Demitre, Carlen, Peter L., Genov, Roman: The 128-channel fully differential digital integrated neural recording and stimulation interface. IEEE Trans. Biomed. Circuits Syst. **4**(3), 149–161 (2010)
9. Islam, M.K., Tuan, N.A., Zhou, Y., Yang, Z.: Analysis and processing of in-vivo neural signal for artifact detection and removal. In: 5th International Conference on BioMedical Engineering and Informatics. IEEE. pp. 437–442 (2012)
10. Delorme, Arnaud, Makeig, Scott: EEGLAB: an open source toolbox for. J. Neurosci. Methods **134**, 9–21 (2004)
11. Keshtkaran, M.R., Yang, Z.: A fast, robust algorithm for power line interference cancellation in neural recording. J. Neural Eng. **11**(2), 026017 (2014)
12. O'Regan, S., Faul, S., Marnane, W.: Automatic detection of EEG artefacts arising from head movements using EEG and gyroscope signals. Med. Eng. Phys. **35**(7), 867–874 (2013)
13. Jafarifarmand, A., Badamchizadeh, M.A.: Artifacts removal in EEG signal using a new neural network enhanced adaptive filter. Neurocomputing **1**(103), 222–231 (2013)
14. Mognon, A., Jovicich, J., Bruzzone, L., Buiatti, M.: ADJUST: an automatic EEG artifact detector based on the joint use of spatial and temporal features. Psychophysiology **48**(2), 229–240 (2011)
15. Burger, C., van den Heever, D.J.: Removal of EOG artefacts by combining wavelet neural network and independent component analysis. Biomed. Sign. Process. Control **1**(15), 67–79 (2015)
16. Hu, J., Wang, C.S., Wu, M., Du, Y.X., He, Y., She, J.: Removal of EOG and EMG artifacts from EEG using combination of functional link neural network and adaptive neural fuzzy inference system. Neurocomputing **3**(151), 278–287 (2015)
17. Schetinin, V., Schult, J.: The combined technique for detection of artifacts in clinical electroencephalograms of sleeping newborns. IEEE Trans. Inf Technol. Biomed. **8**(1), 28–35 (2004)
18. Bhattacharyya, S., Biswas, A., Mukherjee, J., Majumdar, A.K., Majumdar, B., Mukherjee, S., Singh, A.K.: Detection of artifacts from high energy bursts in neonatal EEG. Comput. Biol. Med. **43**(11), 1804–1814 (2013)
19. Shao, S.Y., Shen, K.Q., Ong, C.J., Wilder-Smith, E.P., Li, X.P.: Automatic EEG artifact removal: a weighted support vector machine approach with error correction. IEEE Trans. Biomed. Eng. 336–344 (2008)
20. Shoker, L., Sanei, S., Chambers, J.: Artifact removal from electroencephalograms using a hybrid BSS-SVM algorithm. IEEE Sign. Process. Lett. 721–724 (2005)
21. Lawhern, V., Hairston, W.D., McDowell, K., Westerfield, M., Robbins, K.: Detection and classification of subject-generated artifacts in EEG signals using autoregressive models. J. Neurosci. Methods **208**(2), 181–189 (2012)
22. Schwabedal, J.T., Sippel, D., Brandt, M.D., Bialonski, S.: Automated classification of sleep stages and EEG artifacts in mice with deep learning. (2018). arXiv 1809.08443
23. Yang, B., Duan, K., Fan, C., Hu, C., Wang, J.: Automatic ocular artifacts removal in EEG using deep learning. Biomed. Sign. Process. Control **43**, 148–158 (2018)
24. Sakamoto, Y., Ishiguro, M., Kitagawa, G.: Akaike Information Criterion Statistics. Springer, Dordrecht (1986)
25. Bengtsson, T., Cavanaugh, J.E.: An improved Akaike information criterion for state-space model selection. Comput. Stat. Data Anal. **50**(10), 2635–2654 (2006)
26. Šmídl, V., Anthony, Q.: The Variational Bayes Method in Signal Processing. Springer, New York (2006)

27. Chen, Z., Babacan, S.D., Molina, R., Katsaggelos, A.K.: Variational Bayesian methods for multimedia problems. IEEE Trans. Multimedia **16**(4), 1000–1017 (2014)
28. Drémeau, A., Herzet, C., Daudet, L.: Boltzmann machine and mean-field approximation for structured sparse decompositions. IEEE Trans. Sign. Process. **60**(7), 3425–3438 (2012)
29. Zheng, Y., Fraysse, A., Rodet, Thomas: Efficient variational Bayesian approximation method based on subspace optimization. IEEE Trans. Image Process. **24**(2), 681–693 (2014)
30. Zhao, Q., Hu, B., Shi, Y., Li, Y., Moore, P., Sun, M., Peng, H.: Automatic identification and removal of ocular artifacts in EEG—improved adaptive predictor filtering for portable applications. IEEE Trans. Nanobiosci. 109–117 (2014)
31. Klados, M.A., Papadelis, C., Braun, C., Bamidis, P.D.: REG-ICA: a hybrid methodology combining blind source separation and regression techniques for the rejection of ocular artifacts. Biomed. Sign. Process. Control **6**(3), 291–300 (2011)
32. Li, Y., Ma, Z., Lu, W., Li, Y.: Automatic removal of the eye blink artifact from EEG using an ICA-based template matching approach. Physiol. Measure. **27**(4), 425 (2006)
33. Flexer, A., Bauer, H., Pripfl, J., Dorffner, G.: Using ICA for removal of ocular artifacts in EEG recorded from blind subjects. Neural Netw. **18**(7), 998–1005 (2005)
34. Guerrero-Mosquera, C., Navia-Vázquez, A.: Automatic removal of ocular artefacts using adaptive filtering and independent component analysis for electroencephalogram data. IET Sign. Process. **6**(2), 99–106 (2012)
35. Devuyst, S., Dutoit, T., Stenuit, P., Kerkhofs, M., Stanus, E.: Cancelling ECG artifacts in EEG using a modified independent component analysis approach. EURASIP J. Adv. Sign. Process. **2008**, 1–13 (2008)
36. Roy, V., Shukla, S.: Automatic removal of artifacts from EEG signal based on spatially constrained ICA using daubechies wavelet. Int. J. Mod. Edu. Comput. Sci. (IJMECS) **6**(7), 31–39 (2014)
37. Shoker, L., Sanei, S., Latif, M.A.: Removal of eye blinking artifacts from EEG incorporating a new constrained BSS algorithm. In: Sensor Array and Multichannel Signal Workshop. IEEE. pp. 177–181 (2004)
38. Akhtar, M.T., Mitsuhashi, W., James, C.J.: Employing spatially constrained ICA and wavelet denoising, for automatic removal of artifacts from multichannel EEG data. Sign. Process. **92**(2), 401–416 (2012)
39. James, C.J., Gibson, O.J.: Temporally constrained ICA: an application to artifact rejection in electromagnetic brain signal analysis. IEEE Trans. Biomed. Eng. **50**(9), 1108–1116 (2003)
40. Jung, T.P., Makeig, S., Humphries, C., Lee, T.W., Mckeown, M.J., Iragui, V., Sejnowski, T.J.: Removing electroencephalographic artifacts by blind source separation. Psychophysiology **37**(2), 163–178 (2000)
41. Jung, T.P., Makeig, S., Westerfield, M., Townsend, J., Courchesne, E., Sejnowski, T.J.: Removal of eye activity artifacts from visual event-related potentials in normal and clinical subjects. Clin. Neurophys. **111**(10), 1745–1758 (2000)
42. Sweeney, K.T., McLoone, S.F., Ward, T.E.: The use of ensemble empirical mode decomposition with canonical correlation analysis as a novel artifact removal technique. IEEE Trans. Biomed. Eng. **60**(1), 97–105 (2012)
43. Sweeney, K.T., Ward, T.E., McLoone, S.F.: Artifact removal in physiological signals—practices and possibilities. IEEE Trans. Inf Technol. Biomed. **16**(3), 488–500 (2012)
44. Yong, X., Ward, R.K., Birch, G.E.: Artifact removal in EEG using morphological component analysis. In: International Conference on Acoustics, Speech and Signal Processing. IEEE. 345–348 (2009)
45. Zheng, Y., Fraysse, A., Rodet, T.: Efficient variational Bayesian approximation method based on subspace optimization. IEEE Trans. Image Process. **24**(2), 681–693 (2015)
46. Hunyadi, Borbála, Van Huffel, Sabine, De Vos, Maarten, Clifton, D.A.: The Power of Tensor Decompositions in Biomedical Applications. Machine Learning for Healthcare Technologies, IET (2016)
47. Rankine, L., Stevenson, N., Mesbah, M., Boashash, B.: A nonstationary model of newborn EEG. IEEE Trans. Biomed. Eng. **54**(1), 19–28 (2006)

48. Stevenson, N., Rankine, L., Mesbah, M., Boashash, B.: Newborn EEG seizure simulation using time–frequency signal synthesis. In: APRS Workshop on Digital Image Computing. 145–151 (2005)
49. Oostenveld, R., Fries, P., Maris, E., Schoffelen, J.M.: FieldTrip: open source software for advanced analysis of MEG, EEG, and invasive electrophysiological data. Comput. Intell. Neurosci. (2011)
50. Stephane, M.: A Wavelet Tour of Signal Processing: The Sparse Way. Academic Press, London (1999)
51. Islam, M.K., Rastegarnia, A., Yang, Z.: A wavelet-based artifact reduction from scalp EEG for epileptic seizure detection. IEEE J. Biomed. Health Inf. **20**(5), 1321–1332 (2015)
52. Sweeney, K.T., Ayaz, H., Ward, T.E., Izzetoglu, M., McLoone, S.F., Onaral, B.: A methodology for validating artifact removal techniques for physiological signals. IEEE Trans. Inf Technol. Biomed. **16**(5), 918–926 (2012)
53. Rashed-Al-Mahfuz, M., Islam, M.R., Hirose, K., Molla, M.K.: Artifact suppression and analysis of brain activities with electroencephalography signals. Neural Regeneration Res. **8**(16), 1500 (2013)
54. Molla, M.K., Islam, M.R., Tanaka, T., Rutkowski, T.M.: Artifact suppression from EEG signals using data adaptive time domain filtering. Neurocomputing **15**(97), 297–308 (2012)
55. Ye, Y., Cheng, Y., He, W., Hou, M., Zhang, Z.: Combining nonlinear adaptive filtering and signal decomposition for motion artifact removal in wearable photoplethysmography. IEEE Sens. J. 7133–7141 (2016)
56. Xu, L., Rabotti, C., Zhang, Y., Ouzounov, S., Harpe, P.J., Mischi, M.: Motion-artifact reduction in capacitive heart-rate measurements by adaptive filtering. IEEE Trans. Instrument. Measure. **68**(10), 4085–4093 (2018)
57. Xiong, F., Chen, D., Chen, Z., Dai, S.: Cancellation of motion artifacts in ambulatory ECG signals using TD-LMS adaptive filtering techniques. J. Visual Commun. Image Representation **1**(58), 606–618 (2019)
58. Saeed F., Gazem N., Patnaik S., Saed Balaid A., Mohammed, F.: Motion artifact reduction algorithm using sequential adaptive noise filters and estimation methods for mobile ECG. In: Recent Trends in Information and Communication Technology. IRICT. Springer, New York (2017)
59. Kim, C.S., Sun, J., Liu, D., Wang, Q., Paek, S.G.: Removal of ocular artifacts using ICA and adaptive filter for motor imagery-based BCI. IEEE/CAA J. Automatica Sinica (2017)
60. Quazi, M.H., Kahalekar, S.G.: Artifacts removal from EEG signal: FLM optimization-based learning algorithm for neural network-enhanced adaptive filtering. Biocybernetics Biomed. Eng. **37**(3), 401–411 (2017)
61. Yang, B., Duan, K., Zhang, T.: Removal of EOG artifacts from EEG using a cascade of sparse autoencoder and recursive least squares adaptive filter. Neurocomputing **214**, 1053–1060 (2016)
62. Borowicz, A.: Using a multichannel Wiener filter to remove eye-blink artifacts from EEG data. Biomed. Sign. Process. Control **1**(45), 246–255 (2018)
63. Cohen, M.X.: Analyzing Neural Time Series Data: Theory and Practice. MIT Press, Cambridge (2014)
64. Turnip, A.: Automatic artifacts removal of EEG signals using robust principal component analysis. In: 2nd International Conference on Technology, Informatics, Management, Engineering & Environment. IEEE. pp. 331–334 (2014)
65. Turnip, A., Junaidi, E.: Removal artifacts from EEG signal using independent component analysis and principal component analysis. In: 2nd International Conference on Technology, Informatics, Management, Engineering and Environment. pp. 296–302 (2014)
66. Hamaneh, M.B., Chitravas, N., Kaiboriboon, K., Lhatoo, S.D., Loparo, K.A.: Automated removal of EKG artifact from EEG data using independent component analysis and continuous wavelet transformation. IEEE Trans. Biomed. Eng. **61**(6), 1634–1641 (2013)
67. Castellanos, N.P., Makarov, V.A.: Recovering EEG brain signals: artifact suppression with wavelet enhanced independent component analysis. J. Neurosci. Methods **158**(2), 300–312 (2006)

68. Mahajan, R., Morshed, B.I.: Unsupervised eye blink artifact denoising of EEG data with modified multiscale sample entropy, kurtosis, and wavelet-ICA. IEEE J. Biomed. Health Inf. **19**(1), 158–165 (2014)
69. Zhao, C., Qiu, T.: An automatic ocular artifacts removal method based on wavelet-enhanced canonical correlation analysis. In: Annual International Conference of the IEEE Engineering in Medicine and Biology Society. IEEE. pp. 4191–4194 (2011)
70. Raghavendra, B.S., Dutt, D.N.: Wavelet enhanced CCA for minimization of ocular and muscle artifacts in EEG. World Acad. Sci. Eng. Technol. **57**(6), 1027–1032 (2011)
71. Mammone, N., Morabito, F.C.: Enhanced automatic wavelet independent component analysis for electroencephalographic artifact removal. Entropy **16**(12), 6553–6572 (2014)
72. Calcagno, S., La Foresta, F., Versaci, M.: Independent component analysis and discrete wavelet transform for artifact removal in biomedical signal processing. Am. J. Appl. Sci. **11**(1), 57 (2014)
73. Chen, X., He, C., Peng, H.: Removal of muscle artifacts from single-channel EEG based on ensemble empirical mode decomposition and multiset canonical correlation analysis. J. Appl. Math (2014)
74. Zeng, H., Song, A., Yan, R., Qin, H.: EOG artifact correction from EEG recording using stationary subspace analysis and empirical mode decomposition. Sensors 14839–14859 (2013)
75. Niazy, R.K., Beckmann, C.F., Iannetti, G.D., Brady, J.M., Smith, S.M.: Removal of FMRI environment artifacts from EEG data using optimal basis sets. Neuroimage **28**(3), 720–737 (2005)
76. Nguyen, H.A., Musson, J., Li, F., Wang, W., Zhang, G., Xu, R., Richey, C., Schnell, T., McKenzie, F.D., Li, J.: EOG artifact removal using a wavelet neural network. Neurocomputing **15**(97), 374–389 (2012)
77. Peng, H., Hu, B., Shi, Q., Ratcliffe, M., Zhao, Q., Qi, Y., Gao, G.: Removal of ocular artifacts in EEG—an improved approach combining DWT and ANC for portable applications. IEEE J. Biomed. Health Inf. **17**(3), 600–607 (2013)
78. Navarro, X., Porée, F., Carrault, G.: ECG removal in preterm EEG combining empirical mode decomposition and adaptive filtering. In: International Conference on Acoustics, Speech and Signal Processing (ICASSP). IEEE. pp. 661–664 (2012)
79. Skupch, A.M., Dollfuss, P., Fürbaß, F., Gritsch, G., Hartmann, M.M., Perko, H., Pataraia, E., Lindinger, G., Kluge, T.: Spatial correlation based artifact detection for automatic seizure detection in EEG. In: 35th Annual International Conference of the IEEE Engineering in Medicine and Biology Society (EMBC). IEEE. pp. 1972–1975 (2013)
80. Hesar, H.D., Mohebbi, M.: An adaptive particle weighting strategy for ECG denoising using marginalized particle extended Kalman filter: An evaluation in arrhythmia contexts. IEEE J. Biomed. Health Inf. **21**(6), 1581–1592 (2017)
81. Hesar, H.D., Mohebbi, M.: ECG denoising using marginalized particle extended kalman filter with an automatic particle weighting strategy. IEEE J. Biomed. Health Inf. **21**(3), 635–644 (2016)
82. Warmerdam, G.J., Vullings, R., Schmitt, L., Van Laar, J.O., Bergmans, J.W.: A fixed-lag Kalman smoother to filter power line interference in electrocardiogram recordings. IEEE Trans. Biomed. Eng. **64**(8), 1852–1861 (2016)
83. Daly, I., Scherer, R., Billinger, M., Müller-Putz, G.: FORCe: fully online and automated artifact removal for brain-computer interfacing. IEEE Trans. Neural Syst. Rehabil. Eng. **23**(5), 725–736 (2014)
84. Hallez, H., De Vos, M., Vanrumste, B., Van Hese, P., Assecondi, S., Van Laere, K.: Removing muscle and eye artifacts using blind source separation techniques in ictal EEG source imaging. Clin. Neurophys. **120**(7), 1262–1272 (2009)
85. De Clercq, W., Vergult, A., Vanrumste, B., Van Paesschen, W., Van Huffel, S.: Canonical correlation analysis applied to remove muscle artifacts from the electroencephalogram. IEEE Trans. Biomed. Eng. **53**(12), 2583–2587 (2006)

86. Kolda, T.G., Bader, B.W.: Tensor decompositions and applications. SIAM Rev. **51**(3), 455–500 (2009)
87. Wang, Z., Xu, P., Liu, T., Tian, Y., Lei, X., Yao, D.: Robust removal of ocular artifacts by combining independent component analysis and system identification. Biomed. Sign. Process. Cont. **1**(10), 250–259 (2014)
88. De Vos, M., Deburchgraeve, W., Cherian, P.J., Matic, V., Swarte, R.M., Govaert, P., Visser, G.H., Van Huffel, S.: Automated artifact removal as preprocessing refines neonatal seizure detection. Clin. Neurophys. **122**(12), 2345–2354 (2011)
89. Kothe, C.A., Makeig, S.: BCILAB: a platform for brain–computer interface development. J. Neural Eng. **10**(5), 056014 (2013)
90. Nabian, M., Yin, Y., Wormwood, J., Quigley, K.S., Barrett, L.F., Ostadabbas, S.: An open-source feature extraction tool for the analysis of peripheral physiological data. IEEE J. Transl. Eng. Health Med. **6**, 1–11 (2018)
91. Vidaurre, C., Sander, T.H., Schlögl, A.: BioSig: the free and open source software library for biomedical signal processing. Comput. Intell. Neurosci. (2011)
92. Blechert, J., Peyk, P., Liedlgruber, M., Wilhelm, F.H.: ANSLAB: Integrated multichannel peripheral biosignal processing in psychophysiological science. Behav. Res. Methods **48**(4), 1528–1545 (2016)
93. n.d. Clean_rawdata EEGLAB plugin. Accessed 09 Feb 2020. https://github.com/sccn/clean_rawdata
94. Sedghamiz, H.: BioSigKit: a matlab toolbox and interface for analysis of biosignals. J. Open Sour. Softw. **3**(30), 671 (2018)
95. n.d. BioSPPy. Accessed 09 Feb 2020. https://biosppy.readthedocs.io/en/stable/index.html
96. Silva, I., Moody, G.B.: An open-source toolbox for analysing and processing physionet databases in matlab and octave. J. Open Res. Softw. (2014)
97. Aboy, M., Crespo, C., McNames, J., Bassale, J., Jenkins, L., Goldsteins, B.: A biomedical signal processing toolbox. Proc. Biosignal **2002**(26), 49–52 (2002)
98. McGill, K.C., Lateva, Z.C., Marateb, H.R.: EMGLAB: an interactive EMG decomposition program. J. Neurosci. Methods **149**(2), 121–133 (2005)
99. Chaumon, M., Bishop, D.V., Busch, N.A.: A practical guide to the selection of independent components of the electroencephalogram for artifact correction. J. Neurosci. Methods **30**(250), 47–63 (2015)
100. Nolan, H., Whelan, R., Reilly, R.B.: FASTER: fully automated statistical thresholding for EEG artifact rejection. J. Neurosci. Methods **192**(1), 152–162 (2010)
101. Sameni, R.: OSET: The Open-Source Electrophysiological Toolbox. Accessed 09 Feb 2020. https://gitlab.com/rsameni/OSET. (2012)
102. Gómez-Herrero, G.: Automatic artifact removal (AAR) toolbox v1. 3 (Release 09.12. 2007) for MATLAB. Technical Manual, Tampere University of Technology (2007)
103. Ge, S., Han, M., Hong, X.: A fully automatic ocular artifact removal from EEG based on fourth-order tensor method. Biomed. Eng. Lett. **4**(1), 55–63 (2014)
104. Nicolaou, N., Nasuto, S.J.: Automatic artefact removal from event-related potentials via clustering. J. VLSI Sign. Process. Syst. Sign. Image Video Technol. **48**(1–2), 173–183 (2007)
105. n.d. PRANA® Software Suite. Accessed 09 Feb 2020. https://www.phitools.com/prana.php
106. Rodenhauser, A., Good, W.W., Zenger, B., Tate, J., Aras, K., Burton, B., MacLeod, R.S.: Pfeifer: preprocessing framework for electrograms intermittently fiducialized from experimental recordings. J. Open Sour. Softw. **3**(21), 472 (2018)
107. François, T., Baillet, S., Mosher, J.C., Pantazis, D., Leahy, R.M.: Brainstorm: a user-friendly application for MEG/EEG analysis. Comput. Intell. Neurosci. (2011)
108. Pion-Tonachini, L., Hsu, S.H., Makeig, S., Jung, T.P., Cauwenberghs, G.: Real-time EEG source-mapping toolbox (REST): online ICA and source localization. In: 37th Annual International Conference of the IEEE Engineering in Medicine and Biology Society (EMBC). pp. 4114–4117 (2015)
109. n.d. Bergen fMRI Toolbox. Accessed 09 Feb 2020. http://fmri.uib.no/index.php?option=com_content&view=article&id=53&Itemid=78

110. Viola, F.C., De Vos, M., Hine, J., Sandmann, P., Bleeck, S., Eyles, J., Debener, S.: Semi-automatic attenuation of cochlear implant artifacts for the evaluation of late auditory evoked potentials. Hearing Res. **284**(1–2), 6–15 (2012)
111. Viola, F.C., Thorne, J., Edmonds, B., Schneider, T., Eichele, T., Debener, S.: Semi-automatic identification of independent components representing EEG artifact. Clin. Neurophysiol. **120**(5), 868–877 (2009)
112. Winkler, I., Haufe, S., Tangermann, M.: Automatic classification of artifactual ICA-components for artifact removal in EEG signals. Behav. Brain Funct. **7**(1), 30 (2011)
113. Winkler, I., Brandl, S., Horn, F., Waldburger, E., Allefeld, C., Tangermann, M.: Robust artifactual independent component classification for BCI practitioners. J. Neural Eng. **11**(3), 035013 (2014)
114. n.d. NITRC CleanLine Tool. Accessed 09 Feb 2020. https://www.nitrc.org/projects/cleanline
115. Mohseni, H.R., Ghaderi, F., Wilding, E.L., Sanei, S.: Variational Bayes for spatiotemporal identification of event-related potential subcomponents. IEEE Trans. Biomed. Eng. **57**(10), 2413–2428 (2010)
116. Hubel, D.H., Wiesel, T.N.: Receptive fields, binocular interaction and functional architecture in the cat's visual cortex. J. Physiol. **160**(1), 106 (1962)
117. Fisher, R.S., Vickrey, B.G., Gibson, P., Hermann, B., Penovich, P., Scherer, A., Walker, S.: The impact of epilepsy from the patient's perspective I. Descriptions and subjective perceptions. Epilepsy Res. **41**(1), 39–51 (2000)
118. n.d. Plexon Systems. Accessed 08 Feb 2020. http://www.plexon.com/products/
119. Csicsvari, J., Henze, D.A., Jamieson, B., Harris, K.D., Sirota, A., Barth, P., Wise, K.D., Buzsaki, G.: Massively parallel recording of unit and local field potentials with silicon-based electrodes. J. Neurophysiol. **90**(2), 1314–1323 (2003)
120. O'Regan, S.H.: Artefact detection and removal algorithms for EEG diagnostic systems (2013)
121. Savelainen, A.: Movement artifact detection from electroencephalogram utilizing accelerometer. Helsinki, Finland: M.S. thesis, School of Sci. and Tech., Aalto Univ (2011)
122. Savelainen, A.: An Introduction to EEG Artifacts. School of Sci. Aalto Univ, Finland (2010)
123. Babacan, S.D., Molina, R., Katsaggelos, A.K.: Variational Bayesian super resolution. IEEE Trans. Image Process. **20**(4), 984–999 (2011)
124. Hubel, D.H., Wiesel, T.N.: Receptive fields of single neurones in the cat's striate cortex. J. Physiol. **148**(3), 574 (1959)

Chapter 3
Time-Frequency Analysis in Health Informatics

Itaru Kaneko

Abstract This chapter provides an introductory tutorial on time frequency analysis in health informatics. The chapter begins with basic nature of sampling, Z-transform, Fourier transform, wavelet as conceptual foundation of those are especially important in health informatics. Then we discuss about time-frequency resolutions, windowing, filtering, microphone arrays and transducer arrays, correlation analysis as basic understanding of these techniques are especially useful for health informatics. The last part of the chapter also addresses more advanced techniques and few examples. The chapter should come to be useful for those who consider these techniques for their applications.

Keywords Signal processing · Filter · Fourier transform · Health informatics · Data analysis

3.1 Introduction

Since Joseph Fourier built its foundation in 1822, time-frequency analysis and its theoretical foundation has been well developed and had provided a remarkably diverse and powerful techniques. The reader may access wide selection of textbook for the theories and techniques. Therefore, detail of theory and techniques will not be addressed in this chapter. Instead, we will focus on to provide handy and concise summary of the techniques for those who immediately would like to apply them in health informatics.

The readers are assumed to know basic knowledge of signal processing, i.e. frequency, amplitude, triangular functions, dB, basic concept of frequency spectrum. But the chapter is intended to be understood by readers without prior knowledge of signal processing. When readers apply those techniques in the actual work, readers are suggested to learn fundamentals of signal processing and access various handbooks for the more detail techniques.

I. Kaneko (✉)
Nagoya City University Graduate School of Medical Sciences, 1 Kawasumi Mizuho-Cho, Mizuho-Ku, Nagoya 467-8601, Japan
e-mail: itaru-k@acm.org

M. A. R. Ahad and M. U. Ahmed (eds.), *Signal Processing Techniques for Computational Health Informatics*, Intelligent Systems Reference Library 192,
https://doi.org/10.1007/978-3-030-54932-9_3

In the area of health informatics, time-frequency tool can be applied to many applications relating to time-series of data e.g., Electro Cardio-Meter, speech, body movement and all periodically acquisition of health measurement [1–3]. Through this chapter, we will visit major techniques used in those applications and provides the birds-view scape of the theories and technologies.

3.2 Time Series and Sampling in Health Informatics

The input of time-frequency analysis is time series of data. There are several slightly different methods of the way of acquisition of time series and those methods can be categorized into four (Fig. 3.1).

(a) Sampling of narrow band signal.
(b) Sampling of wide band signal.
(c) Sampling after low pass filter at Nyquist frequency.
(d) Non-uniform sampling.

It is important to understand the nature of time series obtained by different methods.

(a) Sampling of narrow band signal.

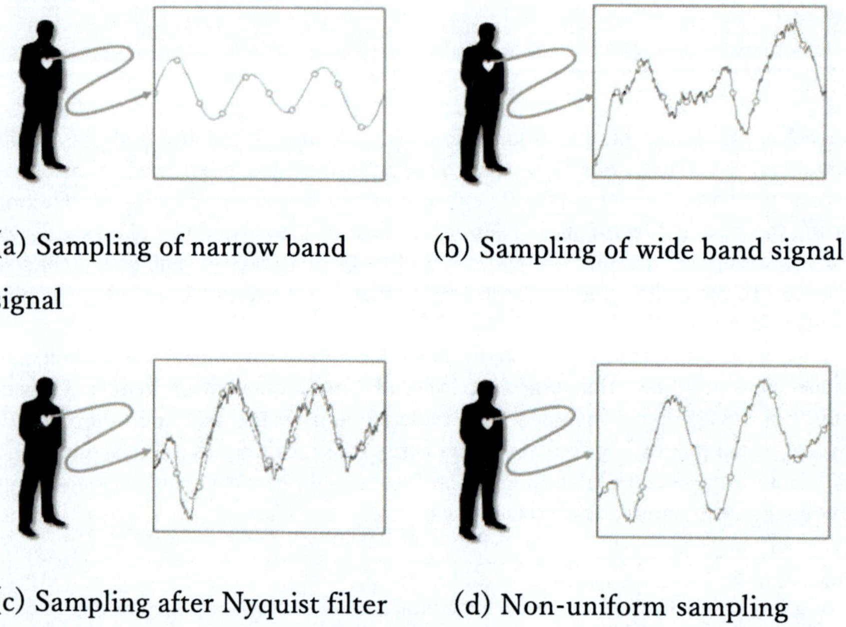

(a) Sampling of narrow band signal
(b) Sampling of wide band signal
(c) Sampling after Nyquist filter
(d) Non-uniform sampling

Fig. 3.1 The four cases of sampling in health informatics

More precisely, it is the sampling of waveform which has very narrow band compared to sampling frequency. This is typical situation of sampling of data which has slow changes compared to sampling frequency. Body motion is an example of such sampling. If bandwidth of source signal is narrow enough there is no problem in sampling and time-frequency analysis.

(b) Sampling of wide band signal

In more precise, it is uniform sampling of waveform which has energy in higher frequency. Some problem may occur if signal contains higher frequency. It is known that half sampling frequency, which is called Nyquist frequency is the limit of frequency accurately represented by the uniform sampled data. Please note that some problem may happen not only for frequency component above Nyquist frequency but even for frequency components near Nyquist frequency.

This is not theoretically preferable way of sampling but may happen with capturing of data which is slower than theoretically preferable measurement period according to the speed of change of data. For example, regular health examination is an example of this type of sampling.

In this case, aliasing may happen so that spectrum in some higher frequency band is not correct because it may contain aliasing noise.

(c) Sampling after low pass filter at Nyquist frequency

More precisely, it is the sampling of waveform after low pass filter at Nyquist frequency. If continuous measurement is available before sampling, low pass filter at Nyquist frequency should take place before the sampling. Almost all digital measurement circuits include such filter. Time frequency analysis perfectly works but only within the limited frequency band. It is also should be pointed out that such filter may distort detailed time domain shape of the signal. Therefore, Nyquist frequency shall be higher enough from the spectrum of measured signal, in case of time domain structure is important.

(d) Non-uniform sampling

More precisely, it is sampling in non-uniform intervals. In some case, sampling interval is not uniform [4]. This may cause great difficulty in time-frequency analysis. Very sophisticated method is necessary but still possible to reconstruct time-frequency information. But this chapter will not cover such method and readers are advised to access more advanced research papers or textbook to study about such method.

In summary, to ensure reliability of time-frequency analysis of health information processing, it is necessary to pay attention to the how time series is obtained. Then it is necessary to appropriately consider the distortions which may be appearing in the frequency spectrum of data.

3.3 Z-Transform

3.3.1 *Introducing Z-Transform*

Z-transform is widely used as a basic tool for the analysis of discrete systems, which is systems processing time series of data. Table 3.1 show processing system and corresponding Z-transform.

Why it is beneficial to define Z-transform this way? The one of the major uses of Z-transform is to define Z-transform representations of digital system. And use such Z-transform representations of digital system as a building blocks to combine and connect to build complex systems and to predict characteristics of such more complex system. Here are several rules to represent and combine Z-transforms which are useful for such purposes.

Table 3.2 shows time series, $x(n)$, $h(n)$, $g(n)$ and their Z-transform those are used in Table 3.3. When we build digital systems by composing complex system using multiple simpler digital systems, it is desirable to be able to induce Z-transform of composed digital system from Z-transform of simpler systems. Table 3.3 shows example to combine Z-transform of various subsystem to derive Z-transform of composed system. Z-transform of $\delta(n)$ will be 1.

As shown in (a) and (b), if 1 is given as an input and Z-transform of digital systems is $H(z)$, Z-transform of output is also $H(z)$. Same for $G(z)$. As shown in (c), if $X(z)$ is given as input to digital system $H(z)$, it gives output $H(z)X(z)$. As shown in (d) and (e), cascading and parallelization of digital system will result multiplication $G(z)H(z)$and addition of $H(z) + G(z)$ in Z-transform domain. As described here, it is possible to induce Z-transform of complex system. And using such mathematical representation and manipulation in Z-transform, it is possible to have better understanding of the theory of designing digital systems.

Table 3.1 Example of Z-transform of time series examples

Time sample	Time series	Z-transform
$x(n)$	$x(1), x(2), x(3), x(4), \ldots$	$X(z) = \sum_{n=1}^{\infty} \left(x(n)z^{-n}\right)$
$\delta(n)$	1, 0, 0, 0, ...	1
$\delta(n-1)$	0, 1, 0, 0, ...	z^{-1}
$u(n)$	1, 1, 1, 1, ...	$\sum_{n=1}^{\infty} z^{-n}$

Table 3.2 Example time series, $x(n)$, $h(n)$, $g(n)$, and their Z-transforms

Example	Time series	Z-transform
$x(n)$	[2,1,0,0,0, ...]	$X(z) = 2 + z^{-1}$
$h(n)$	[1, – 1,0,0,0, ...]	$H(z) = 1 - z^{-1}$
$g(n)$	[2, – 1,0,0, ...]	$G(z) = 2 - z^{-1}$

Table 3.3 Calculation of Z-transforms combining given Z-transforms

	Time domain representations	Z-transforms	How to calculate resulting Z-transforms
(a)	$\delta(n) \rightarrow \boxed{h(n)} \rightarrow h(n)$	$1 \rightarrow \boxed{H(z)} \rightarrow Y_1(z)$	$Y_1(z) = H(z) \cdot 1$ $= 1 - z^{-1}$
(b)	$\delta(n) \rightarrow \boxed{g(n)} \rightarrow g(n)$	$1 \rightarrow \boxed{G(z)} \rightarrow Y_2(z)$	$Y_2(z) = G(z) \cdot 1G(z) \cdot 1$ $= 2 - z^{-1}$
(c)	$x(n) \rightarrow \boxed{h(n)} \rightarrow y_3(n)$	$X(z) \rightarrow \boxed{H(z)} \rightarrow Y_3(z)$	$Y_3(z) = H(z)X(z)$ $= 2 - z^{-1} - z^{-2}$
(d)	$x(n) \rightarrow \boxed{h(z)} \rightarrow \boxed{g(z)} \rightarrow y_4(n)$	$X(z) \rightarrow \boxed{H(z)} \rightarrow \boxed{G(z)} \rightarrow Y_4(n)$	$Y_3(z) = G(z)H(z)X(z)$ $= 4 - 4z^{-1} - z^{-2} - z^{-3}$

(continued)

Table 3.3 (continued)

	Time domain representations	Z-transforms	How to calculate resulting Z-transforms
(e)	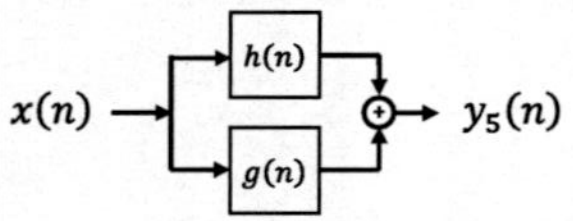	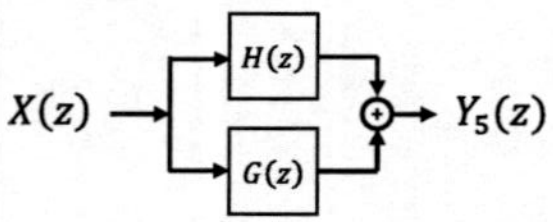	$Y_4(z) = (H(z) + G(z))X(z)(H(z) + G(z))X(z)$ $= 6 - z^{-1} - 2z^{-2} = 6 - z^{-1} - 2z^{-2}$

3.3.2 Understanding Benefit of Z-Transform

But why Z-transform should be defined such way? And what does Z mean? In many applications, there are linearity in the operation of signal. So easy part of the requirement is linearity. Thus, the calculation of Z-transform is better to follow the mathematical rule in regular mathematical expression. Single sample should be represented by number that represents magnitude of that sample itself.

We also need notation of delay. So, let us represent single sample delay as D. Now, if we have series of samples such as [1–3] 1 comes immediately, 3 is one sample later and 2 is two sample later, it should be represented as $1 + 3D + 2DD$. D shown here is not regular value but means one sample delay. But fortunately, D will follow same rules as regular variable. If we develop such notation and change D with Z, we will eventually get notation same as Z-transform.

This is far from theoretically precise definition. But reader could get basic understanding of Z transform and progress to more theoretical expression of Z-transform in various textbook for Z-transform.

Z-transform will give sophisticated theoretical framework to give precise theoretical view in the designing digital system, their combination, and characteristics of composed system. If you are not using Z-transform, only way to estimate behavior of digital system is, to calculate its behavior sample by samples. But using Z-transform, it is possible to predict various important nature of digital systems which have complex network even there are many feedbacks and complex connections.

Important concept with the Z-transforms of the signal processing system is nature of response and stability of the output. Table 3.4 shows block diagram and Z-transform, for finite impulse response filter and infinite impulse response filter. In (a), finite impulse response filter, there is no feedback and because $B(z)$ is polynomial of z, $Y(z)$ is polynomial of z. In (b), infinite impulse response filter, there is feedback and Z-transform will be fractions of polynomial of z. This means, if we convert $Y(z)$ to polynomial of z, which is Taylor expansion of the fractions of polynomial of z, $Y(z)$ must have infinite series of terms. And this means impulse response will not terminate in finite duration. Therefore, we may know, IIR filter must have infinite impulse response. And if $Y(z)$ became infinite in some z, it means $Y(z)$ can be divergent.

Table 3.4 Z-transform of finite and infinite response filter

(a)	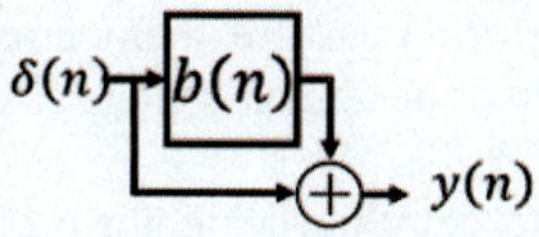	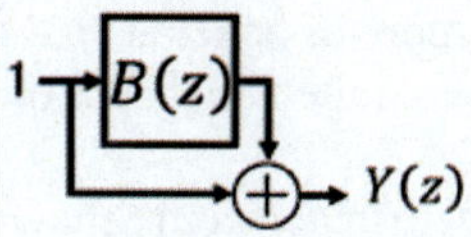	$Y(z) = 1 + B(z)$
(b)	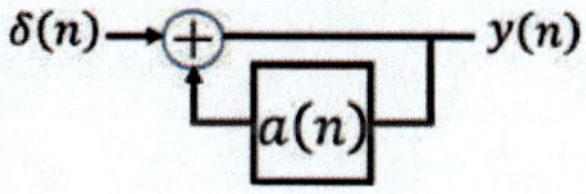	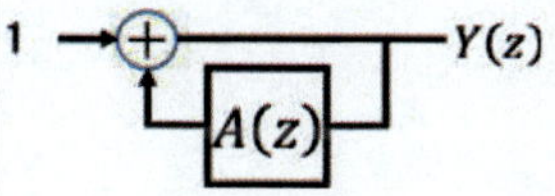	$Y(z) = A(z)Y(z) + 1$ $Y(z) = \frac{1}{1-A(z)}$

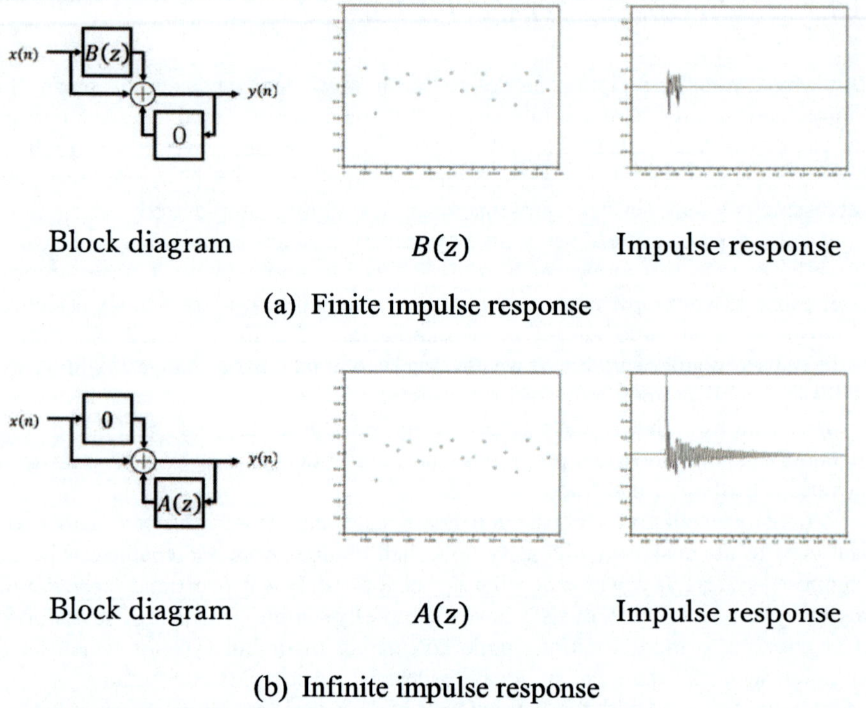

Fig. 3.2 Example of filters which has infinite response and finite response

Figure 3.2 shows an example of filters and their responses which has infinite response and finite response. Digital systems, which has feedback, has infinite response and if there is no feedback, response is finite.

Figure 3.3 shows diverging filter and stable filter. If filter is diverging, filter's output will be diverging to infinite after specific input. Please note that magnitude and shape of impulse response $A(z)$ is not necessary to be special for diverging response.

This can be understood by the fact that value of X multiplied by H has infinite in some value of domain.

And by designing signal processing without such infinite, it is possible to design stable digital signal processing, i.e. it is possible to avoid to divergence with any limited input. There are far more of benefits in Z-transform than already mentioned above and Z-transform is used quite widely for the area of design of digital systems which uses time series.

Z-transform is quite useful to understand behavior, structure and designing method of digital systems.

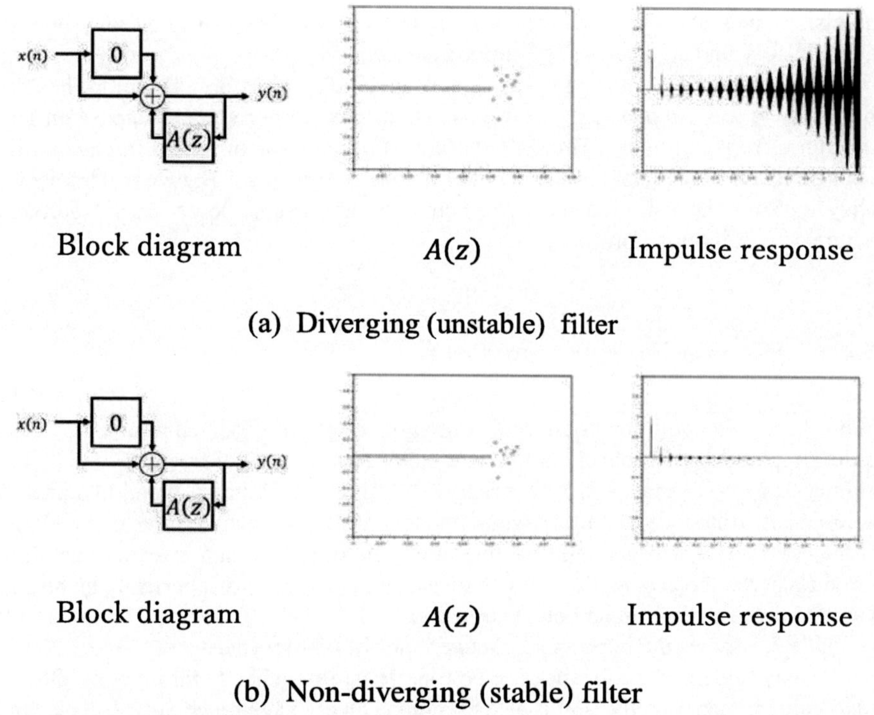

Fig. 3.3 Example of diverging filter and stable filter

However, Z-transform is not a tool to analyze characteristics of time series, just like Fourier Transform is used. Z-transform is not used to analyze signal itself. But it is quite useful to understand frequency domain characteristics of digital systems such as filters.

3.4 Fourier Transform and Wavelets

Fourier transform is the transform from time series to the frequency spectrum. It has incredibly old root back to the Fourier series in the book by Joseph Fourier in 1822. But extraordinary explosion of the application of Fourier transform took place after Fast Fourier Transform had been invented by James Cooley and John Tukey. Then Fourier transform became one of most powerful tools for the computation.

Basic functionality of Fourier transform is to map time series to the series of samples in frequency domain. However, it can be applied to many other different purposes. It is not only for time-frequency analysis, but it is also useful for the high-efficient computing such as fast calculating of cross correlation as well as arbitral precision calculation to calculate long digits of π. Readers can find many books about history and application of Fourier transform.

Since we would like to show just how to use Fourier transform as tool for health informatics, this chapter will not discuss about how to introduce discrete Fourier transform from continuous Fourier transform (Fourier transform defined on continuous time). Or we will not discuss about Fast Fourier Transform. But we will immediately introduce the definition of discrete Fourier transform and show several important nature of Fourier transforms.

3.4.1 Discrete Fourier Transform

Table 3.5 shows definition of discrete Fourier transform (DFT). Definition of DFT is quite simple. Reader probably notice that there is more order of freedom with $X(k)$ compared to $x(i)$ because $X(k)$ consists of N values which has real and imaginary component. But since $X(k)$ has symmetry for given $x(i)$, actual order of freedom is the same. And it also should be noted that this transform and inverse transform provides perfect reconstruction. Which means, we can reconstruct perfectly identical value of time series from its Fourier transform.

Table 3.6 shows the important characteristics of Fourier transform.

We may find many applications of Fourier transform in health informatics. Other than time frequency analysis, it is also used in medical image processing. But also in the time frequency domain signal, many applications use Fourier transform [5–12].

Table 3.5 Definition of Fourier transform

$X = \mathcal{F}(x)$	$X(k) = \sum_{n=0}^{N-1} x(i)e^{\frac{-j2\pi kn}{N}}$
$x = \mathcal{F}^{-1}(X)$	$x(n) = \frac{1}{N}\sum_{n=0}^{N-1} X(n)e^{\frac{j2\pi kn}{N}}$

Table 3.6 The important characteristics of Fourier transform

$y(n) = a_1x_1(n) + a_2x_2(n)$	$Y(k) = a_1X_1(k) + a_2X_2(k)$
$y(n) = x_1(n) \cdot x_2(n)$	$Y(k) = \frac{1}{N}\sum_{l=0}^{N-1} X_1(l)X_2((k-l) \bmod N)$
$y(n) = \sum_{m=0}^{N-1} x_1(m)x_2((n-m) \bmod N)$	$Y(k) = X_1(k) \cdot X_2(k)$

3.4.2 *Wavelet*

Wavelet is "multi resolution" analysis using mother wavelet which is a waveform with its amplitude decrease to zero as distant from the center of the wave which may have various shape for different purposes. Wavelet has various advantages and disadvantages compared to the Fourier transform.

Those differences are more understandable after explanation of various time-frequency characteristics of different time windowing combined with Fourier transform. Therefore, following section will explain nature of Fourier transform with different windowing and then revisit wavelets.

Wavelet can be used for restoration and analysis of biomedical signals [13, 14].

3.5 Time-Frequency Resolution

To appropriately apply time frequency analysis, it is important to understand limitation in resolution in time domain or frequency domain for various circumstances. The important and basic law of such limitation is called uncertainty relation. Uncertainty relation is tradeoff between bandwidth and sharpness in location of the localized signal.

Figure 3.4 shows uncertainty relation. The signal, which is narrowly distributed in time, must have wide frequency bandwidth. The signal which has narrow bandwidth must have long duration in time.

Frequency resolution of the Fourier transform of slice of signal having duration time T is 1/T. For an example, as shown in Fig. 3.4a, if the given signal is $x(t) = e^{-\left(\frac{t}{0.5}\right)^2} \sin(2\pi 100t)$ which has time domain duration around 2 s, then frequency resolution is around 1 Hz as shown in (b). If given the signal is $y(t) = e^{-\left(\frac{t}{0.01}\right)^2} \sin(2\pi 100t)$, which has very short duration time 10 ms, as shown in (c), frequency resolution will be broader, around 100 Hz as shown in (d).

However, precision to identify frequency of sinusoidal signal is not limited to the 1/T. There is well known technique called zero padding as shown in Fig. 3.5. Figure 3.5 (c) shows 17 Hz sinusoidal signal having 100 ms length. Because frequency resolution is 10 Hz, (d) does not show peak at 17 Hz. By adding zeros to original waveform and make it longer signal, you may increase frequency resolution. For example, with 0.1 s slice of 17 Hz by adding zeros to be 1 s signal, 1 Hz frequency resolution can be obtained, as shown in (e) and (f).

Please note that the resulting frequency response has peak at the place of frequency line, however there will be many side robes. You can ignore side robe in this case. And note that, this technique is depending on the nature of single frequency line signal and not applicable to the signals which have more complex frequency spectrum.

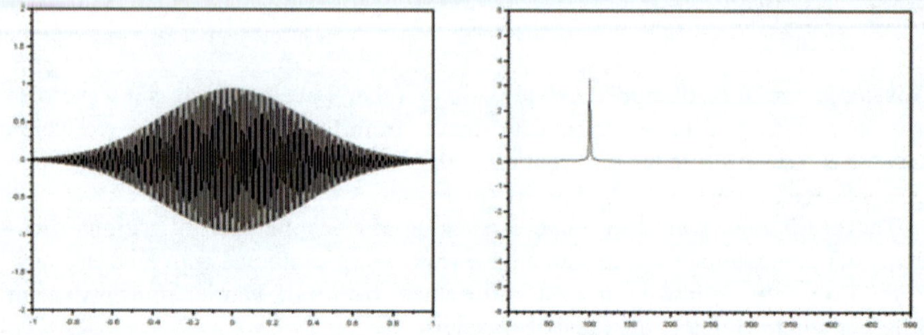

(a) $x(t) = e^{-\left(\frac{t}{0.5}\right)^2} sin(2\pi 100t)$ (b) Frequency spectrum of $x(t)$

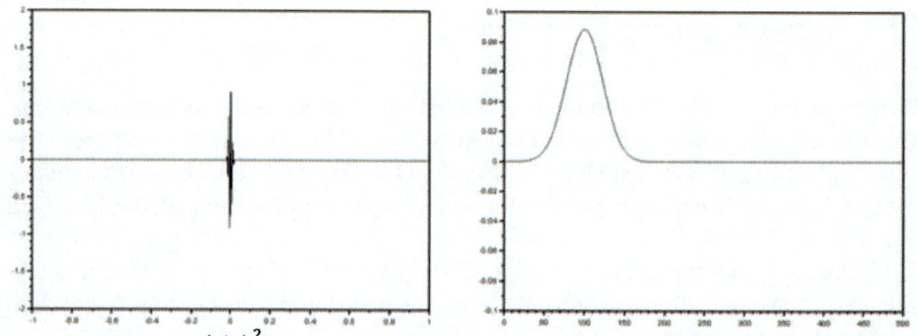

(c) $y(t) = e^{-\left(\frac{t}{0.01}\right)^2} sin(2\pi 100t)$ (d) Frequency spectrum of $y(t)$

Fig. 3.4 Uncertainty relation

3.6 Windowing and Filtering

To analyze signal both in time domain and frequency domain, the technique called windowing is used.

Here we show concept of time windowing. Smooth shaped time window will be multiplied to the waveform and limited time region will be selected. Then such signal will be analyzed by Fourier transform.

If length of time window is t1, since windowed signal has duration t1, frequency resolution of Fourie transform is limited to f = 1/t1. If shape of window is sharp, that causes anti focusing effect in the result of Fourier transform. So, sharper (narrow) time window result lower frequency resolution. Figure 3.6 shows time windowing and Fourier transform results in different frequency resolution by various time windowing. There are several parameters those need to be considered for the best result of such windowed signal. But most important factor is width of time window and frequency resolution.

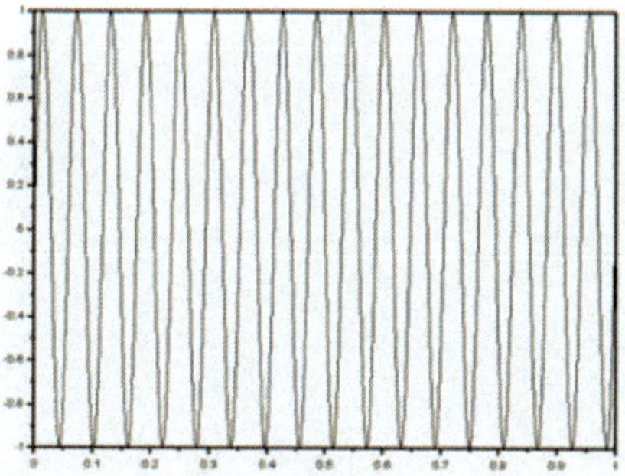

(a)17Hz 1sec sinusoidal signal

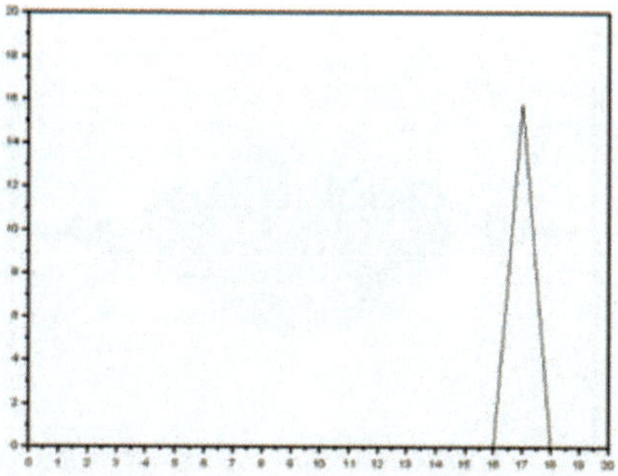

(b)Peak at 17Hz in frequency spectrum

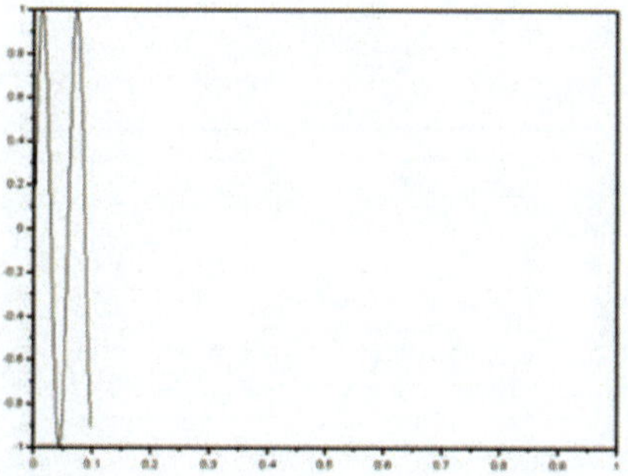

(c)17Hz 100ms sinusoidal signal

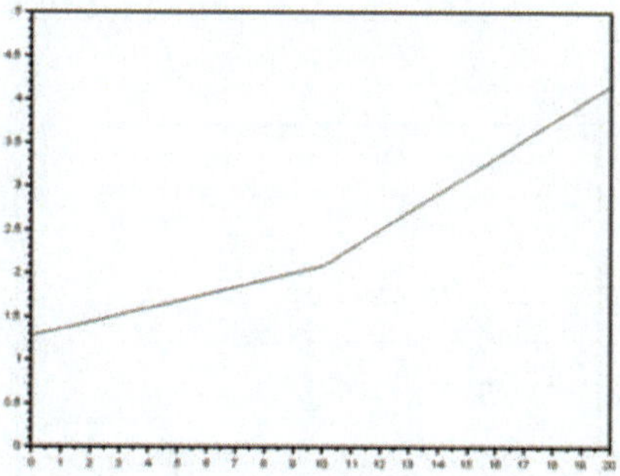

(d) Spectral reslution is 10Hz.

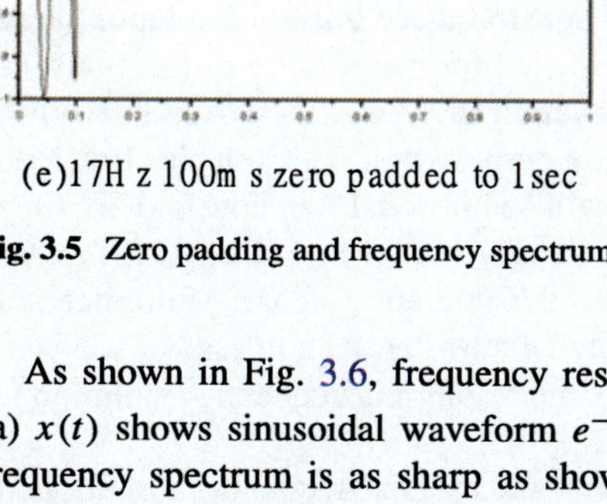

(e)17Hz 100ms zero padded to 1sec

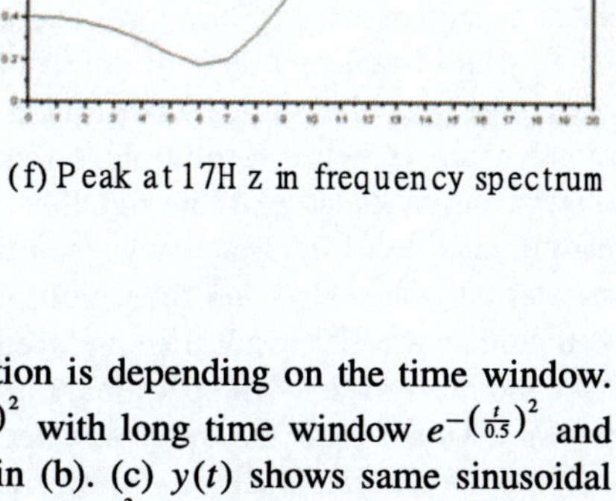

(f) Peak at 17Hz in frequency spectrum

Fig. 3.5 Zero padding and frequency spectrum

As shown in Fig. 3.6, frequency resolution is depending on the time window. (a) $x(t)$ shows sinusoidal waveform $e^{-(\frac{t}{0.5})^2}$ with long time window $e^{-(\frac{t}{0.5})^2}$ and frequency spectrum is as sharp as shown in (b). (c) $y(t)$ shows same sinusoidal signal $in(2\pi 100t)$ with short time window $e^{-(\frac{t}{0.01})^2}$ and frequency spectrum is as

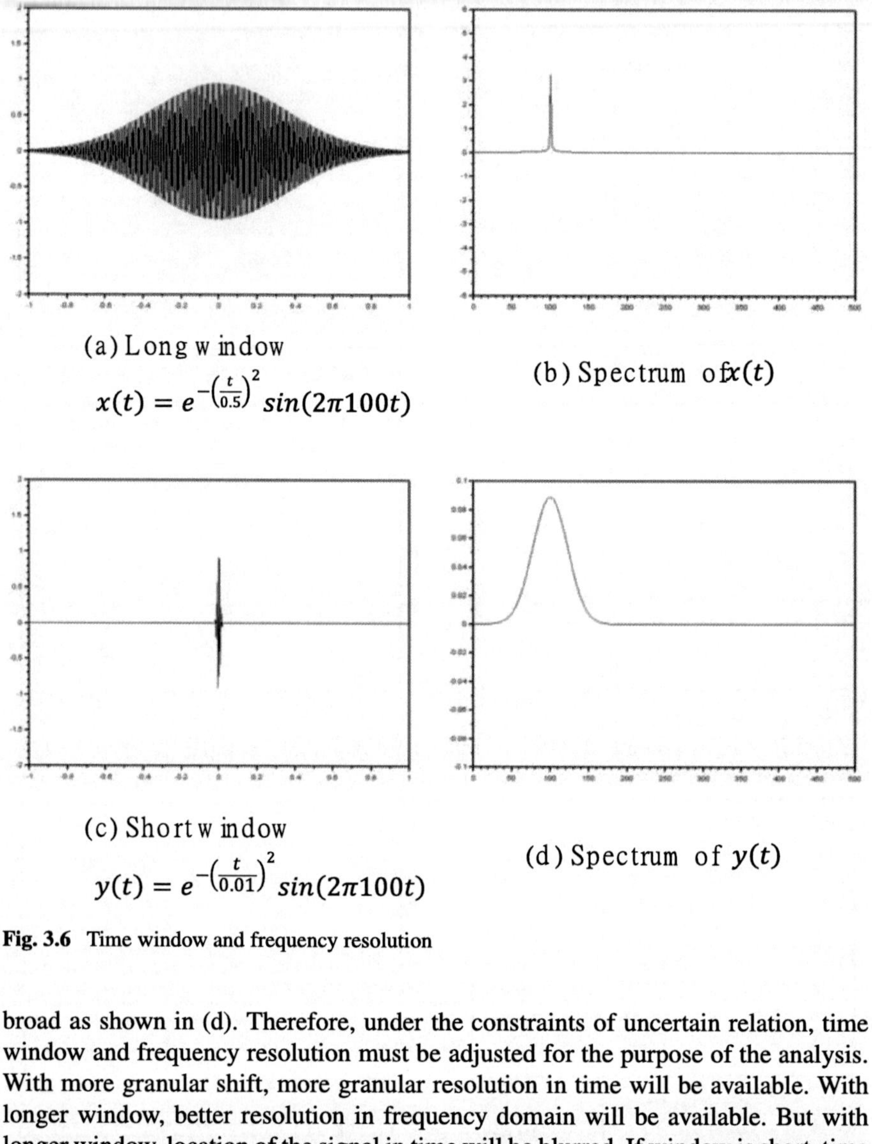

Fig. 3.6 Time window and frequency resolution

broad as shown in (d). Therefore, under the constraints of uncertain relation, time window and frequency resolution must be adjusted for the purpose of the analysis. With more granular shift, more granular resolution in time will be available. With longer window, better resolution in frequency domain will be available. But with longer window, location of the signal in time will be blurred. If window is short, time resolution is better, but frequency resolution will be worse. In case of wavelet, mother wavelet will be scaled and then multiplied to the reference signal. Multiplication with mother wavelet result time and frequency windowing. And in case of wavelet, since mother wavelet will be scaled, ratio of time resolution/frequency resolution is constant. This is basic nature of wavelet.

If mother wavelet is same as Fourier Transform Kernel for frequency f_1 multiplied with time window w_1, in case of Fourier transform, frequency resolution and time resolution are constant. In contrast, wavelet will give anti proportional ratio between time and frequency resolutions.

3.7 Microphone Arrays and Transducer Arrays

Thanks to the development of microfabrication technology and MEMS (Micro-electromechanical system) technology, microphone array or transducer array can be widely used today. When there are finite number of sound source, it is possible to separate and locate individual sound source if we can use more microphones than number of sound source. The technique is called sound source separation and sound source localization. But to derive satisfactory result using these techniques, it is important to limit echo and reverb under certain level, i.e. have enough noise margin, SNR in other words, from background echo and reverb to the direct signal from sound source to the microphones.

Even for signal having much echo, it is still possible to separate direct sound from room reverberation using technique called non-negative matrix factorization. Thanks to the advancement of MEMS sensors and expansion of the area of IoT (internet of things) applications, there are rapid and massive development of the use of microphone array and array sensors. User may find variety of research topics in this area [15–18].

3.8 Correlation

Correlation can be explained as kind of similarity which is numerically defined. Mathematically, it is simply the closeness of two vectors in vector space. If two vectors align perfectly, correlation is 1. If two vectors are orthogonal, correlation becomes zero. These situations are exactly same with correlation of two time series. Correlation 1 means full alignment of two waveform. Correlation 0 means no alignment at all. Please note that correlation is single scalar value representing similarity of two time series.

It is more interesting to think about calculating correlation after one waveform y slide against x. If amount of slide of one waveform against another can be given as t and correlation is defined as a function of such slide t, which may be explained as $R_{xy}(t)$, then it is called correlation function. $R_{xy}(t)$ is function of t.

If $R_{xy}(3) = 1$, it means two waveforms x and y are identical when x slide as offset 3 against y. Correlation function of waveform with waveform itself is called autocorrelation function. For an example, $R_{xx}(t)$ means correlation between x and x itself when x slide as offset t against another x. And if $R_{xx}(2) = 1$, it means that x perfectly matches itself when it slides amount of 2 that also means x is cyclic waveform which has cycle of 2.

If waveform is periodical with interval T, autocorrelation will be 1 for all $t = nT$. And here, autocorrelation function will link to frequency structure. When waveform is periodical, autocorrelation and frequency distribution have structure like comb. Correlation function is quite useful tool to examine relation of two waveforms.

You may simply calculate correlation function of two waveforms to determine whether if there is any relation between two waveforms. If any non-zero value over noise level did not found, two waveforms likely have no relation. And correlation function is highly sensitive for small similarity of waveform.

As show in Fig. 3.7, exceedingly small similarity can be detected by calculating

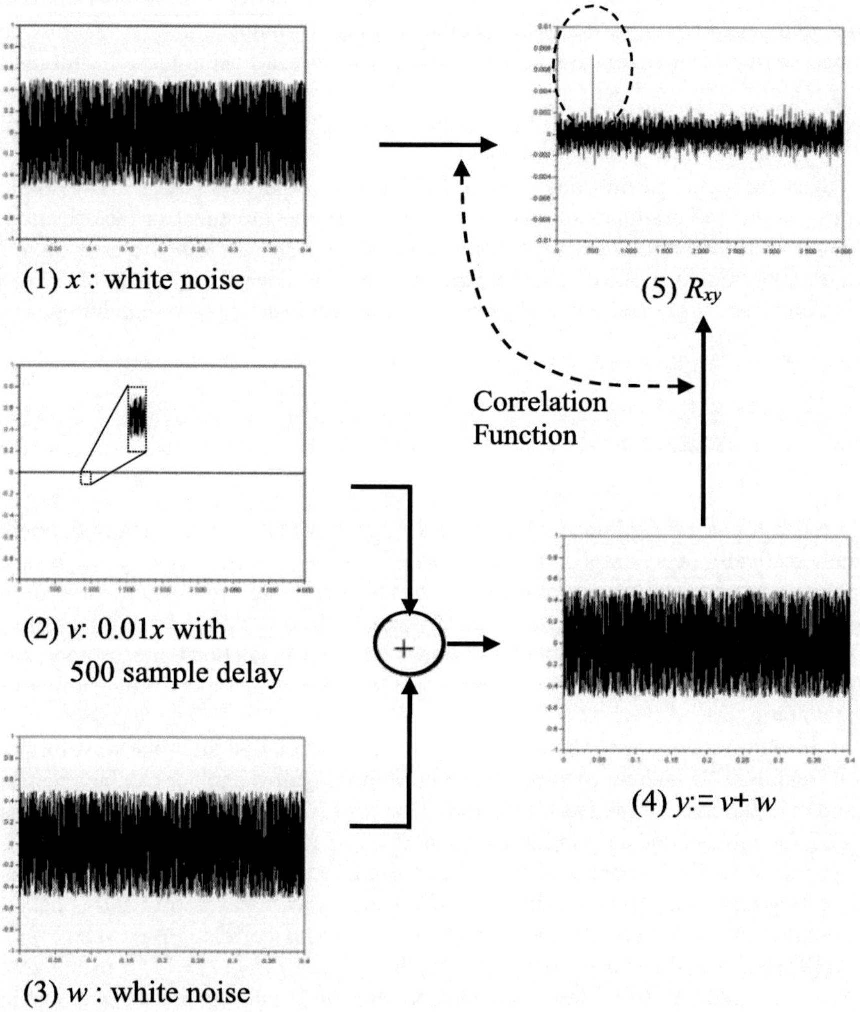

Fig. 3.7 Correlation function of signal which contain 1% of correlated signal

correlation function. In this figure, (1) x and (3) w are independent random signal. (2) $v = 0.01x$ is part of (1) which has only 1% of magnitude and 500 samples in duration, which is also 1% of the whole signal. Therefore (4) $y = v + w$ contains portion of x which has 1% in magnitude and about 1% in duration, which means 0.01% of whole signal. But (5) R_{xy} has very clear peak as marked by dash ellipse.

Correlation function can be calculated through Fourier transform to save computational power. Since correlation is one of most sensitive primary method of statistical evaluation of the signal, it is often used for the statistical analysis and estimation [19–21].

3.9 More Advanced Techniques

3.9.1 Mode Decomposition and Variational Mode Decompression

Mode decomposition is developed after 1990s. Mode is amplitude modulation, frequency modulation components of the signal. And mode decomposition decompose signal to modes which can be more precisely represents the components those consists signals compared to the sinusoidal signal.

Empirical mode decomposition (EMD) is proposed by Huan on 1996. Using EMD, time series can be decomposed into a finite and often small number of 'mode' functions [22]. And this decomposition process consists with well-behaved Hilbert transforms.

While empirical mode decomposition was used longtime until 2010s as major method for mode decomposition [23], it is limited by their ad hoc nature and did not allow backward error correction, thus incapable to nicely cope with noise. And Variational mode decomposition appeared later around 2010s [24]. Variational mode decomposition will determine the relevant bands adaptively and estimate corresponding mode concurrently and outperform empirical mode decomposition in terms of noise resilience.

$$U_k(t) = A_k(t)cos(\phi_k(t))$$

3.10 Examples

This chapter provides three examples of the time frequency analysis in the health informatics. The examples are not covering all the techniques, but they must be useful to give some idea how time frequency analysis can be applied in this application area.

3.10.1 Body Movement

Body movement can be measured as part of health information independently or as an associated information with another measurement [25].

Accelerometers and gyro sensors are typical sensors used for body movement. Sampling frequency of those are typically quite high compared to the body motion. Therefore, it is beneficial to subsample it for reduction of data. But in such a case, it should be recalled that subsample may cause aliasing if there are frequency component greater than Nyquist frequency. To avoid aliasing, sampling function should be applied instead of simple sub sampling.

3.10.2 Ultrasound Imaging

Ultrasound imaging is a method to imaging tissues using extremely high frequency sound, around 10 MHz [26]. Using linear transducer array and by scanning beam of ultrasound along with drawing image of echo, 2-dimensional image can be obtained. This is called A mode. It is also possible to use 2D array, receiving 2D image. Drawing 2D distribution of echo as 2D image and reflect amplitude of echo as brightness of dots, better imaging can be obtained compared to A mode. This is called B mode. It is also useful to detect frequency shift of echo. Such shift is caused by Doppler Effect. And imaging using it is called Doppler imaging.

3.10.3 Null Beamforming

In some application, it is preferable to receive signals from one direction and block waveform from another direction. For an example, there is a case of some strong noise source exists in one side of the sensor. In such case, technique called null beamforming can be used. Null beamforming is a kind of beamforming and it blocks waveform from one specific direction [27]. Using longitudinal microphone array, it is possible to cover large area as null by beamforming. Figure 3.8 shows a possible longitudinal microphone array configuration to suppress heartbeat. Using null beamforming, sensitivity to x_1 will be zero and enough gain to x_2 is maintained.

3.11 Conclusion

This chapter begins with the summary of basic and modern time-frequency analysis techniques. The explanation is intended to be understood without readers much background of signal processing. In the later part of the chapter addresses some modern

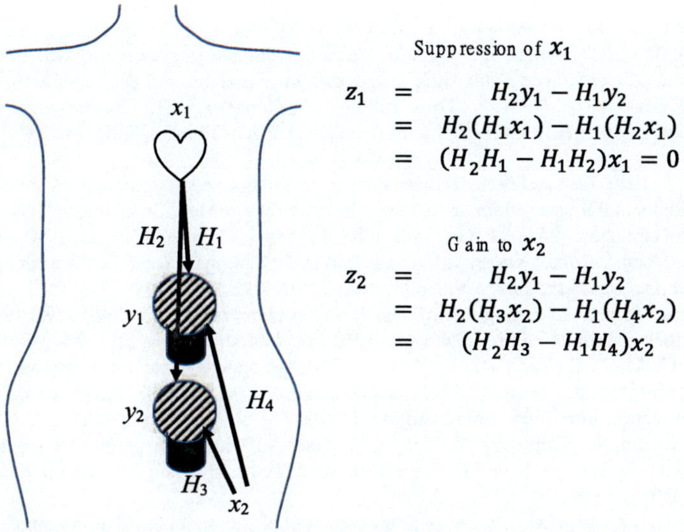

Fig. 3.8 Possible longitudinal microphone array configuration to suppress heartbeat

techniques and practical techniques. In some type of application, time-frequency analysis is especially useful technique to detect small amount of similarity and separate signal from noise. Therefore, it is quite useful for the feature detection and noise removal. Although some conceptual understanding of frequency analysis is important to appropriately apply these techniques for the real applications. The author hope that reader will find charm of frequency analysis and value to spend pain to learn more about this area. It should come in useful as quick introduction to time-frequency analysis for those who is new to this area and consider these techniques for their application.

References

1. Cerutti, S.: In the spotlight: biomedical signal processing. IEEE Rev. Biomed. Eng. **1** (2008)
2. Logier, R., Dassonneville, A., Delmar, G., Vasseur, C.: PhysioTrace: an efficient toolkit for biomedical signal processing. In: 2005 IEEE Engineering in Medicine and Biology 27th Annual Conference (2005)
3. Carmel, S., Macy, A.J.: Physiological signal processing laboratory for biomedical engineering education. In: 2005 IEEE Engineering in Medicine and Biology 27th Annual Conference (2005)
4. Li, Y., Zhao, D., Serdijn, W.A.: A sub-microwatt asynchronous level-crossing ADC for biomedical applications. IEEE Trans. Biomed. Circ. Syst. **7**(2), 149–157 (2013)
5. Varaleshmi, K., Venkatalakshmi, B.: Optimal FFT for wearable wireless medical devices. In: 2015 Global Conference on Communication Technologies (2015)
6. Tang, S.N., Jan, F.C., Cheng, H.W., Lin, C.K., Wu, G.Z.: Multimode memory-based FFT processor for wireless display FD-OCT medical systems. IEEE Trans. Circ. Syst. I Regul. Pap. **61**(12), 3394–3406 (2014)

7. Taki, H., Taki, K., Sakamoto, T., Yamakawa, M., Shiina, T., Sato, T.: High range resolution medical acoustic vascular imaging with frequency domain interferometry. In: 2010 Annual International Conference of the IEEE Engineering in Medicine and Biology (2010)
8. Riaz, F., Hassan, A., Nisar, R., Dinis-Ribeiro, M., Coimbra, M.T.: Content-adaptive region-based color texture descriptors for medical images. IEEE J. Biomed. Health Inf. **21**(1), 162–171 (2015)
9. Nayak, J., Bhat, P.S., Acharya, R., Niranjan, U.C.: Simultaneous storage of medical images in the spatial and frequency domain: a comparative study. BioMed. Eng. OnLine **3**(1), 17 (2004)
10. Cedillo-Hernandez, Manuel, Garcia-Ugalde, Francisco, Nakano-Miyatake, Mariko, Perez-Meana, Hector: Robust watermarking method in DFT domain for effective management of medical imaging. Sign. Image Video Process. **9**, 1163–1178 (2015)
11. Sezan, M.I., Stark, H.: Tomographic image reconstruction from incomplete view data by convex projections and direct Fourier inversion. IEEE Trans. Med. Imaging **3**(2), 91–98 (1984)
12. Zhang, G., Ma, Z.M., Tong, Q., He, Y., Zhao, T.: Shape feature extraction using fourier descriptors with brightness in content-based medical image retrieval. In: 2008 International Conference on Intelligent Information Hiding and Multimedia Signal Processing (2008)
13. Ng, J., Prager, R., Kingsbury, N., Treece, G., Gee, A.: Wavelet restoration of medical pulse-echo ultrasound images in an EM framework. IEEE Trans. Ultrason. Ferroelectr. Freq. Control **54**(3), 550–568 (2007)
14. Serbes, G., Gulcur, H.O., Aydin, N.: Directional dual-tree rational-dilation complex wavelet transform. In: 2014 36th Annual International Conference of the IEEE Engineering in Medicine and Biology Society (2014)
15. Boutry, C.M., Nguyen, A., Lawal, Q.O., Chortos, A., Rondeau-Gagné, S., Bao, Z.: A sensitive and biodegradable pressure sensor array for cardiovascular monitoring. Adv. Mate. **27**(43), 6954–6961 (2015)
16. Cikach Jr., F.S., Dweik, R.A.: Cardiovascular biomarkers in exhaled breath. Prog. Cardiovasc. Dise. **55**(1), 34–43 (2012)
17. Song, J.K., Son, D., Kim, J., Yoo, Y.J., Lee, G.J., Wang, L., Choi, M.K., Yang, J., Lee, M., Do, K., Koo, J.H.: Wearable force touch sensor array using a flexible and transparent electrode. Adv. Funct. Mater. **27**(6), 1605286 (2017)
18. Wei, H., Denga, Y., He, Y.: Visual colorimetric sensor array for discrimination of antioxidants in serum using MnO2 nanosheets triggered multicolor chromogenic system. Biosens. Bioelectr. **91**, 15 (2017)
19. Xu, W., Chang, C., Hung, Y.S., Kwan, S.K., Fung, P.C.: Order statistics correlation coefficient as a novel association measurement with applications to biosignal analysis. IEEE Trans. Sign. Process. **55**(12), 5552–5563 (2007)
20. Gao, J., Hu, J., Tung, W.W.: Facilitating joint chaos and fractal analysis of biosignals through nonlinear adaptive filtering. In: ASME 2011 Dynamic Systems and Control Conference and Bath/ASME Symposium on Fluid Power and Motion Control (2011)
21. Maki, Y., Sano, G., Kobashi, Y., Nakamura, T., Kanoh, M., Yamada, K.: Estimating subjective assessments using a simple biosignal sensor. In: 2012 IEEE International Conference on Fuzzy Systems (2011)
22. Huang, N.E., Shen, Z., Long, S.R., Wu, M.C., Shih, H.H., Zheng, Q., Yen, N.C., Tung, C.C., Liu, H.H.: The empirical mode decomposition and the Hilbert spectrum for nonlinear and non-stationary time series analysis. Math. Phys. Eng. Sci. **454**(1971), 903–995 (1971)
23. Flandrin, P., Rilling, G., Goncalves, P.: Empirical mode decomposition as a filter bank. IEEE Sign. Process. Lett. **11**(2), 112–114 (2004)
24. Dragomiretskiy, K., Zosso, D.: Variational mode decomposition. IEEE Trans. Sign. Process. **62**(3), 531–544 (2014)
25. Kaneko, I., Yoshida, Y., Yuda, E.. Improvements of the analysis of human activity using acceleration record of electronic cardiographs. Sign. Image Process. Int. J. (SIPIJ) **10**(5) (2019)

26. Nishimura, R.A., Edwards, W.D., Warnes, C.A., Reeder, G.S., Holmes, D.R., Tajik, A.J., Yock, P.G.: Intravascular ultrasound imaging: in vitro validation and pathologic correlation. J. Am. Coll. Cardiol. **16**(1), 145–154 (1990)
27. Krim, H., Viberg, M.: Two decades of array signal processing research: the parametric approach. IEEE Sign. Process. Maga. **13**(4), 67–94 (1996)

Chapter 4
Complexity Analysis in Health Informatics

Mosabber Uddin Ahmed

Abstract Complexity can be interpreted as a manifestation of the intricate entwining or inter-connectivity of elements within a system and between a system and its surroundings. Complex adaptive systems (CAS) are comprised of multiple subsystems that exhibit nonlinear deterministic & stochastic characteristics, and are regulated hierarchically. Examples of CAS include stock markets, human heart or brain, weather and climate systems, internet etc. A system's complexity usually reflected in the dynamical fluctuations of the output generated by the free-running conditions. In this chapter, the definitional controversies for complexity are introduced and signal properties associated with complexity are reviewed. We then introduce some criteria used to classify complexity measures in the literature, and finally some representative complexity measures used in health informatics are described.

Keywords Complexity · Long-range correlation · Multiscale entropy · Dynamical systems · Information-theoretic measures · Chaos-theoretic measures · Random fractal-theoretic measures · Randomness

4.1 What is Complexity?

The concept of complexity and the study of complex adaptive systems originated from a whole chain of interdisciplinary approaches, from the theory of nonlinear dynamical systems to information theory, statistical mechanics, biology, sociology, ecology, economics and others. Researchers in those areas have been trying to define complexity, nonetheless, no all-encompassing definition has emerged as yet.

Murray Gell-Mann, the winner of 1969 Nobel Prize in physics, traces the meaning of complexity to the root of the word. The English word *complex* is derived from the Latin word *complexus*, meaning 'entwined' or 'braided together [1]. Similarly, the Oxford Dictionary defines something as 'complex' if it is 'made of (usually several)

[1] http://www.necsi.edu/guide/concepts/complexity.html.

M. U. Ahmed (✉)
University of Dhaka, Dhaka 1000, Bangladesh
e-mail: mosabber.ahmed@du.ac.bd

M. A. R. Ahad and M. U. Ahmed (eds.), *Signal Processing Techniques for Computational Health Informatics*, Intelligent Systems Reference Library 192,
https://doi.org/10.1007/978-3-030-54932-9_4

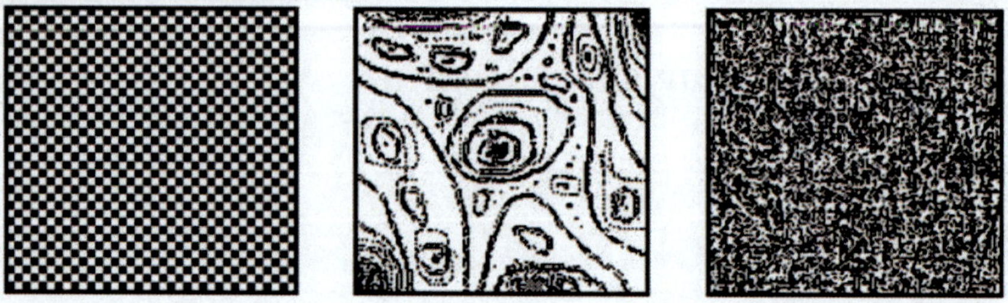

Fig. 4.1 An illustration of complexity: Left panel displays a completely ordered pattern, middle panel displays a complex pattern and right panel displays a completely random pattern [2]

closely connected parts'. New England Complex Systems Institute (NECSI[1]) defines complexity as: (1) 'the (minimal) length of a description of the system'. (2) 'the (minimal) amount of time it takes to create the system'. On the other hand, Grassberger [2] positioned complexity somewhere between order and disorder. He considered three patterns similar to those in Fig. 4.1 and described that human identifies the pattern in the middle as the most complex since it seems to have more "structure." On the contrary, the pattern on the right has no rules as it is generated using a random number generator though at the level of each pixel, however, the amount of information required to objectively and fully describe this pattern is greatest. This agrees with the notion that living organism should be more complex than, for example, both perfect crystals and ideal gases.

Besides, the following definitions are taken from the existing literature of complexity science featuring many key figures in this field:

1. 'To us, complexity means that we have structure with variations' [3].
2. 'Complexity starts when causality breaks down' [4].
3. 'The term describe phenomena, structures, aggregates, organisms, or problems that share some common themes: (1) They are inherently complicated or intricate; (2) they are rarely completely deterministic; (3) mathematical models of the system are usually complex and involve non-linear, ill-posed, or chaotic behavior; (4) the systems are predisposed to unexpected outcomes (so-called emergent behavior)' [5].
4. 'An ill-defined term that means many things to many people. Complex things are neither random nor regular, but hover somewhere in between. Intuitively, complexity is a measure of how interesting something is' [6].
5. 'Complexity is that property of a model which makes it difficult to formulate its overall behavior in a given language, even when given reasonably complete information about its atomic components and their inter-relations' [7].
6. 'Complexity = integration of observer and trinity of factors (size, variety, rules)' [8].
7. 'Complexity can then be characterized by lack of symmetry or "symmetry breaking", by the fact that no part or aspect of a complex entity can provide sufficient information to actually or statistically predict the properties of the others parts' [9].

From the above definitions, it can be concluded that:

- There is still no agreed-upon definition, much less a theoretically rigorous formalization of complexity.
- Complexity is contextual and domain-specific. It is pretty much in the eye of the beholder.
- None of the definitions or approaches in the complexity literature are mutually exclusive.
- Neither perfect disorder nor perfect order are complex, rather complexity lies between order and disorder, or, using a recently fashionable expression, "on the edge of chaos".
- Complexity is a comparative/relative measure rather than an absolute measure, as we want to be able to say frequently "X is more complex than Y which is, in turn, more complex than Z".

4.2 Manifestation of Complexity

There are numerous attributes or characteristics associated with complexity. The following attributes are neither exhaustive list nor are they individually necessary and/or sufficient conditions for complexity.

Nonlinearity. Nonlinearity means that the superposition principle does not hold. Though often considered to be essential for complexity, it is not a necessary condition for complexity as there are complex systems studied in game theory and quantum dynamics which are in the domain of linear dynamics [10].

Feedback. Feedback is an important necessary condition for complexity. It ensures adaptability and self-organization in complex systems. For example, Malthusian population dynamics rely on positive feedback for explosive growth and negative feedback, due to resource shortages, for population decline [11]. However, the existence of feedback in a system is not sufficient for complexity as it requires the individuals to be part of a large enough group for exhibiting complexity [10].

Spontaneous order. This arises from the combined effect of a very large number of uncoordinated interactions between elements. Notions related to order include symmetry, organization, periodicity, determinism and pattern. Admitting the fact that complexity lies in between total order and absolute randomness, it is a necessary condition for a complex system that it exhibits some kind of spontaneous order. For example, spontaneous order can be easily seen in the flocking behavior of birds or in swarm behavior of shoals of fishes [12].

No central control. There is no single centralized control in a complex system. Control is distributed throughout the system and local decisions are made by parts or modules (elements) within overall system. As the control is distributed/self-organized, the system is robust and stable under perturbations. For example, the order observed in the swarming behavior of birds (fishes) are stable and robust despite the individual and erratic motions of its members or the perturbations in the system by the wind (ocean current) or the random elimination of some of the members of the swarm. This is due to the lack of central control in the system. However, it is not sufficient for complexity as non-complex systems may have no control or order at all [10].

Emergence. It is associated with the properties of 'wholes' (or more complex situations) that cannot be defined through the properties of the 'parts' (or simpler situations) as concisely summarized by Aristotle in the Metaphysics: "The whole is more than the sum of its parts". It is some kind of global property which arises from the aggregate behavior of individuals, something that could not have been predicted from understanding each particular individual. It is in contrast to the reductionist approach. Emergent behavior seems to be ubiquitous in nature. For example, in the brain, consciousness is an emergent phenomenon, which comes from the interaction of the brain cells. However, it is not sufficient, for example, an ideal gas exhibits emergent order but is not a complex system [12, 13].

Hierarchical organization. Complexity arises when many levels of organization forms a hierarchy of system and sub-system. The complex system exhibits a variety of levels of structure and various kinds of symmetry, order and periodic behavior through interaction within and across levels. Examples include ecosystem, brain, cosmos etc. [14].

Numerosity. System should consists of a large number of parts and the individual parts should be engaged in many linear/non-linear interactions to constitute complexity. All of the above properties emerges only if the system consists of a large number of parts [13].

Self-similarity. A special kind of scale invariance in which the parts closely resemble the whole. If the parts are identical re-scaled replica, the fractal is exact. If they show the same statistical properties at different scales, the fractal is statistical. Mathematical fractals such as the Cantor set or the Mandelbrot tree are exact whereas most natural fractal objects like Pial arterial tree running along the brain cortex of the cat or coastline are statistical as shown in Fig. 4.2 [15]. The self-similarity can also be distinguished as spatial self-similarity and temporal self-similarity. Most of the complex fluctuations in respiration, heart rate variability, human gait etc. possesses temporal self-similarity and their self-similarity is statistical. However, self-similarity need to be differentiated from self-affinity. Self-similar objects are isotropic as the scaling is identical in all directions whereas for self-affine objects scaling is anisotropic. For example, physiological signals are self-affine temporal structures because the units of their amplitude is not time as shown in Fig. 4.3 [15].

Long-range correlation. A hallmark of physiologic systems is their extraordinary complexity resulting from the long-range correlations extending exponentially over many spatio-temporal scales. For example, the inter beat interval (IBI) time series from healthy subjects shows long-range correlations extending to thousands of heartbeats. This multiscale complexity appears to degrade in characteristic ways with

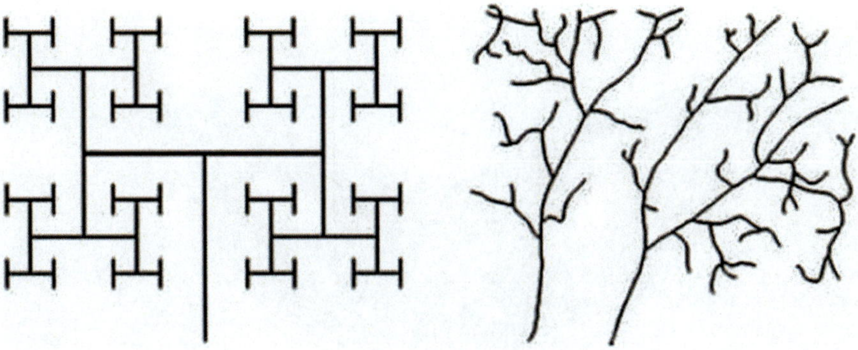

Fig. 4.2 Spatial fractals: Left panel displays Mandelbrot tree, an exact fractal and right panel displays Pial arterial network, a statistical fractal [15]

Fig. 4.3 Fractals: Left panel displays a tree-like fractal which is self-similar and right panel displays heart rate fluctuation process which is self-affine [16]

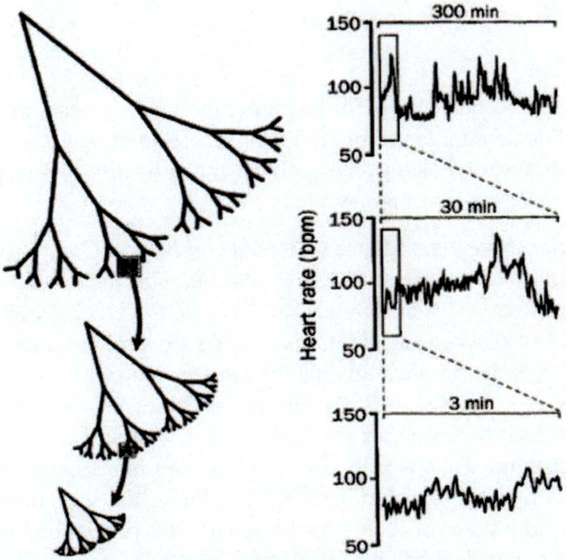

aging and disease, reducing the adaptive capacity of the individual. As a result, this fractal breakdown and associated complexity loss can be quantified and have potential applications to diagnostic and prognostic assessment [17].

Far from equilibrium. This phenomenon illustrates how systems that are forced to explore their space of possibilities will create different structures and new patterns of relationships. This notion is also related to physiologic complexity. Under healthy conditions, living systems which are open dissipative systems (as there are mass, energy, entropy, and information fluxes across their boundaries) operates far from equilibrium. On the contrary, maximum equilibrium is reached when a living system

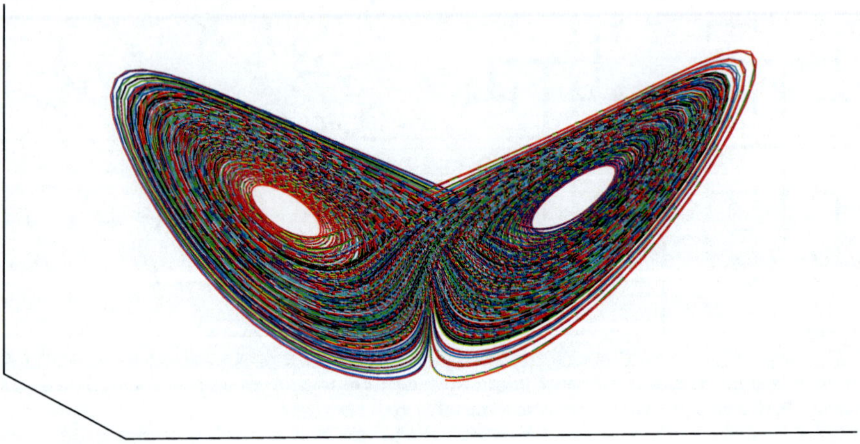

Fig. 4.4 Lorenz attractor

approaches death. For example, the healthy heart rate dynamics exhibits irregular fluctuations far from equilibrium. Regularity in the heartbeat interval is a sign of disease indicating insensitivity and inflexibility and thus inability to adapt to the changing environment [15].

Sensitive dependence on initial conditions. Complexity also arises due to the sensitive dependence on initial conditions. This means that small differences in the initial state of a system can lead to dramatic differences in its long-term dynamics (popularly known as the 'butterfly effect'). Edward Lorenz was among the first to study this dependency by simulating the long term evolution of weather using a simplified version of the Navier-Stokes equations. By slightly varying initial values of temperature, pressures and other parameters, he found solutions showing new type of behavior patterns as shown in Fig. 4.4. The consequences of this discovery were profound as limited precision in measuring the initial state precludes accurate predictions of future states of such systems. Long-term prediction and control of complex systems are therefore believed to be very hard or impossible [12].

State of paradox. Complexity arises from dynamics combining both order and chaos which supports the idea of bounded instability or the edge of chaos characterized by a state of paradox: stability and instability, competition and cooperation, order and disorder [12].

Co-evolution. With co-evolution, elements in a system can change not only based on their interactions with one another but also with the environment. Additionally, patterns of behavior can change over time. For example, evolution of species occurs with respect to their environment as well as their relationship to other species. Stuart Kauffman described co-evolution with the concept of fitness landscapes [12]. The fitness landscape is an n-dimensional function made of many maxima/minima.

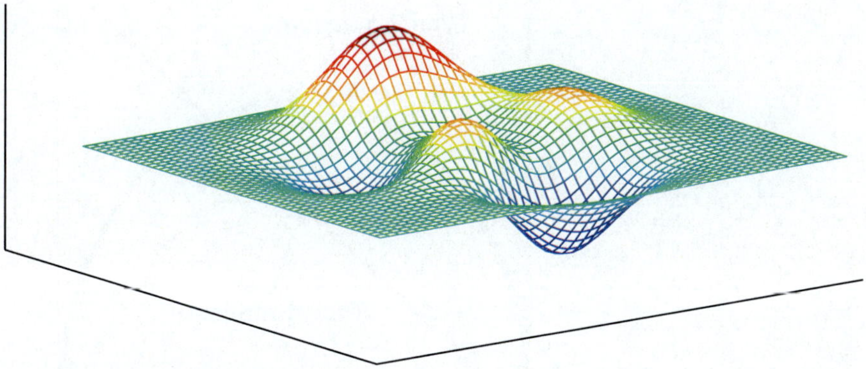

Fig. 4.5 Three dimensional fitness landscape

Each of them corresponds to a potential of fitness/unfitness. The higher a maximum/minimum is, the greater the fitness/unfitness it represents. Figure 4.5, shows a three dimensional fitness landscape. The evolution of a system can be thought of as a voyage across the fitness landscape with the aim of discovering the global maximum. The system can get stuck on the first maximum it approaches if the strategy is incremental improvement. If the system changes its strategy, other interconnected systems will respond and thus changes the shape of the fitness landscape dynamically.

4.3 Classification of Complexity Measures

As with the definitions, there are again several approaches regarding classification of complexity measures. Some of the approaches are described below.

From the perspective contrasting complexity and randomness. In this perspective, measures of complexity are grouped into two types: Type 1 measures monotonically increase with increasing disorder or randomness in the system whereas Type 2 measures behave as globally convex function of randomness and exhibit highest complexity for systems with intermediate order or regularity. This is depicted in Fig. 4.6. Example of Type 1 measures include Algorithmic complexity [18], various generalized entropies, approximate entropy (ApEn) [19], sample entropy (SampEn) [20] etc. On the other hand, effective measure complexity (EMC) [2], ϵ-machine complexity [21], fluctuation complexity [22], multiscale entropy (MSE) [23] etc. belongs to the Type 2 measures.

From the perspective contrasting determinism and stochasticity. In this view, complexity measures are classified either as deterministic or statistical. All determin-

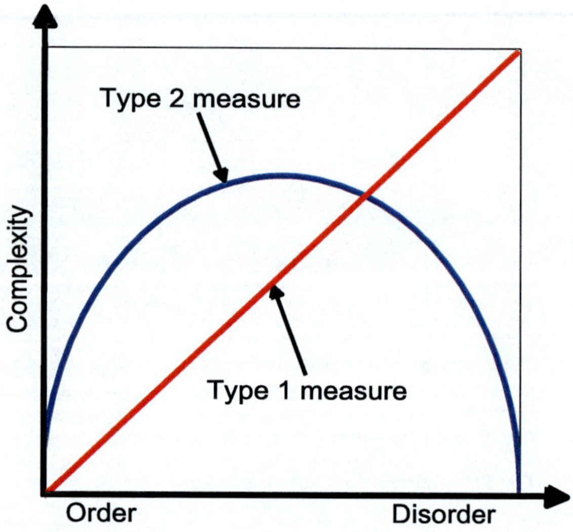

Fig. 4.6 Complexity versus randomness

istic measures are essentially measures of randomness and increases monotonically with the increase of randomness whereas all statistical measures are convex function of randomness.

From the perspective of dynamical systems. In this view, complexity measures are classified in the context of dynamical systems so that the measures can distinguish between order and chaos. The four-fold scheme is based on the dichotomous notions of structure and dynamics as well as homogeneous partitions and generating partitions. Structural aspects are related with the appearance of state probabilities (with respect to the partition) in the definition of the measure while dynamical measures contain transition probabilities in addition [24].

From philosophical perspective. This scheme is epistemologically inspired and assigns ontic and epistemic levels of description to deterministic and statistical measures respectively. It turns out that this scheme distinguishes measures of complexity precisely in the same manner as Type 1 and Type 2. In other words, ontic measures are actually Type 1 measures whereas epistemic measures are Type 2 measures [25].

From the perspective of the way statistics is implemented. Complexity measures can be classified according to the way statistics is implemented in each of these measures. In this perspective, convex measures, in contrast to monotonic measures, are meta-statistically formalized. In other words, they use second-order statistics in the sense of 'statistics of statistics'. For example, fluctuation complexity is the standard deviation (second-order) of a net mean information flow (first-order), effective measure complexity (EMC) is the convergence rate (second-order) of a difference of entropies (first-order) etc. [25].

From the perspective of computability. In this context, complexity measures can be classified as computable or non-computable. Example of computable measures are statistical complexity, effective measure complexity (EMC) etc. On the other hand algorithmic complexity, effective complexity [26] etc. are non-computable.

From the perspective of difficulty. In this scheme, 42 complexity measures are grouped according to the answer of three questions that are frequently posed when attempting to quantify complexity of something under study [27]:

- How hard is it to describe?
- How hard is it to create?
- What is its degree of organization?

In the category of 'difficulty of description', there are algorithmic complexity, generalized entropies etc. In the category of 'difficulty of creation', there are computational complexity, logical depth etc., whereas effective complexity, effective measure complexity (EMC) etc. belong to the category of 'degree of organization'.

4.4 Representative Complexity Measures

As there are a great number of complexity measures in the literature and still new measures are enriching this list, it is almost impossible to review all these measures. In developing complexity measures, there have been contributions from a diverse set of fields including Thermodynamics, Information Theory, Statistical Mechanics, Control Theory, Applied Mathematics, Operations Research etc. In the following, we categorize complexity measures according to those broad field from which they are originated and describe some representative measures.

4.4.1 Information-Theoretic Complexity Measures

Most of information-theoretic complexity measures are based on either Shannon entropy or its derivatives. Claude Shannon was the first to show the connection between thermodynamical entropy and information-theoretic entropy [28]. Though it was derived as a measure of randomness or uncertainty in a system, it has been used as a measure of complexity by subsequent authors. This type of measure requires data to be first categorized into binary or another fixed number of bins ('symbols'). Complexity measures are then based on the probability (p_x) of observing symbol x in the data, as well as on second order probabilities such as the frequency of observing symbol x next to symbol y or of observing particular sequences of symbols of length L in the series (known as L-words). The measures can be of Type 1 or Type 2 as defined previously in Fig. 4.6.

4.4.1.1 Shannon Entropy

Shannon entropy [28] is a measure of the average amount of information in a transmitted message or the difficulty of guessing a message passing through a channel, given the range of possible messages. Let X be a discrete random variable on a finite set $X = \{x_1, x_2, \ldots, x_n\}$, with probabilities $p(x_i) = Pr(X = x_i)$. Then the entropy $H(X)$ of X is defined as $H(X) = -\sum_{i=1}^{n} p(x_i) \log p(x_i)$. The logarithm is usually taken to the base 2, in which case the entropy is measured in 'bits', or to the base e, in which case $H(X)$ is measured in 'nats'. In the case of transmitted messages, these probabilities are the probabilities that a particular message was actually transmitted and the term $-\log p(x_i)$ is defined as the information content of the message x_i. For the case of equal probabilities (i.e. each message is equally probable), the Shannon entropy is highest.

4.4.1.2 Kolmogorov-Sinai Entropy

This is related to measures of partitions in dynamical systems. Suppose a phase space is divided into D-dimensional hypercubes of content ϵ^D. Let $P_{i_0,i_1,\ldots,i_n}$ be the probability that a trajectory is in hypercube i_0 at $t = 0$, i_1 at $t = T$, i_2 at $t = 2T$, etc. and define

$$K_n = h_K = -\sum_{i_0,i_1,\ldots,i_n} P_{i_0,i_1,\ldots,i_n} \ln P_{i_0,i_1,\ldots,i_n} \tag{4.1}$$

where $K_{n+1} - K_n$ is the information needed to predict which hypercube the trajectory will be in at $(n+1)T$ given trajectories up to nT. The Kolmogorov-Sinai (KS) entropy is then defined by

$$K \equiv \lim_{T\to 0} \lim_{\epsilon\to 0^+} \lim_{n\to\infty} \frac{1}{nT} \sum_{n=0}^{n-1} (K_{n+1} - K_n) \tag{4.2}$$

The KS-entropy can be interpreted as highest average amount of information that the system can produce per step relative to a coding and is thus related to the Shannon entropy. A positive KS-entropy is often linked to chaos. Moreover, the sum of all the positive Lyapunov exponents gives an estimate of the Kolmogorov-Sinai entropy according to Pesin's theorem [29].

4.4.1.3 Correlation Entropy

Correlation entropy/K2 entropy is a lower bound of KS entropy. Historically, it is developed to classify deterministic systems by rates of information generation and was not developed for statistical applications.

Grassberger & Procaccia [30] first defined the correlation sum for a collection of delay embedding vectors X_n of dimension m as the fraction of all possible pairs of vectors which are closer than a given distance ϵ in the Euclidean norm sense. The basic formula is

$$C(m,\epsilon) = \frac{2}{N(N-1)} \sum_{i=1}^{N} \sum_{j=i+1}^{N} \Theta(\epsilon - \|X_i - X_j\|) \tag{4.3}$$

where Θ is a Heaviside step function. In the limit, for an infinite amount of data ($N \rightarrow \infty$) and for small ϵ, $C(m,\epsilon)$ scales like a power law, that is $C(\epsilon) \propto \epsilon^{D_2}$, where the correlation dimension D_2 is defined by

$$\begin{aligned} d(N,\epsilon) &= \frac{\partial \ln C(\epsilon, N)}{\partial \ln \epsilon} \\ D_2 &= \lim_{\epsilon \rightarrow 0} \lim_{N \rightarrow \infty} d(N,\epsilon) \end{aligned} \tag{4.4}$$

when the embedding dimension m exceeds the box-dimension of the attractor. Since we do not know the box-dimension a priori, we need to check for convergence of the estimated values of D_2 in m.

While correlation dimension characterizes the dependence of ϵ on the correlation sum inside the scaling range, the correlation entropy characterizes the m-dependence. The number of ϵ-neighbors of an m-dimensional delay vector is an estimate of the local probability density, and in fact it is a kind of joint probability—all m-components of the neighbor have to be similar to those of the actual vector simultaneously. Thus, when increasing m, joint probabilities covering larger time spans get involved. The scaling of these joint probabilities is related to the correlation entropy, h_2, such that $C(m,\epsilon) \propto \epsilon^{D_2} e^{-m h_2}$, where the correlation entropy is calculated as:

$$h_2(m,\epsilon) = \ln \frac{C(m,\epsilon)}{C(m+1,\epsilon)} \tag{4.5}$$

As for the scaling in ϵ, also the dependence on m is valid only asymptotically for large m, which cannot be attained due to the lack of data points. So, a so called scaling range of ϵ values is sought for which h_2 is nearly constant (convergent) for large m (which is extrapolated from different h_2 versus m plot). As correlation entropy is defined by some limiting procedure, we are in trouble if we have a finite sample instead of a full distribution: N is limited by the sample size, and the range of meaningful choices for ϵ is limited from below by the finite accuracy of the data and by the inevitable lack of near neighbors at small length scales [31].

4.4.1.4 Approximate Entropy

Pincus [19] introduced approximate entropy (ApEn) as a regularity statistic with fixed m and ϵ to distinguish between finite, noisy, possibly stochastic, or composite deterministic and stochastic data sets. It represents the conditional probability that sequences that are close to each other for m consecutive data points will still be close to each other when one more data point is known. Though approximate entropy was constructed along similar lines to the correlation entropy, it had a different focus: to provide a widely applicable, statistically valid entropy formula. The motivation behind approximate entropy was that, if joint probability measures for reconstructed dynamics that describe each of two systems are different, then their marginal probability distributions on a fixed partition, given by aforementioned conditional probabilities are probably different too. Typically, one need orders of magnitude fewer points to accurately estimate these marginal probabilities as compared to the number of points needed to accurately reconstruct the "attractor" measure defining the process. As a result, approximate entropy is applicable to noisy, typically short, real-world time series and, unlike the correlation entropy, it can distinguish between different correlated stochastic processes. Approximate entropy is routinely used in computational health informatics for disease diagnosis and prognosis [32, 33].

4.4.1.5 Sample Entropy

Sample entropy (SampEn) is a modification of the Approximate Entropy introduced by Richman et al. [20]. It reduces the bias of ApEn by excluding self-matches, i.e., vectors are not compared to themselves. Moreover, it is largely independent of time series length and displays relative consistency over a wide range of operating conditions. Sample entropy is the most widely used complexity estimate in health informatics [34, 35]. Recently, some modifications of sample entropy have also been proposed [36–38].

4.4.1.6 Multiscale Entropy

Costa et al. [23] proposed multiscale entropy (MSE) which calculates SampEn across multiple time scales. As multiscale entropy is based on SampEn, it measures the degree of randomness (or inversely, the degree of orderliness) of a time series. But unlike KS entropy or sample entropy, which are based on a 'one step difference' (e.g., $H_{n+1} - H_n$) and hence do not account for features related to structure and organization of scales other than the shortest one, multiscale entropy analysis focuses on quantifying the interrelationship of entropy and scale thus associating complexity with the ability of living systems to adjust to an ever-changing environment which requires integrative multiscale functionality. The scales in MSE method are generated using the so called 'coarse-graining' method. A review on MSE and its derivatives can be found in [39].

4.4.1.7 Fourier Entropy

To calculate Fourier entropy, first the power spectral density (PSD) of a time series is computed and then normalized to produce a probability-like distribution. Afterwards, the Shannon entropy of this normalized PSD is calculated which is known as spectral entropy or Fourier entropy. The Fourier entropy measures the extent to which the power spectrum of the signal is concentrated (or not) into a given (narrow) frequency range. Low entropy values correspond to narrow-band (mono-frequency) activity characterizing highly ordered (regularized) signal and thus lower complexity. On the contrary, high entropy values reflect a wide-band (multi-frequency) activity in the signal and correspond to higher complexity.

4.4.1.8 Wavelet Entropy

This complexity measure is related to the number of wavelet components needed to fit a signal [40]. In contrast to spectral entropy, it is capable of detecting changes in a nonstationary signal due to the localization characteristics of the wavelet.

4.4.1.9 Effective Measure Complexity

Grassberger [2] introduced Effective Measure Complexity (EMC) of a pattern as the asymptotic behavior of the amount of information that must be stored in order to make an optimal prediction about the next symbol to the level of granularity. EMC can be seen as the difficulty of predicting the future values of a stationary series, as measured by the size of regular expression of the required model. It can capture structure in sequences that range over multiple scales. For a random string, EMC is zero while for structured or correlated string, it increases linearly with the correlation.

4.4.1.10 GeoEntropy

GeoEntropy [41] is based on the theory of regionalized variables. The concept of regionalized variables is central to geo-statistics which concerns with spatially distributed properties. Such a variable is usually a characteristic of certain phenomenon, as metal grades, for example, are characteristics of mineralization. The degree of spatial variability of a regionalized variable is usually expressed by a semi-variogram. Based on the semi-variogram, GeoEntropy yields an analytical procedure for estimating the parameter m and r that are used to compute SampEn/MSE.

4.4.1.11 Correntropy

Correntropy [42] is a nonlinear similarity measure between two random variables. It generalizes the autocorrelation function to nonlinear spaces. If $\{x_t, t \epsilon, T\}$ is a strict stationary stochastic process with an index set T, then the correntropy function is defined as $V(s,t) = E\{\langle \phi(x_s), \phi(x_t) \rangle\}$, where ϕ is a nonlinear mapping from the input space to the feature space. It makes use of the 'kernel trick' to define the inner product of the nonlinear mappings as a positive-definite Mercer kernel: $K(x_s, x_t) = \langle \phi(x_s), \phi(x_t) \rangle$. Though it is not a direct complexity measure, it is used to detect nonlinearity in the signal and thus measures complexity.

4.4.2 *Algorithmic Complexity Measures*

Apart from the various information-theoretic measures of complexity, some measures are algorithmic in nature and are applied on strings or other data structures. For these measures, complexity relates to a generative process or description rather than to an actually existing physical system or dynamical process.

4.4.2.1 Algorithmic Information Complexity (AIC)

This measure was developed independently by Solomonoff, Kolmogorov, and Chaitin and also known as Kolmogorov-Solomonoff-Chaitin complexity. Though it is the most influential among algorithmic complexity measures, it is not computable. It is defined as the minimum possible length of a description in some language. For a string of symbols, it is the length of the shortest program to produce the string as an output. Highly regular, periodic or monotonic strings may be computed by programs that are short because the description can be greatly compressed without loss of meaning and as a result, they are less complex. On the other hand, the complexity of a truly random string is highest since it cannot be compressed at all and the shortest program that outputs that string will have to contain the string itself. However, incompressible strings (those whose programs are not shorter than themselves) are indistinguishable from random strings [43].

4.4.2.2 Logical Depth

Logical depth [44] is defined as the minimum necessary effort or computational cost (time and memory) required for creating and running a shortest program that can reproduce a given object. Thus it is a combination of both storage and computational power. A random string is incompressible and hence the shortest program that can reproduce it is a simple copying program. Consequently, both random strings and very simple ones have a low logical depth as the computation time for both is very small. On the other hand, strings which have structure and regularity, in addition to some randomness, are logically deep as they require longer time to compute. Similar to AIC, this measure is not computable.

4.4.2.3 Topological Complexity

Crutchfield and Young extended the concept of algorithmic information complexity by defining complexity as the minimal size of a model representation of a system that can statistically reproduce the observed data within a specified tolerance. This definition takes into account both the minimal size and the fixed hierarchy or structural rules of a system. One disadvantage of this definition is that it could not provide a unique measure of complexity for a system because there may not be necessarily a minimal model for the system or users may construct different models of the same system [8].

4.4.2.4 Computational Complexity

It is the asymptotic difficulty in computing the output relative to the size of the input in terms of computational resources (typically time or storage space), given the specification of the problem. The degree of complexity of a problem depends on the level of detail used to describe it. As a result, it is a measure of the effort required to obtain an agreed amount of details of information [7].

4.4.2.5 Arithmetic Complexity

Arithmetic complexity is defined as the minimum number of arithmetic operations needed to complete a task. Though it is not a general concept of complexity, it is practically important for making computational algorithms more efficient [7].

4.4.2.6 Lempel-Ziv (LZ) Complexity

It is a major compression scheme in Unix systems which approximates the algorithmic complexity of a given string. It asymptotically approaches Shannon entropy. This scheme is also the basis for compression of TIFF images and ZIP files, where it is referred to as LZW (Lempel-Ziv-Welch) compression [10].

4.4.2.7 Effective Complexity

Effective complexity was introduced by Gell-Mann [26] as a statistical measure of complexity based on Kolmogorov complexity. It is defined as the length of a concise description of the regularities (as contrasted to the degree of randomness) of a system or bit string. It is a statistical measure of complexity as it is the shortest description, not of the entity itself, but of the ensemble in which the entity is embedded as a typical member. It is a Type 2 measure and also not computable.

4.4.3 Chaos-Theoretic Complexity Measures

These type of measures are based on the basic properties of chaotic system like the aperiodic and highly erratic behavior of trajectories of chaotic dynamical systems or their sensitive dependence on initial conditions.

4.4.3.1 Lyapunov Exponent

It characterizes the rate of divergence (or convergence) of two neighboring trajectories in the phase space and thus measures the instability (or stability) of generic trajectories against infinitesimal perturbations. Though it is not a direct complexity measure, it can be interpreted as a measure of the rate at which the system generates new information. Besides, the maximal Lyapunov exponent (the largest of the spectrum of Lyapunov exponents), is related to a notion of predictability for a dynamical system and thus can measure complexity [31].

4.4.3.2 Attractor Dimension

Various attractor dimensions like information dimension, box-counting dimension, generalized dimension etc. can also be used as complexity measures. The higher the dimension of the attractor, the more complex the dynamical system associated with the attractor is.

4.4.3.3 Permutation Entropy

This complexity measure has aspects of both dynamical systems and information theory measures because complexity is estimated as the entropy of the distribution of permutations of groups of time samples. At first, each member of the group is given a sequence number from 1 to n. Then the n members of each group are placed in ascending order and the new order of the sequence numbers for each group is noted. The new order serves as a bin number into which the total matches of that order among all of the groups is stored. The result is a histogram of number of occurrences of each sequence order which is further normalized to a probability distribution and finally the entropy of that probability distribution is calculated. Permutation entropy (PermEn), thus, measures the local order structure of the time series in phase space.

The use of ordinal statistics (rank) makes PermEn robust to noise embedded in phase space. It is an extremely fast and robust measure and used for measuring complexity for real-world time series [45]. Recent extensions of permutation entropy used in health informatics are documented in [46–50].

4.4.4 *Random Fractal-Theoretic Complexity Measures*

Complexity measures based on random fractal theory differ from those based on chaos theory in the sense that in chaos theory complexity is assumed to be generated by nonlinear deterministic interactions of the system components with only a few degrees of freedom, where noise or intrinsic randomness does not play an important role. On the contrary, random fractal theory assumes that the dynamics of the system are inherently random. These measures also relate complexity with the long-range correlation and scaling behavior of the system. Complexity measures from this field includes Hurst parameter, spectral index calculated from power spectral density, α-parameter of detrended fluctuation analysis (DFA) method etc [15].

4.5 Conclusion

There is no denying the fact that there are numerous complexity measures used in computational health informatics. To cover all those measures in a single chapter is a daunting task. We have tried to decipher in this chapter the notion of complexity, its different manifestation, its way of classification and finally have presented some representative complexity measures that are routinely used in health informatics. We hope that the systematic analysis of different complexity measures covered in this book will further our understandings of complexity and help us to choose the appropriate complexity measures in health informatics.

References

1. Gell-Mann, M.: Let's call it plectics. Complexity **1**(5) (1995/96)
2. Grassberger, P.: Toward a quantitative theory of self-generated complexity. Int. J. Theor. Phys. **25**, 907–938 (1986)
3. Goldenfeld, N., Kadanoff, L.P.: Simple lessons from complexity. Science **284**(5411), 87–89 (1999)
4. Editorial. No man is an island. Nat. Phys. **5**(1), 1–1 (2009)
5. Foote, R.: Mathematics and complex systems. Science **318**(5849), 410–412 (2007)
6. Flake, G.W: The Computational Beauty of Nature: Computer Explorations of Fractals, Chaos, Complex Systems, and Adaptation. MIT Press, Cambridge, MA, USA (1998)
7. Edmonds, B.: Syntactic Measures of Complexity. Ph.D. thesis, University of Manchester, Manchester, UK (1999)

8. Xing, J., Manning, C.A.: Complexity and automation displays of air traffic control: Literature review and analysis. Final Report DOT/FAA/AM-05/4. Civil Aerospace Medical Institute, Federal Aviation Administration, Oklahoma City, OK 73125, Apr 2005
9. Heylighen, F.: The growth of structural and functional complexity during evolution. In: Heylighen, F., Bollen, J., Riegler, A. (eds.) The Evolution of Complexity, pp. 17–44. Kluwer Academic Publishers, Dordrecht (1999)
10. Ladyman, J., Lambert, J., Wiesner, K.: What is a complex system? Eur. J. Philos. Sci. 1–35 (2012). https://doi.org/10.1007/s13194-012-0056-8
11. Manson, S.M.: Simplifying complexity: a review of complexity theory. Geoforum **32**(3), 405–414 (2001)
12. Couture, M.: Complexity and Chaos—state-of-the-art: overview of theoretical concepts. In: Technical Memorandum DRDC Valcartier TM 2006-453, Defence R&D Canada-Valcartier, Aug 2007
13. Anderson, P.W.: More is different. Science **177**(4047), 393–396 (1972)
14. Simon, H.A.: The architecture of complexity. Proc. Am. Philos. Soc. **106**(6), 467 (1962)
15. Eke, A., Herman, P., Kocsis, L., Kozak, L.R.: Fractal characterization of complexity in temporal physiological signals. Physiol. Meas. **23**(1), R1–R38 (2002)
16. Goldberger, A.L.: Non-linear dynamics for clinicians: Chaos theory, fractals, and complexity at the bedside. Lancet **347**(9011), 1312–1314 (1996)
17. Goldberger, A.L., Amaral, L.A.N., Hausdorff, J.M., Ivanov, P.C., Peng, C.-K., Stanley, H.E.: Fractal dynamics in physiology: alterations with disease and aging. Proc. Natl. Acad. Sci. U.S.A. **99**(Suppl 1), 2466–2472 (2002)
18. Kolmogorov, A.N.: Three approaches to the quantitative definition of information. Prob. Inf. Trans. **1**(1), 3–11 (1965)
19. Pincus, S.M.: Approximate entropy as a measure of system complexity. Proc. Natl. Acad. Sci. U.S.A. **88**(6), 2297–2301 (1991)
20. Richman, J.S., Moorman, J.R.: Physiological time-series analysis using approximate entropy and sample entropy. Am. J. Physiol. Heart Circ. Physiol. **278**(6), H2039–2049 (2000)
21. Crutchfield, J.P., Young, K.: Inferring statistical complexity. Phys. Rev. Lett. **63**, 105–108 (1989). Jul
22. Bates, J.E., Shepard, H.K.: Measuring complexity using information fluctuation. Phys. Lett. A **172**(6), 416–425 (1993)
23. Costa, M., Goldberger, A.L., Peng, C.-K.: Multiscale entropy analysis of complex physiologic time series. Phys. Rev. Lett. **89**(6), 068102 (2002)
24. Wackerbauer, R., Witt, A., Atmanspacher, H., Kurths, J., Scheingraber, H.: A comparative classification of complexity measures. Chaos Solit. Fract. **4**(1), 133–173 (1994)
25. Atmanspacher, H., Räth, C., Wiedenmann, G.: Statistics and meta-statistics in the concept of complexity. Phys. A **234**(34), 819–829 (1997)
26. Gell-Mann, M., Lloyd, S.: Information measures, effective complexity, and total information. Complexity **2**(1), 44–52 (1996)
27. Lloyd, S.: Measures of complexity: a nonexhaustive list. IEEE Control Syst. Mag. **21**(4), 7–8 (2001)
28. Shannon, C.E.: A mathematical theory of communication. Bell Syst. Tech. J. **27**(2093), 379–423, 623–656 (1948)
29. Frigg, R., Werndl, C.: Entropy–A guide for the perplexed. In: Beisbart, C., Hartmann, S. (eds.) Probabilities in Physics, Chapter 5, pp. 115–142. Oxford University Press, Oxford, UK (2011)
30. Grassberger, P., Procaccia, I.: Estimation of the Kolmogorov entropy from a chaotic signal. Phys. Rev. A **28**, 2591–2593 (1983)
31. Kantz, H., Schreiber, T.: Nonlinear Time Series Analysis. Cambridge University Press, Cambridge, UK (2000)
32. Bansal, T., Haji, G.S., Rossiter, H.B., Polkey, M.I., Hull, J.H.: Exercise ventilatory irregularity can be quantified by approximate entropy to detect breathing pattern disorder. Respirat. Physiol. Neurobiol. **255**, 1–6 (2018)

33. Udhayakumar, R.K., Karmakar, C., Palaniswami, M.: Approximate entropy profile: a novel approach to comprehend irregularity of short-term HRV signal. Nonlinear Dyn. **88**(2), 823–837 (2017)
34. Martínez-Cagigal, V., Santamaría-Vázquez, E., Hornero, R.: Asynchronous control of p300-based brain? Computer interfaces using sample entropy. Entropy **21**(3) (2019)
35. Jia, Y., Huaguang, G.: Identifying nonlinear dynamics of brain functional networks of patients with schizophrenia by sample entropy. Nonlinear Dyn. **96**(4), 2327–2340 (2019). Jun
36. Liao, F., Jan, Y.-K.: Using modified sample entropy to characterize aging-associated microvascular dysfunction. Front. Physiol. **7**, 126 (2016)
37. Marwaha, P., Sunkaria, R.K.: Complexity quantification of cardiac variability time series using improved sample entropy (I-SampEn). Aust. Phys. Eng. Sci. Med. **39**(3), 755–763 (2016)
38. Porta, A., Bari, V., De Maria, B., Cairo, B., Vaini, E., Malacarne, M., Pagani, M., Lucini, D.: On the relevance of computing a local version of sample entropy in cardiovascular control analysis. IEEE Trans. Biomed. Eng. **66**(3), 623–631 (2019)
39. Humeau-Heurtier, A.: The multiscale entropy algorithm and its variants: a review. Entropy **17**(5), 3110–3123 (2015)
40. Rosso, O.A., Blanco, S., Yordanova, J., Kolev, V., Figliola, A., Schürmann, M., Basar, E.: Wavelet entropy: a new tool for analysis of short duration brain electrical signals. J. Neurosci. Methods **105**(1), 65–75 (2001)
41. Pham, T.D.: Geoentropy: a measure of complexity and similarity. Pattern Recogn. **43**(3), 887–896 (2010)
42. Santamaria, I., Pokharel, P.P., Principe, J.C.: Generalized correlation function: definition, properties, and application to blind equalization. IEEE Trans. Signal Process. **54**(6), 2187–2197 (2006)
43. Li, M., Vitányi, P.M.B.: An Introduction to Kolmogorov Complexity and Its Applications. Springer, New York, USA (2008)
44. Bennett, C.H.: Logical depth and physical complexity. In: Herken, R. (ed.) A Half-Century Survey on the Universal Turing Machine, pp. 227–257. Oxford University Press, Oxford (1988)
45. Bandt, C., Pompe, B.: Permutation entropy: a natural complexity measure for time series. Phys. Rev. Lett. **88**(17), 174102 (2002)
46. Azami, H., Escudero, J.: Amplitude-aware permutation entropy: illustration in spike detection and signal segmentation. Comput. Methods Programs Biomed. **128**, 40–51 (2016)
47. Bandt, C.: A new kind of permutation entropy used to classify sleep stages from invisible EEG microstructure. Entropy **19**(5), 197 (2017). Apr
48. Tao, M., Poskuviene, K., Alkayem, N., Cao, M., Ragulskis, M.: Permutation entropy based on non-uniform embedding. Entropy **20**(8), 612 (2018). Aug
49. Li, C., Shang, P.: Multiscale Tsallis permutation entropy analysis for complex physiological time series. Phys. A **523**, 10–20 (2019)
50. Chen, Z., Yaan, L., Liang, H., Jing, Y.: Improved permutation entropy for measuring complexity of time series under noisy condition. Complexity **1–12**(03), 2019 (2019)

Chapter 5
Entropy Analysis in Health Informatics

Anne Humeau-Heurtier

Abstract This chapter aims at presenting entropy measures that are now widely used in health informatics. Entropy measures have been introduced in 1990s and are derived from the theory of chaos. The traditional entropy-based analysis methods evaluate the degree of regularity of signals. We therefore present, first, the very well-known entropy measures used in the biomedical field: their theoretical background is detailed and some medical applications are presented. Then, more and very recent entropy measures are exposed and some of their used in health informatics are listed. This is performed from two points of view: for time series (uni-dimensional data) and for images (bi-dimensional data).

Keywords Entropy · Irregularity · Biomedical application · Time series · Image · Texture

5.1 Introduction

Output signals of a biological system exhibit complex fluctuations that contain information on underlying interacting components that regulate the system. These components react across several spatial and temporal scales. The study of these complex fluctuations helps in interpreting the behavior of the system: the complexity of a biological system reveals its capacity to adjust in ever-changing situations. Therefore, data coming from a healthy system should have a higher complexity than those coming from a pathologic one [1].

Nonlinear methods have shown their ability to capture physiological information that were not caught by traditional linear methods. Among the nonlinear approaches, several entropy measures have been introduced in the 1990s. They are derived from the theory of chaos. The traditional entropy-based analysis methods evaluate the degree of regularity. Uncorrelated random signals (white noise) are unpredictable but their structure is not complex. As they are unpredictable, the traditional entropy

A. Humeau-Heurtier (✉)
Univ Angers, LARIS—Laboratoire Angevin de Recherche en Ingénierie des Systèmes, 62 Avenue Notre-Dame du Lac, 49000 Angers, France
e-mail: anne.humeau@univ-angers.fr

M. A. R. Ahad and M. U. Ahmed (eds.), *Signal Processing Techniques for Computational Health Informatics*, Intelligent Systems Reference Library 192,
https://doi.org/10.1007/978-3-030-54932-9_5

methods give the highest entropy values to these data: the more random the signal, the greater its entropy. This is why these methods give higher entropy values to some pathologic systems that give erratic outputs than to healthy systems that are regulated by multiple interacting components. However, random time series have no structure. They are therefore not complex. Complexity is different from irregularity. This is the reason why multiscale entropy methods have been developed: to better describe the complexity of physiological data [2]. These measures consider the entropy of the signals at different time scales of the time series through a coarse-graining procedure, most of the time. The results are consistent with the fact that fully ordered and fully random signals are not complex; however correlated random time series (colored noise) are more complex than uncorrelated random time series (white noise).

In what follows, we first detail the widely used uni-dimensional entropy measures in health informatics (approximate entropy, sample entropy, fuzzy entropy, and permutation entropy) and give examples of their use in the biomedical field. We then expose very recent entropy-based measures proposed in health informatics. This is performed first for the 1D-case (time series) and then the extensions to the bi-dimensional case that exist are presented. We do not mention the multiscale approaches that have been derived from these entropy-based methods: we focus on the entropy measures only.

5.2 Approximate Entropy, Sample Entropy, Fuzzy Entropy, and Permutation Entropy: The Widely Used Uni-dimensional Entropy Measures in Health Informatics

5.2.1 *Approximate Entropy*

5.2.1.1 Concept

Approximate entropy (*ApEn*) quantifies the irregularity of time series [3, 4]. It evaluates the unpredictability of fluctuations patterns: the more repetitive patterns in the signal, the more predictable the signal, and thus the less irregular it is. The algorithm to compute *ApEn* for a time series $\mathrm{u} = \{u(i), 1 \leq i \leq N\}$ of N samples is the following [3]:

1. State space reconstruction

Define an embedding dimension m (m will be the length of compared runs) and a threshold parameter r. Form a sequence of vectors $\mathrm{X}_m(i)$ defined as:

$$\mathbf{X}_m(i) = \{u(i), u(i+1), \ldots, u(i+m-1)\}, \quad 1 \leq i \leq N-m+1. \tag{5.1}$$

2. Ranking similar vectors

Compute the distance $d[\mathrm{X}_m(i), \mathrm{X}_m(j)] = d^m_{i,j}$ between $\mathrm{X}_m(i)$ and $\mathrm{X}_m(j)$ ($1 \leq i, j \leq N-m+1$). This distance is computed as:

$$d_{i,j}^{m} = \max(|u(i+k) - u(j+k)|, 0 \le k \le m-1). \tag{5.2}$$

Compute, for a given i, C_i^m(r) as:

$$C_i^m(r) = \frac{\text{number of vectors } X_m(j) \text{ within } r \text{ of } X_m(i)}{N-m+1}. \tag{5.3}$$

Compute $\Phi^{(m)}(r)$ as the average of the natural logarithm of the functions $C_i^m(r)$:

$$\Phi^{(m)}(r) = \frac{1}{N-m+1} \sum_{i=1}^{N-m+1} \ln\left[C_i^m(r)\right]. \tag{5.4}$$

3. Repeat steps (1) and (2) for dimension (*m* + *1*). This leads to the computation of $\Phi^{(m+1)}(r)$.
4. Computation

   Compute *ApEn* as:

$$ApEn(m, r, N) = \Phi^{(m)}(r) - \Phi^{(m+1)}(r), \tag{5.5}$$

$$ApEn(m, r, N) = \frac{1}{N-m+1} \sum_{i=1}^{N-m+1} \ln\left[C_i^m(r)\right] - \frac{1}{N-m} \sum_{i=1}^{N-m} \ln\left[C_i^{m+1}(r)\right]. \tag{5.6}$$

ApEn is in fact a biased estimator because it counts self-matches (i.e., the distance between $X_m(i)$ and itself is taken into account) [5]: self-matches are counted in the computation of *ApEn* or else log-of-zero situations may appear. This is why a corrected *ApEn* (*cApEn*) has been proposed [6].

5.2.1.2 Application in Health Informatics

ApEn was recently used on ventilation, during an incremental cardiopulmonary exercise test, to obtain a quantitative way to detect breathing pattern disorder [7]. In 2017, Udhayakumar et al. proposed an approach based on *ApEn* to evaluate the impact of aging on heart rate variability (HRV) from short-term HRV signals [8]. In 2016, *ApEn* on electroencephalography (EEG) time series was used as an evaluation criteria of cognitive workload [9].

5.2.2 *Sample Entropy*

5.2.2.1 Concept

As seen above, in the *ApEn* algorithm the self-match of vectors is counted to escape the occurrence of ln(0) in the formulation. This leads to two drawbacks for *ApEn*: (i) *ApEn* is heavily dependent on the data length; (ii) *ApEn* lacks relative consistency [5]. To get over these drawbacks, Richman and Moorman proposed the sample entropy (*SampEn*) in 2000 [5].

SampEn is the negative natural logarithm of the conditional probability that two vectors (in the state space representation) that are similar for m points remain similar at the next point [5]. Its definition for a time series $\mathrm{u} = \{u(i), 1 \leq i \leq N\}$ of N samples is the following [5]:

1. State space reconstruction

Define an embedding dimension m (m will be the length of compared runs) and a threshold parameter r. Form a sequence of vectors $\mathrm{X}_m(i)$ defined as:

$$\mathbf{X}_m(i) = \{u(i), u(i+1), \ldots, u(i+m-1)\}, \quad 1 \leq i \leq N-m+1. \tag{5.7}$$

2. Ranking similar vectors

Keeping the same definition of distance as in *ApEn*, i.e.:

$$d_{i,j}^m = \max(|u(i+k) - u(j+k)|, 0 \leq k \leq m-1), \tag{5.8}$$

define $B_i^m(r)$ as [5]:

$$B_i^m(r) = \frac{\text{number of vectors } \mathrm{X}_m(j) \text{ within } r \text{ of } \mathrm{X}_m(i)}{N-m-1} \tag{5.9}$$

where $1 \leq j \leq N-m$, and $j \neq i$ to exclude self-matches.

Then, compute $\mathrm{B}^m(r)$, the probability that two sequences will be considered as similar for m points, as:

$$\mathrm{B}^m(r) = \frac{1}{N-m} \sum_{i=1}^{N-m} B_i^m(r). \tag{5.10}$$

In the same way, define $A_i^m(r)$ as

$$A_i^m(r) = \frac{\text{number of vectors } \mathrm{X}_{m+1}(j) \text{ within } r \text{ of } \mathrm{X}_{m+1}(i)}{N-m-1}, \tag{5.11}$$

where j ranges from 1 to $N-m$, and $j \neq i$.

Then, compute $A^m(r)$, the probability that two sequences will be considered as similar for *m + 1* points, as:

$$\mathrm{A}^m(r) = \frac{1}{N-m} \sum_{i=1}^{N-m} A_i^m(r). \tag{5.12}$$

3. Computation

Compute *SampEn* as:

$$SampEn(m, r, N) = -\ln\left[\frac{A^m(r)}{B^m(r)}\right]. \tag{5.13}$$

In the definition of *SampEn*, the similarity of vectors relies on the Heaviside function. Therefore, the contributions of all the data points inside the boundary are treated in the same way. The data points just outside the boundary are not taken into account. The distances $d_{i,j}^m$ that are greater than the tolerance *r* are not considered in the computation of $\mathrm{B}^m(r)$ and $A^m(r)$. The distances $d_{i,j}^m$ that are lower than the tolerance are treated equally. Therefore, *SampEn* may rise or fall dramatically for slight changes of the tolerance *r*.

5.2.2.2 Application in Health Informatics

In 2019, authors proposed to examine the regularity of EEG signals with *SampEn* to identify control and non-control states; they also assessed the efficacy of the multi-scale approach of *SampEn* to provide asynchronous control in P300-based brain-computer interfaces systems [10]. In 2019 also, Jia and Gu used blood oxygen level-dependent (BOLD) signals to study if *SampEn* of dynamic functional connectivity is modified in patient with schizophrenia and if this modification is related to symptoms of schizophrenia [11]. From their results, the authors showed that patients with schizophrenia have a significantly higher *SampEn* compared to the one of the healthy subjects at different levels of the brain; this is mainly due to a significantly higher *SampEn* in the visual cortex of the patients. Moreover, they also showed that *SampEn* values of the visual cortex are significantly and positively correlated with the illness duration or the symptom severity scores [11]. *SampEn* has also recently been of use for finger movement recognition using electromyography (EMG) [12].

5.2.3 *Fuzzy Entropy*

5.2.3.1 Concept

As mentioned above, the Heaviside function θ used in *ApEn* and *SampEn* behaves as a a two-state classifier that determines if two vectors as "similar" or "dissimilar":

$$\theta(z) = \begin{cases} 1, \text{ if } z \geq 0, \\ 0, \text{ if } z < 0. \end{cases}$$

There is not intermediate states. However, in the real physical world, boundaries between classes are not "strict": it is not easy to say if an input pattern belongs totally to a class [13].

In 2007, Chen et al. imported the concept of "fuzzy sets" and used the family of exponential function $\exp\left(-\frac{(d_{i,j})^n}{r}\right)$ as the fuzzy function in the computation of vectors' similarity ($d_{i,j}$ is the distance between $X_m(i)$ and $X_m(j)$ and is defined below) [13]. The family of exponential function possesses the following properties: (i) is continuous; therefore the similarity does not change abruptly; (ii) is convex so that self-similarity is the maximum.

Thus, the definition of fuzzy entropy (*FuzzyEn*) for a time series $u = \{u(i), 1 \leq i \leq N\}$ of N samples is the following [13]:

1. State space reconstruction

Define an embedding dimension m (m will be the length of compared runs) and a threshold parameter r. Form a sequence of vectors $X_m(i)$ defined as:

$$\begin{aligned} \mathbf{X}_m(i) =& \{u(i), u(i+1), \ldots, u(i+m-1)\} - u_0(i), \\ & 1 \leq i \leq N - m + 1. \end{aligned} \tag{5.14}$$

where $u_0(i)$ is defined as:

$$u_0(i) = \frac{1}{m} \sum_{j=0}^{m-1} u(i+j). \tag{5.15}$$

2. Ranking similar vectors

Define the distance $d[X_m(i), X_m(j)] = d_{i,j}^m$ as:

$$d_{i,j}^m = \max(|(u(i+k) - u_0(i)) - (u(j+k) - u_0(j))|, 0 \leq k \leq m-1) \tag{5.16}$$

Compute the similarity degree $D_{i,j}^m$ between $X_m(i)$ and $X_m(j)$ through a fuzzy function $\mu\big(d_{i,j}, n, r\big)$ as:

$$D_{i,j}^m(n, r) = \mu\big(d_{i,j}^m, n, r\big), \tag{5.17}$$

where the fuzzy function $\mu\left(d_{i,j}^{m}, n, r\right)$ is the exponential function defined as:

$$\mu\left(d_{i,j}^{m}, n, r\right) = \exp\left(-\frac{\left(d_{i,j}^{m}\right)^{n}}{r}\right). \tag{5.18}$$

Define ϕ^m—the probability that two vector sequences will match—as:

$$\phi^{m}(n,r) = \frac{1}{N-m}\sum_{i=1}^{N-m}\left(\frac{1}{N-m-1}\sum_{j=1, j\neq i}^{N-m} D_{i,j}^{m}(n,r)\right). \tag{5.19}$$

In the same way, from the vector sequence $\{X_{m+1}(i)\}$, compute the function ϕ^{m+1} as:

$$\phi^{m+1}(n,r) = \frac{1}{N-m}\sum_{i=1}^{N-m}\left(\frac{1}{N-m-1}\sum_{j=1, j\neq i}^{N-m} D_{i,j}^{m+1}(n,r)\right). \tag{5.20}$$

3. Computation

Compute *FuzzyEn* as:

$$FuzzyEn(m, n, r, N) = \ln\left(\phi^{m}(n,r)\right) - \ln\left(\phi^{m+1}(n,r)\right). \tag{5.21}$$

Therefore, in *FuzzyEn* the vectors similarity is fuzzily defined on the basis of a function and its shapes. A Gaussian function, a bell-shaped function, a Sigmoid function, or any kind of fuzzy membership function is suitable to assess the similarities between the two vectors; however, the membership function should show the following two properties [14]: (i) continuity, to avoid abrupt change of the similarity; and (ii) convexity, so that self-similarity is maximized.

In 2013, Liu et al. proposed another fuzzy entropy measure—the so-called fuzzy measure entropy (*FuzzyMEn*) [15]. Indeed, one drawback of *FuzzyEn* is that it deals with the local characteristics of the sequence only. The *FuzzyMEn* algorithm for a time series $\mathrm{u} = \{u(i), 1 \le i \le N\}$ of N samples is the following [15]:

1. State space reconstruction

Define an embedding dimension m (m will be the length of compared runs) and two threshold parameters r_L and r_F. Form a sequence of vectors $X_m(i)$ defined as:

$$X_m(i) = \{u(i), u(i+1), \ldots, u(i+m-1)\}, \quad 1 \le i \le N-m+1, \tag{5.22}$$

and define $u_0(i)$ the mean value of the sequence segment $X_m(i)$. Then, form a local sequence of vectors $XL_m(i)$ defined as:

$$\begin{aligned}\mathrm{XL}_m(i) =& \{u(i) - u_0(i), u(i+1) - u_0(i), \ldots, u(i+m-1) - u_0(i)\} \\ & 1 \leq i \leq N - m + 1.\end{aligned} \tag{5.23}$$

and a global sequence of vectors $\mathrm{XF}_m(i)$ defined as:

$$\begin{aligned}\mathrm{XF}_m(i) =& \{u(i) - u_{mean}, u(i+1) - u_{mean}, \ldots, u(i+m-1) - u_{mean}\} \\ & 1 \leq i \leq N - m + 1.\end{aligned} \tag{5.24}$$

where u_{mean} is the mean value of the sequence $\mathbf{u}$.

2. Ranking similar vectors

Define the distance $dL_m(i, j)$ between the local sequence of vectors $\mathbf{XL}_m(i)$ and $\mathrm{XL}_m(j)$ as:

$$dL_m(i, j) = d[\mathrm{XL}_m(i), \mathrm{XL}_m(j)] = \max(|(u(i+k) - u_0(i)) - (u(j+k) - u_0(j))|), \tag{5.25}$$

where $0 \leq k \leq m - 1$. In the same way, define the distance $dF_m(i, j)$ between the global sequence of vectors $\mathrm{XF}_m(i)$ and $\mathrm{XF}_m(j)$ as:

$$dF_m(i, j) = d[\mathrm{XF}_m(i), \mathrm{XF}_m(j)] = \max(|(u(i+k) - u_{mean}) - (u(j+k) - u_{mean})|), \tag{5.26}$$

where $0 \leq k \leq m - 1$.

Compute the similarity degree $DL^m_{i,j}$ between $\mathrm{XL}_m(i)$ and $\mathrm{XL}_m(j)$ through a fuzzy function $\mu_L(dL_m(i, j), n_L, r_L)$ as:

$$DL^m_{i,j}(n_L, r_L) = \mu_L(dL_m(i, j), n_L, r_L), \tag{5.27}$$

where the fuzzy function $\mu_L(dL_m(i, j), n_L, r_L)$ is the exponential function defined as:

$$\mu_L(dL_m(i, j), n_L, r_L) = \exp\left(-\left(\frac{dL_m(i, j)}{r_L}\right)^{n_L}\right). \tag{5.28}$$

Compute also the similarity degree $DF^m_{i,j}$ between $\mathrm{XF}_m(i)$ and $\mathrm{XF}_m(j)$ through a fuzzy function $\mu_F(dF_m(i, j), n_F, r_F)$ as:

$$DF^m_{i,j}(n_F, r_F) = \mu_F(dF_m(i, j), n_F, r_F), \tag{5.29}$$

where the fuzzy function $\mu_F(dF_m(i, j), n_F, r_F)$ is the exponential function defined as:

$$\mu_F(dF_m(i, j), n_F, r_F) = \exp\left(-\left(\frac{dF_m(i, j)}{r_F}\right)^{n_F}\right). \tag{5.30}$$

Define ϕL^m—the probability that two vector sequences $\{XL_m(i)\}$ will match—as:

$$\phi L^m(n_L, r_L) = \frac{1}{N-m}\sum_{i=1}^{N-m}\left(\frac{1}{N-m-1}\sum_{j=1, j\neq i}^{N-m} DL_{i,j}^m(n_L, r_L)\right). \quad (5.31)$$

In the same way, from the vector sequence $\{XL_{m+1}(i)\}$, compute the function ϕL^{m+1} as:

$$\phi L^{m+1}(n_L, r_L) = \frac{1}{N-m}\sum_{i=1}^{N-m}\left(\frac{1}{N-m-1}\sum_{j=1, j\neq i}^{N-m} DL_{i,j}^{m+1}(n_L, r_L)\right). \quad (5.32)$$

Do the same for vector sequences $\{XF_m(i)\}$ and vector sequences $\{XF_{m+1}(i)\}$ as:

$$\phi F^m(n_F, r_F) = \frac{1}{N-m}\sum_{i=1}^{N-m}\left(\frac{1}{N-m-1}\sum_{j=1, j\neq i}^{N-m} DF_{i,j}^m(n_F, r_F)\right), \quad (5.33)$$

$$\phi F^{m+1}(n_F, r_F) = \frac{1}{N-m}\sum_{i=1}^{N-m}\left(\frac{1}{N-m-1}\sum_{j=1, j\neq i}^{N-m} DF_{i,j}^{m+1}(n_F, r_F)\right). \quad (5.34)$$

3. Computation

Compute the fuzzy local measure entropy *FuzzyLMEn* and the fuzzy global measure entropy *FuzzyFMEn* as:

$$\begin{aligned} FuzzyLMEn(m, n_L, r_L, N) =& \ln\left(\phi L^m(n_L, r_L)\right) - \\ & \ln\left(\phi L^{m+1}(n_L, r_L)\right), \end{aligned} \quad (5.35)$$

and

$$\begin{aligned} FuzzyFMEn(m, n_F, r_F, N) =& \ln\left(\phi F^m(n_F, r_F)\right) - \\ & \ln\left(\phi F^{m+1}(n_F, r_F)\right). \end{aligned} \quad (5.36)$$

Finally, compute *FuzzyMEn* as:

$$\begin{aligned} FuzzyMEn(m, n_L, r_L, n_F, r_F, N) =& FuzzyLMEn(m, n_L, r_L, N) \\ & + FuzzyFMEn(m, n_F, r_F, N). \end{aligned} \quad (5.37)$$

Compared to *FuzzyEn*, *FuzzyMEn* uses the fuzzy local measure entropy and also the fuzzy global measure entropy. Therefore, *FuzzyMEn* integrates both local and global characteristics and can quantify the entire complexity in a time series [15].

5.2.3.2 Application in Health Informatics

In 2018, Acharya et al. used *FuzzyEn* to automatically detect coronary artery disease using electrocardiogram (ECG) signals [16]. From the authors' results, *FuzzyEn* of coronary artery disease ECGs is higher than that of controls' recordings [16]. In 2017, Tibdewal et al. worked on EEG signals recorded in epileptic and non-epileptic subjects [17]. For this purpose, they used different kinds of entropy measures (*ApEn*, *SampEn*, *FuzzyEn* among others). The authors reported that *FuzzyEn* outperforms the other entropy measures to discriminate epileptic from non-epileptic EEG recordings [17]. Other authors used *FuzzyEn* to inspect epileptic seizures based on *FuzzyEn* [18]. The authors have shown that *FuzzyEn* leads to higher classification accuracy values compared to *SampEn*-based techniques [18].

5.2.4 Permutation Entropy

5.2.4.1 Concept

Permutation entropy (*PermEn*) relies on the order relations of samples from a signal [19]. From a conceptual point of view, *PermEn* is simple, robust to artifacts, and fast in terms of computation time.

For a time series $u = \{u(i), 1 \leq i \leq N\}$ of N samples, *PermEn* is computed as follows [19]:

1. State space reconstruction

   Define an embedding dimension m. Form a sequence of vectors $X_m(i)$ defined as:

$$X_m(i) = \{u(i), u(i+1), \ldots, u(i+m-1)\}, \quad 1 \leq i \leq N-m+1. \tag{5.38}$$

2. Arrangement of the vectors

   Arrange each $X_m(i)$ in an increasing order with integer indices from 0 to *m-1*:

$$\{u(i+j_1-1), u(i+j_2-1), \ldots, u(i+j_m-1)\}. \tag{5.39}$$

   For different samples, there are $m!$ symbol sequences π_i (the so-called "motifs").

3. Count of the occurrences

   Count the occurrences $f(\pi_i)$ of the order pattern *i*, for i = 1, 2, ..., $m!$. Then, count the relative frequency $p(\pi_i)$ for each π_i as:

$$p(\pi_i) = \frac{f(\pi_i)}{N-m+1}. \tag{5.40}$$

4. Computation

Compute *PermEn* as follows:

$$PermEn(n, N) = -\sum_{\pi_i=1}^{\pi_i=m!} p(\pi_i)\ln(\pi_i). \tag{5.41}$$

5.2.4.2 Application in Health Informatics

In 2018, Cuesta-Frau et al. used *PermEn* to reveal changes between glucose records of healthy and possible diabetic subjects [20]. In 2018 also, Yang et al. investigated the predictability of an epileptic seizure from intracranial EEG [21]. For this purpose, they used a model based on *PermEn* and nonlinear support vector machine. Zanin et al. proposed a kinematic analysis based on *PermEn* to compare the dynamics of cerebral palsy subjects and matched controls [22].

5.3 The Most Recent Uni-dimensional Entropy Measures Proposed for Health Informatics

As mentioned above, *SampEn* is one of the entropy measures that is the most used in health informatics to quantify irregularity of signals. Its extension to different time scales has also been proposed to quantify complexity of data (multiscale entropy approach, *MSE*). *MSE* has drawbacks and several variants have been published to overcome its limitations. In 2015, a review paper reported the variants of *MSE* [23]. In what follows, only the irregularity measures that have been published from 2015 and for which applications in the biomedical field exist are therefore presented.

5.3.1 Modified Sample Entropy

In 2016, Liao and Jan proposed to modify the *SampEn* definition to be able to correctly deal with oversampled data [24]. For this purpose, they included a lag between successive data points of the vectors that are compared. This lag value was equal to the first minimum of the auto-mutual information function of the time series. When applied on simulated data, the modified *SampEn* shows consistent results for several sampling frequency values while *SampEn* does not. They applied this new measure to skin blood flow time series. Their results showed that skin blood flow is significantly different between baseline and the maximal dilation periods obtained by a thermal stimulus, and between young and older subjects [24].

5.3.2 Local Version of Sample Entropy

SampEn is computed globally and, therefore, may not show reliably the local behavior in the neighborhood of a specific pattern [25]. This is why Porta et al. proposed in 2019 a local version of *SampEn*, the so-called *LSampEn* [25]. This new version of *SampEn* has the advantage of having the local approach of *ApEn* and the robustness of *SampEn*.

The authors studied several physiological signals (such as ECG, plethysmographic arterial pressure,...) on subjects while they were on a bicycle ergometer. From a theoretical point of view, their results show (among others) that *LSampEn* is more robust than *SampEn* in describing deterministic periodic or nonlinear features when additive noise is present and that *LSampEn* and *SampEn* are equivalent in presence of a stochastic linear process [25]. From experimental data, their results lead to the conclusion that *LSampEn* is able to show the decrease of complexity of heart period time series during incremental bicycle ergometer exercise. This may be a hallmark of the sympathetic activation [25].

5.3.3 Range Entropy

In 2018, Omidvarnia et al. proposed the range entropy (*RangeEn*) as a measure that is more robust to nonstationary signal changes and more linearly related with the Hurst exponent than *ApEn* and *SampEn*: *RangeEn* is more robust to changes in signal amplitude and more sensitive to self-similarity in the data [26]. For this purpose, they proposed an updated version of the distance function in the algorithms of *ApEn* and *SampEn*. The authors applied their new measure on epileptic EEG datasets and showed interesting results in the differentiation between normal and epileptic brain states.

5.3.4 Normalized Fuzzy Entropy

In 2018, Liu et al. proposed the normalized fuzzy entropy for atrial fibrillation detection based on short-term RR time series [27]. The normalized fuzzy entropy uses a fuzzy function for vector similarity determination. Moreover, for entropy approximation, it uses density estimate instead of probability estimate. It also uses a flexible distance threshold parameter and subtracts the natural log of mean RR intervals to adjust for heart rate [27]. The authors applied the normalized fuzzy entropy measure to HRV data to classify atrial fibrillation and non-atrial fibrillation rhythms. The results obtained were compared with those given by *SampEn*, *FuzzyMEn*, and coefficient of sample entropy. The authors showed that the normalized fuzzy entropy achieves the highest area under receiver operating characteristic curve values [27].

5.3.5 Centered and Average Fuzzy Entropy

In 2018, Girault and Humeau-Heurtier proposed the so-called centered and averaged *FuzzyEn* to improve the precision of *FuzzyEn* [28]. For this purpose, the authors proposed to increase the number of samples that are used in the computation of the entropy measure while the length of the signal is unchanged [28]. When applied to fetal heart rate time series, the measure shows that the normal fetuses present a significantly higher entropy value than the pathological fetuses. Moreover, the results show that the new measure may be more interesting for classification purposes than *FuzzyEn* [28].

5.3.6 Permutation Entropy's Derivatives

In 2016, Bian et al. applied the weighted-permutation entropy (*WPermEn*)—proposed by Fadlallah et al. in 2013 [29]—to detect amnestic mild cognitive impairment in diabetes patients from resting-state EEG data [30]. *WPermEn* is an improvement of *PermEn* that takes into account the amplitude information of signals: *WPermEn* assigns different weights to adjacent vectors that present the same permutation pattern but have variations in amplitude that are not similar. The authors showed that the values of *WPermEn* in the right temporal region are significantly lower in the amnestic mild cognitive impairment group before Bonferoni correction, but no significant difference was observed when using *PermEn* even before the correction [30].

In 2016 also, Azami and Escudero introduced the amplitude-aware *PermEn* (*AAPermEn*) [31]. *AAPermEn* aims at overcoming two drawbacks of *PermEn* that are: (i) the mean value of amplitudes and the differences between neighboring samples are not considered; (ii) the case of two samples with equal amplitude values is not precisely determined in the definition of *PermEn*. By opposition to *PermEn*, *AAPermEn* is sensitive to variations in the amplitude, but also to the frequency, of the signals. The authors showed the performance of their algorithm for signal segmentation and spike detection applications (EEG and neural signal) [31]. The authors also mentioned that *AAPermEn* is more flexible than *WPermEn*.

In 2017, Bandt introduced a new version of *PermEn* interpreted as "distance to white noise" [32]. Bandt proposed to use this new entropy measure on EEG time series to classify sleep depth (the deeper the sleep, the more the EEG signal deviates from white noise) [32].

In 2018, Tao et al. proposed a new visualization scheme for *PermEn* that is based on non-uniform attractor embedding of the signal [33]. The authors showed the power of their algorithm on synthetic data and EEG signals [33].

In 2019, Li and Shang proposed the Tsallis permutation entropy [34]. In their work, the authors replaced the Shannon entropy used in the standard *PermEn* by the Tsallis entropy, in order to obtain a method with better computational accuracy and effectiveness. The authors applied their new measure on EEG time series of different physical conditions [34].

In 2019 also, Chen et al. proposed the improved *PermEn* (*IPE*) that, contrary to *PermEn*, takes into account the information of amplitude and fluctuations of signals but also tackles the limitation of equal values [35]. When applied to biomedical data, the authors showed that *IPE* is able to correctly differentiate HRV signals [35].

Other methods derived from *PermEn* have been proposed (see, e.g., [36–39]) but are not listed herein: the corresponding seminal papers did not apply the new measure to biomedical data.

5.3.7 Distribution Entropy

In 2015 Li et al. proposed the distribution entropy (*DistEn*) to improve the robustness in the complexity evaluation of short-term RR interval signals [40]. As mentioned above, in *SampEn* the probability of similar vectors is computed. In *DistEn*, the Shannon entropy of all distances $d^m_{i,j}$, ($1 \leq i, j \leq N - m$, where N is the number of samples in the time series under study and m is the embedding dimension) is estimated: the empirical probability density function of the distance matrix $d^m_{i,j}$ (except the main diagonal) is estimated by an histogram approach using a fixed number of bins B and then *DistEn* is computed as [40]:

$$DistEn(m, B) = -\frac{1}{\log_2(B)} \sum_{t=1}^{B} p_t \log_2(p_t), \tag{5.42}$$

where p_t ($t = 1, 2, \ldots, B$) is the probability of each bin. The authors showed that *DistEn* has relatively lower sensitivity to the predetermined parameters (compared to *SampEn* and *FuzzyEn*) and shows stability in the quantification of the complexity even for very short time series [40].

5.3.8 Fuzzy Distribution Entropy

In 2018, Zhang et al. proposed the fuzzy *DistEn* (*fDistEn*) for automated seizure detection [41]. For this purpose, they based their work on *DistEn* but they proposed (i) the use of the fuzzy membership function (as in *FuzzyEn*): an exponential function is used on the distance matrix $d^m_{i,j}$ before computing the histogram analysis; (ii) the baseline removal (as in *FuzzyEn*) to remove the impact of baseline during the state space reconstruction procedure. Using *fDistEn* in an automated seizure detection scheme, the authors goal was to automatically differentiate various kinds of EEG combinations [41].

5.3.9 *Dispersion Entropy*

In 2016, Rostaghi and Azami proposed the dispersion entropy (*DispEn*) as a new irregularity measure for signals that overcomes *SampEn* and *PermEn* limitations [42]. In *DispEn*, the signal under study (u $= \{u(i), 1 \leq i \leq N\}$ of N samples) is first filtered by a normal cumulative distribution function to treat outliers. The resulting time series is mapped into c classes that gives a series z^c. Afterwards, each set $y_m(i)$ (where m is the pattern length) of consecutive samples in z^c from i to $i + m - 1$ ($y_m(i) = [z^c(i), z^c(i + 1), z^c(i + 2), \ldots, z^c(i + m - 1)], i = 1, 2, \ldots, N-m+1$), that represents a dispersion pattern, is used to determine the probability distribution for all possible dispersion patterns $p(y_m(i))$ (through the computation of the probability of occurrence of each dispersion pattern $y_m(i)$ in z^c). *DispEn* is then computed as the Shannon entropy of $p(y_m(i))$: $DispEn(m, c) = -\sum_{i=1}^{c^m} p(y_m(i)) \log(p(y_m(i)))$ [42]. In the biomedical field, the authors used this measure to process focal and non-focal EEG signals as well as to analyze the regularity of blood pressure signals [42]. The results show that *DispEn* outperforms *PermEn* to discriminate different groups of dataset and has a lower computation time than *SampEn* and *PermEn* [42].

5.3.10 *Increment Entropy*

To outperform existing entropy measures in change detection of time series, Liu et al. proposed increment entropy (*IncrEn*) in 2016 [43]. *IncrEn* is defined as the Shannon entropy of words that are computed from each increment: a word is composed of two letters, one for the sign and the other for its magnitude. The authors applied *IncrEn* to detect epileptic EEGs containing a seizure. Their results show that *IncrEn* is better than *SampEn* and *PermEn* for seizure detection [43].

5.3.11 *Cosine Similarity Entropy*

In 2017, Chanwimalueang and Mandic introduced the cosine similarity entropy (*CSE*) to overcome some limitations of *SampEn* [44]: *SampEn* requires long data segments for reliable estimation; moreover, *SampEn* is sensitive to spikes and erratic peaks in time series, and leads an uncontrollable range of entropy values [44]. In *SampEn*, the Chebyshev distance and the standard conditional probability are used. In *CSE*, the Chebyshev distance is changed by the angular distance and Shannon entropy is used instead of the standard conditional probability [44]. In their work, the authors applied the multiscale approach of *CSE* to HRV data and three cardiovascular conditions were studied: normal sinus rhythm, congestive heart failure, and atrial fibrillation [44]. The results show that, even though the multiscale approach of *CSE* leads to results that are in contrast to the results from the multiscale approach of *SampEn* and *FuzzyEn*, the measure is able to separate the three cardiac conditions.

5.3.12 Bubble Entropy

In 2017, Manis et al. proposed the bubble entropy, an entropy measure based on *PermEn* where the vectors in the embedding space are ranked according to the bubble sort algorithm and the number of swaps necessary for each vector are counted [45]. The advantage of the bubble entropy is that it is almost free of parameters. Using synthetic data and Holter recordings, the authors showed that their algorithm presents increased stability and discriminating power compared to other entropy measures [45].

5.3.13 Entropy of Entropy

In 2017, Hsu et al. proposed a new complexity measure – the so-called entropy of entropy (*EoE*) [46]. It consists of two steps: (i) the Shannon entropy is used to characterize the "state" of a system within a time window ("information" contained in that time period); (ii) the Shannon entropy is used to characterize the degree of the "changing" of the states. The authors applied *EoE* to cardiac interbeat interval time series and showed that the *EoE* value is significantly higher for the healthy than the pathologic groups. From the results they obtained, they show that the overall accuracy of *EoE* method is higher than that of the multiscale *SampEn* method, and that *EoE* can be applied to relatively short time series [46].

5.4 Bi-dimensional Entropy Measures in Health Informatics

Recently, some entropy measures have been adapted to analyze irregularity of bidimensional data (images). Their applications to the biomedical field are very promising [47]. We therefore present below the entropy measures for which an extension to 2D data has already been proposed.

5.4.1 Bi-dimensional Approximate Entropy

In 2016, Moore proposed an extension of *ApEn* to bi-dimensional data ($ApEn_{2D}$) and applied his algorithm to X-ray computed tomography (CT) used in image guided radiotherapy for cancer [48]. When applied to CT and cone beam CT (CBCT) images, the results showed that $ApEn_{2D}$ is able to reveal challenging threshold structures in a consistently calibrated manner [48].

5.4.2 Bi-dimensional Sample Entropy

In 2011, Yeh et al. [49] and later in 2016 Silva et al. [50] extended the *SampEn* algorithm to the 2D case ($SampEn_{2D}$) as a measure of irregularity in pixel patterns. The results showed that $SampEn_{2D}$ can be useful to quantify texture features and can discriminate rat sural nerve images by age groups with high accuracy [50]. Extensions to a multiscale approach have also been proposed [49, 51, 52]. The results showed that this multiscale approach can reveal the statistical differences of paired comparisons from reactive lymphadenopathy and five categories of lymphomas [49] and is also interesting for cardiac histological images studies [51, 52].

5.4.3 Bi-dimensional Fuzzy Entropy

In 2018 Segato dos Santos et al. proposed the multiscale fuzzy sample entropy for colored images [53]. In their work, each pixel of a colour image on the RGB colour standard was defined as an *n*-dimensional vector analyzed from the Minkowski distance (for the comparison between vectors). The authors quantified and classified hematoxylin and eosin (H&E) histological images of colorectal cancer (benign and malignant groups). Very recently, Hilal et al. proposed another multiscale fuzzy entropy measure and found interesting results when applied on dermoscopic images to detect pseudoxanthoma elasticum [54].

5.4.4 Bi-dimensional Distribution Entropy

In 2017, Azami et al. introduced the bi-dimensional version of *DistEn* ($DistEn_{2D}$) to deal with small-sized textures [55]: $DistEn_{2D}$ overcomes the problem of undefined $SampEn_{2D}$ values for small-sized textures. Moreover, the time needed to obtain the entropy values is less than the one of $SampEn_{2D}$ especially for small-sized images. Even if no biomedical application is proposed in [55], $DistEn_{2D}$ can surely be of interest to process medical images.

5.4.5 *Bi-dimensional Dispersion Entropy*

In 2019, Azami et al. proposed an extension to the 2D-case of *DispEn* ($DispEn_{2D}$) [56]. The goal was to propose an irregularity measure of images that overcomes some drawbacks of $SampEn_{2D}$: undefined values for small-sized images and computation time. The authors showed that $DispEn_{2D}$ can be of interest for the classification of cardiac histological image datasets (myocardial infarction *vs* sham surgery procedures) [56].

5.4.6 *Others*

The bi-dimensional entropy measures presented above are quite recent but very promising to analyze texture of images. Let's note that the bi-dimensional version of *PermEn* ($PermEn_{2D}$) has also been proposed but used in a different way: the authors used the complexity-entropy-causality plane as a complexity measure for two-dimensional patterns [57–59]. Moreover, *ApEn* and *FuzzyEn* have also been extended for 3D data [60–62] but are not presented herein. The readers can refer to the corresponding papers.

5.5 Conclusion

This chapter aimed at presenting well-known entropy measures and more recent ones as well as some of their use in health informatics. The field of applications is very large and this is probably why new entropy-based measures are still developed to overcome drawbacks of the existing ones. More recently, extensions to bi-dimensional data have been proposed. They are very promising in health informatics. They surely deserve attention for the future.

References

1. Costa, M., Goldberger, A.L., Peng, C.K.: Multiscale entropy analysis of biological signals. Phys. Rev. E **71**(2), Article id. 021906 (2005)
2. Costa, M., Goldberger, A.L., Peng, C.K.: Multiscale entropy analysis of complex physiologic time series. Phys. Rev. Lett. **89**(6), Article id. 068102 (2002)
3. Pincus, S.M.: Approximate entropy as a measure of system complexity. Proc. Natl. Acad. Sci. **88**(6), 2297–2301 (1991)
4. Pincus, S.M., Goldberger, A.L.: Physiological time-series analysis: what does regularity quantify? Am. J. Physiol. Heart Circ. Physiol. **266**(4), H1643–H1656 (1994)
5. Richman, J.S., Moorman, J.R.: Physiological time-series analysis using approximate entropy and sample entropy. Am. J. Physiol. Heart Circ. Physiol. **278**(6), H2039–H2049 (2000)

6. Porta, A., Gnecchi-Ruscone, T., Tobaldini, E., Guzzetti, S., Furlan, R., Montano, N.: Progressive decrease of heart period variability entropy-based complexity during graded head-up tilt. J. Appl. Physiol. **103**(4), 1143–1149 (2007)
7. Bansal, T., Haji, G.S., Rossiter, H.B., Polkey, M.I., Hull, J.H.: Exercise ventilatory irregularity can be quantified by approximate entropy to detect breathing pattern disorder. Respir. Physiol. Neurobiol. **255**, 1–6 (2018)
8. Udhayakumar, R.K., Karmakar, C., Palaniswami, M.: Approximate entropy profile: a novel approach to comprehend irregularity of short-term HRV signal. Nonlinear Dyn. **88**(2), 823–837 (2017)
9. Li, X., Jiang, Y., Hong, J., Dong, Y., Yao, L.: Estimation of cognitive workload by approximate entropy of EEG. J. Mech. Med. Biol. **16**(06), 1650077 (2016)
10. Martinez-Cagigal, V., Santamaria-Vazquez, E., Hornero, R.: Asynchronous control of P300-based brain-computer interfaces using sample entropy. Entropy **21**(3), Article id. 230 (2019)
11. Jia, Y., Gu, H.: Identifying nonlinear dynamics of brain functional networks of patients with schizophrenia by sample entropy. Nonlinear Dyn. **96**, 2327–2340 (2019)
12. Phukan, N., Kakoty, N.M.: Sample entropy based selection of wavelet decomposition level for finger movement recognition using EMG. In: Progress in Advanced Computing and Intelligent Engineering (pp. 61–73). Springer, Singapore (2019)
13. Chen, W., Wang, Z., Xie, H., Yu, W.: Characterization of surface EMG signal based on fuzzy entropy. IEEE Trans. Neural Syst. Rehabil. Eng. **15**(2), 266–272 (2007)
14. Xie, H.B., Chen, W.T., He, W.X., Liu, H.: Complexity analysis of the biomedical signal using fuzzy entropy measurement. Appl. Soft Comput. **11**(2), 2871–2879 (2011)
15. Liu, C., Li, K., Zhao, L., Liu, F., Zheng, D., Liu, C., Liu, S.: Analysis of heart rate variability using fuzzy measure entropy. Comput. Biol. Med. **43**(2), 100–108 (2013)
16. Acharya, U.R., Hagiwara, Y., Koh, J.E.W., Oh, S.L., Tan, J.H., Adam, M., San Tan, R.: Entropies for automated detection of coronary artery disease using ECG signals: A review. Biocybern. Biomed. Eng. **38**(2), 373–384 (2018)
17. Tibdewal, M.N., Dey, H.R., Mahadevappa, M., Ray, A., Malokar, M.: Multiple entropies performance measure for detection and localization of multi-channel epileptic EEG. Biomed. Signal Process. Control **38**, 158–167 (2017)
18. Xiang, J., Li, C., Li, H., Cao, R., Wang, B., Han, X., Chen, J.: The detection of epileptic seizure signals based on fuzzy entropy. J. Neurosci. Methods **243**, 18–25 (2015)
19. Bandt, C., Pompe, B.: Permutation entropy: a natural complexity measure for time series. Phys. Rev. Lett. **88**(17), 174102 (2002)
20. Cuesta-Frau, D., Miro-Martinez, P., Oltra-Crespo, S., Jordan-Nunez, J., Vargas, B., Vigil, L.: Classification of glucose records from patients at diabetes risk using a combined permutation entropy algorithm. Comput. Methods Programs Biomed. **165**, 197–204 (2018)
21. Yang, Y., Zhou, M., Niu, Y., Li, C., Cao, R., Wang, B., Yan, P., Ma, Y., Xiang, J.: Epileptic seizure prediction based on permutation entropy. Front. Computat. Neurosci. **12**, Article id. 55 (2018)
22. Zanin, M., Gomez-Andres, D., Pulido-Valdeolivas, I., Martin-Gonzalo, J., Lopez-Lopez, J., Pascual-Pascual, S., Rausell, E.: Characterizing normal and pathological gait through permutation entropy. Entropy **20**(1), Article id. 77 (2018)
23. Humeau-Heurtier, A.: The multiscale entropy algorithm and its variants: A review. Entropy **17**(5), 3110–3123 (2015)
24. Liao, F., Jan, Y.K.: Using modified sample entropy to characterize aging-associated microvascular dysfunction. Front. Physiol. **7**, Article 126 (2016)
25. Porta, A., Bari, V., De Maria, B., Cairo, B., Vaini, E., Malacarne, M., Pagani, M., Lucini, D.: On the relevance of computing a local version of sample entropy in cardiovascular control analysis. IEEE Trans. Biomed. Eng. **66**(3), 623–631 (2019)
26. Omidvarnia, A., Mesbah, M., Pedersen, M., Jackson, G.: Range entropy: A bridge between signal complexity and self-similarity. Entropy **20**(12), 962 (2018)
27. Liu, C., Oster, J., Reinertsen, E., Li, Q., Zhao, L., Nemati, S., Clifford, G.D.: A comparison of entropy approaches for AF discrimination. Physiol. Meas. **39**(7), Article 074002 (2018)

28. Girault, J.M., Humeau-Heurtier, A.: Centered and averaged fuzzy entropy to improve fuzzy entropy precision. Entropy **20**(4), Article id. 287 (2018)
29. Fadlallah, B., Chen, B., Keil, A., Principe, J.: Weighted-permutation entropy: a complexity measure for time series incorporating amplitude information. Phys. Rev. E **87**(2), Article id. 022911 (2013)
30. Bian, Z., Ouyang, G., Li, Z., Li, Q., Wang, L., Li, X.: Weighted-permutation entropy analysis of resting state EEG from diabetics with amnestic mild cognitive impairment. Entropy **18**(8), Article id. 307 (2016)
31. Azami, H., Escudero, J.: Amplitude-aware permutation entropy: illustration in spike detection and signal segmentation. Comput. Methods Programs Biomed. **128**, 40–51 (2016)
32. Bandt, C.: A new kind of permutation entropy used to classify sleep stages from invisible EEG microstructure. Entropy **19**(5), Article id. 197 (2017)
33. Tao, M., Poskuviene, K., Alkayem, N., Cao, M., Ragulskis, M.: Permutation entropy based on non-uniform embedding. Entropy **20**(8), Article id. 612 (2018)
34. Li, C., Shang, P.: Multiscale Tsallis permutation entropy analysis for complex physiological time series. Physica A **523**, 10–20 (2019)
35. Chen, Z., Li, Y., Liang, H., Yu, J.: Improved permutation entropy for measuring complexity of time series under noisy condition. Complexity **2019**, Article id. 1403829 (2019)
36. Watt, S.J., Politi, A.: Permutation entropy revisited. Chaos, Soliton Fract **120**, 95–99 (2019)
37. Wang, X., Si, S., Wei, Y., Li, Y.: The optimized multi-scale permutation entropy and its application in compound fault diagnosis of rotating machinery. Entropy **21**(2), Article id. 170 (2019)
38. Chen, S., Shang, P., Wu, Y.: Weighted multiscale Rényi permutation entropy of nonlinear time series. Physica A **496**, 548–570 (2018)
39. Yin, Y., Shang, P.: Weighted permutation entropy based on different symbolic approaches for financial time series. Physica A **443**, 137–148 (2016)
40. Li, P., Liu, C., Li, K., Zheng, D., Liu, C., Hou, Y.: Assessing the complexity of short-term heart beat interval series by distribution entropy. Med. Biol. Eng. Compu. **53**(1), 77–87 (2015)
41. Zhang, T., Chen, W., Li, M.: Fuzzy distribution entropy and its application in automated seizure detection technique. Biomed. Signal Process. Control **39**, 360–377 (2018)
42. Rostaghi, M., Azami, H.: Dispersion entropy: a measure for time-series analysis. IEEE Signal Process. Lett. **23**(5), 610–614 (2016)
43. Liu, X., Jiang, A., Xu, N., Xue, J.: Increment entropy as a measure of complexity for time series. Entropy **18**(1), 22 (2016)
44. Chanwimalueang, T., Mandic, D.: Cosine similarity entropy: self-correlation-based complexity analysis of dynamical systems. Entropy **19**(12), Article 652 (2017)
45. Manis, G., Aktaruzzaman, M.D., Sassi, R.: Bubble entropy: an entropy almost free of parameters. IEEE Trans. Biomed. Eng. **64**(11), 2711–2718 (2017)
46. Hsu, C., Wei, S.Y., Huang, H.P., Hsu, L., Chi, S., Peng, C.K.: Entropy of entropy: measurement of dynamical complexity for biological systems. Entropy **19**(10), 550 (2017)
47. Humeau-Heurtier, A.: Texture feature extraction methods: a survey. IEEE Access **7**, 8975–9000 (2019)
48. Moore, C.J.: A threshold structure metric for medical image interrogation: the 2D extension of approximate entropy. In: 2016 20th International Conference Information Visualisation (IV) (pp. 336–341). IEEE (July, 2016)
49. Yeh, J.R., Lin, C.W., Shieh, J.S.: An approach of multiscale complexity in texture analysis of lymphomas. IEEE Signal Process. Lett. **18**(4), 239–242 (2011)
50. Silva, L.E.V., Senra Filho, A.C.S., Fazan, V.P.S., Felipe, J.C., Junior, L.M.: Two dimensional sample entropy: assessing image texture through irregularity. Biomed. Phys. Eng. Express **2**(4), 045002 (2016)
51. Silva, L.E., Duque, J.J., Felipe, J.C., Murta Jr., L.O., Humeau-Heurtier, A.: Two-dimensional multiscale entropy analysis: applications to image texture evaluation. Sig. Process. **147**, 224–232 (2018)

52. Humeau-Heurtier, A., Omoto, A.C.M., Silva, L.E.: Bi-dimensional multiscale entropy: relation with discrete Fourier transform and biomedical application. Comput. Biol. Med. **100**, 36–40 (2018)
53. dos Santos, L.F.S., Neves, L.A., Rozendo, G.B., Ribeiro, M.G., do Nascimento, M.Z., Tosta, T.A.A.: Multidimensional and fuzzy sample entropy (SampEnMF) for quantifying H&E histological images of colorectal cancer. Comput. Biol. Med. **103**, 148–160 (2018)
54. Hilal, M., Berthin, C., Martin, L., Azami, H., Humeau-Heurtier, A.: Bidimensional multiscale fuzzy entropy and its application to pseudoxanthoma elasticum. IEEE Trans. Biomed. Eng. (in press) (2019)
55. Azami, H., Escudero, J., Humeau-Heurtier, A.: Bidimensional distribution entropy to analyze the irregularity of small-sized textures. IEEE Signal Process. Lett. **24**(9), 1338–1342 (2017)
56. Azami, H., da Silva, L.E.V., Omoto, A.C.M., Humeau-Heurtier, A.: Two-dimensional dispersion entropy: an information-theoretic method for irregularity analysis of images. Sig. Process. Image Commun. **75**, 178–187 (2019)
57. Sigaki, H.Y., Perc, M., Ribeiro, H.V.: History of art paintings through the lens of entropy and complexity. Proc. Natl. Acad. Sci. **115**(37), E8585–E8594 (2018)
58. Zunino, L., Ribeiro, H.V.: Discriminating image textures with the multiscale two-dimensional complexity-entropy causality plane. Chaos, Soliton. Fract. **91**, 679–688 (2016)
59. Ribeiro, H.V., Zunino, L., Lenzi, E.K., Santoro, P.A., Mendes, R.S.: Complexity-entropy causality plane as a complexity measure for two-dimensional patterns. PLoS ONE **7**(8), e40689 (2012)
60. Moore, C., Marchant, T.: The approximate entropy concept extended to three dimensions for calibrated, single parameter structural complexity interrogation of volumetric images. Phys. Med. Biol. **62**(15), 6092 (2017)
61. Marchant, T., Murphy, M., Madden, G., Moore, C.: Quantifying structure regularity in fluorescence microscopy cell images using a novel multi-dimensional approximate entropy metric. In: 2011, 18th IEEE International Conference on Image Processing (pp. 3085–3088). IEEE (September, 2011)
62. Gaudêncio, A.S.F., Vaz, P.G., Hilal, M., Cardoso, J.M., Mahé, G., Lederlin, M., Humeau-Heurtier, A.: Three-dimensional multiscale fuzzy entropy: validation and application to idiopathic pulmonary fibrosis. IEEE J. Biomed. Health Inf. (in press) (2020)

Chapter 6
Image Processing in Health Informatics

Allam Shehata, Mahmoud Salem, and Md Atiqur Rahman Ahad

Abstract There is no doubt that the image has become the most common source of information in all ways as it carries a huge amount of natural descriptions about the corresponding scene. Recently, biomedical images-based applications have received more attention from the image processing and health informatics research communities. Principally, biomedical image processing has become interesting in its multidisciplinary nature. The medical image processing can be executed in 2D, 3D or even multi-dimensional images to extract useful information. These images serve in the ultimate goals of clinical activities such as monitoring, diagnosis, localization, and treatment. Nowadays, there is an inevitable need to get a concrete surgery system to help and automate the clinical workflow to solve in a shorter period. As well, providing the medical images in high quality and fascinating storage may contribute in such surgery systems. Therefore, in this chapter, we shortly cover core principal medical image processing techniques, image enhancement, and compression. We consider to cover these techniques as they handle the most two challenges in biomedical imaging, which are image quality and image storage/transmission. We focus on three main types of medical images: magnetic resonance imaging (MRI), X-ray/computed tomography (CT), and Ultrasound images. Furthermore, we report the usage of image processing-based techniques in the recent medical imaging systems and technologies.

A. Shehata (✉) · M. A. R. Ahad
Institute of Scientific and Industrial Research, Osaka University, Suita, Japan
e-mail: allam@am.sanken.osaka-u.ac; allam@eri.sci.eg

M. A. R. Ahad
e-mail: atiqahad@du.ac.bd

A. Shehata
Informatics Department, Electronics Research Institute, Cairo, Egypt

M. Salem
Faculty of Engineering, Ain Shams University, Cairo, Egypt
e-mail: g16091591@eng.asu.edu.eg

M. A. R. Ahad
Department of Electrical and Electronic Engineering,
University of Dhaka, Dhaka, Bangladesh

M. A. R. Ahad and M. U. Ahmed (eds.), *Signal Processing Techniques for Computational Health Informatics*, Intelligent Systems Reference Library 192,
https://doi.org/10.1007/978-3-030-54932-9_6

Keywords 2D/3D Image processing · Mesh analysis · Computer topography (CT) · Diagnosis diseases · Magnetic resonance imaging (MRI)

6.1 Introduction

Over the last century, a lot of advancements have been emerged in medical image processing techniques, which introduced core innovations and achievements for medical imaging and health informatics systems. These achievements created unprecedented opportunities for noninvasive diagnostic and treatment. Because of that, medical imaging as well as vision-based systems have become an integral part of healthcare and health informatics systems [1]. The medical image processing field has attracted many researchers as one of the key areas of innovation. Medical imaging incorporates image processing, algorithmic developments for various applications, systems and devices, and methodologies. In this chapter, we try to present the most well-known key areas of advancements/trends in the medical image processing techniques, principally, medical enhancement and medical image compression, considering the context of specific imaging modalities such as X-ray imaging, Computed Tomography (CT) imaging, Magnetic Resonance Imaging (MRI), and Ultrasound imaging.

The outline of the chapter is organized as follow: Sect. 6.1.1 covers the methodologies of the three medical imaging systems (MRI, X-ray/CT, and Ultrasound), their benefits and risks on human health. Section 6.2 discuses the recently applied image enhancement techniques on various medical images. As well, the recent advancement of applying the image compression algorithms on the medical images are reported in Sect. 6.3 aiming at handling the massive demand on the remote medication. In Sect. 6.4, we summarize the involvement of image processing techniques in the new medical technologies such as additive manufacturing and the Internet of Things (IoT). The conclusion and the key challenges that still face the medical imaging-based systems are reported in Sect. 6.5.

6.1.1 *Medical Imaging Acquisition*

Generally speaking, medical image is an image that needs special devices to capture and representation. This image is used to reveal the internal structures of the human body that are hidden by the skin and bones mainly for diagnose and treating disease tasks. Compared to the traditional image capturing systems which use CMOS, CCD, and thermal lenses, the medical image capturing system depend on MRI, X-ray/CT, or Ultrasound signals. In the following sections, we introduce a brief explanation about the methodologies of these medical image capturing systems and report their benefits and risks on the human health.

6.1.2 *Magnetic Resonance Imaging (MRI)*

The MRI image is mainly captured based on an expensive machine, which uses a strong magnetic field to produce images of any parts of the body that can not be deciphered by other sensors easily, as shown in Fig. 6.1. To produce the MRI images, there is no need for radiation that is used in the case of CT or X-ray, which makes it widely used for medical diagnosis. It is worth noting that the MRI-based scanners can capture the images in a very fine-tuned manner. According to [2], 30 millions MRI scans are done in the USA per year where 6.6 million cases among them are related to head scans. MRI, functional MRI, S-MRI, etc. are widely explored in different disease analyses [3–5]. The MRI scan is an incredibly effective and accurate method for the whole body scanning and disease findings. In most of the cases, it is often used when the other tests become less effective to provide adequate information for accurate diagnosis and correct treatment.

Merits of MRI
Generally speaking, because no radiation is used during MRI scan, there are no big risks of exposure on the patient body.

- MRI images can be taken for any body part at a variety of imaging directions.
- MRI can provide smarter soft-tissue contrast compared to other modalities like CT scanning.
- It can smartly distinguish among water, fat, muscle, and various other soft tissues, compared with CT scanning.
- MRI data can be very useful in some cases where other imaging systems fails. For example, disease like *Craniosynostosis* (where an infant's skull does not allow to grow the brain and hence doctors need to cut/reshape the skull to allow the brain to grow). Doctors need to do MRI as well as CT scanning of the brain and skull to understand the watermarks or any disturbances on the growth of a brain. There are other cases, where proper fusions between MRI and CT scans may bring a better understanding of a disease.

MRI Risks on Human Health

- Because of the involvement of the strong and static magnet, a magnetic field (that changes with time), and radio-frequency energy may harm the patient 's health.

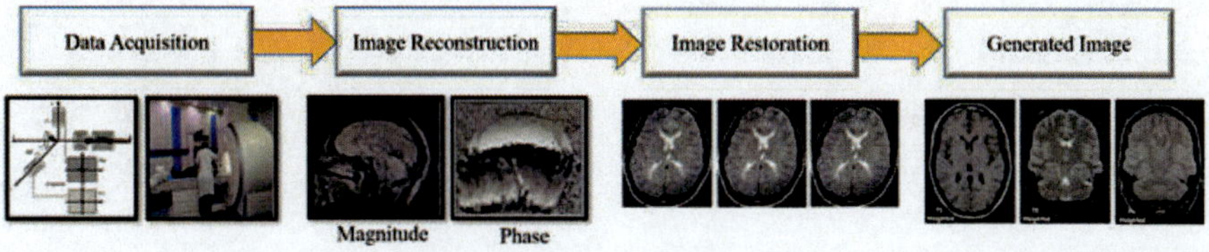

Fig. 6.1 MR study of the head and abdomen: Three different weighted MRI scans are shown on the right-most part. After data acquisition, image reconstruction and image restoration steps are followed before generating any MR image

- MRI scan may fail in the presence of internal metallic objects such as bullets or keys, as well as surgical clips, pins, plates attached, etc.
- MRI scan is not advised for pregnant patients due to the potential of a harmful increase in the temperature of the amniotic fluid.
- It also is not advised for patients with epilepsy.
- During MRI scanning, the magnetic fields produce continuous noises. For some patients, especially young children, it becomes difficult to remain normal. Any movement of the body may produce less accurate imaging. Also, one may feel uncomfortable during MRI. As the MRI scanning continues for several minutes, even to 20–30 minutes, the noise sources can be annoying—even may be detrimental for the hearing problem to some patients having hearing difficulties. However, the cases are not so high and not to worry much.

6.1.3 X-Ray/Computer Tomography (CT) Imaging

The X-ray image is formed by recording X-ray beam properties using a set of X-ray detectors. The CT terminology refers to a computerized control algorithm applied to produce narrow beams of X-ray around the patients in order to capture cross-sectional images/scans for the human body is so-called slices. After that, all of these slices are concatenated together to reconstruct a 3D image, which can be identified and can allow extractions of 3D features of abnormalities such as tumors (see Fig. 6.2).

To produce an X-ray image, the anatomical region through a single projection plane is imaged onto the detector as shown in Fig. 6.2. As well, the several projections at different angles produce the 3D CT image [6]. It is worth noting that CT scan images provide more-detailed information than X-rays do. CT scan are particularly well-suited to quickly examine people with internal injures or broken.

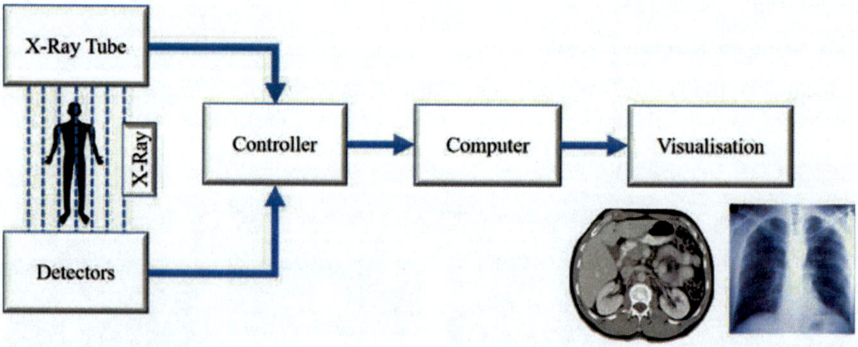

Fig. 6.2 X-ray/CT imaging system

X-Ray/CT Merits

X-ray and CT scanning are very widely explored in the medical domain. Though CT scanning is an expensive approach similar to MRI scanning, both are used millions of times in different hospitals around the world. Some of the important benefits of CT scanning are mentioned below:

- It is a painless method, as well as, almost a non-invasive approach to scan the body parts with in-depth imaging that is not possible otherwise (except MRI scanning that can be assistive in a similar fashion).
- CT scan is essential to monitor after major surgery or therapy.
- It is an essential approach for the treatment of various surgeries, the operation of tumors, blockages related to blood, and so on.
- Not noisy like MRI scanning.
- It also takes less time to accomplish any scanning than the same by an MRI machine.

Risks on Human Heath

However, compare to the MRI scanning, X-rays and CT scanning have some detrimental impacts on health if these are done for a longer period in many times. Physicians usually do not recommend it unless something is genuinely essential for the treatment. The ionization radiation may damage body cells or may damage DNA. However, the impact is not so high considering the benefits of treatment. Therefore, there should not be any worry to deal with after doctor recommendations.

- Too much radiation continuously for a longer period can damage cells and it may cause cancer too. However, the modern machines are much superior and unless anyone is in bad luck due to malfunctioning a machine, or non-expert deals and make mistakes, then there is no danger.
- Repetition may cause hair loss or irritation in skins in rare cases.
- CT scanning expensive, similar to MRI scanning.

6.1.4 Ultrasound Imaging

The ultrasound image is formed based on using high-frequency sound waves. These sound waves are then used to produce a dynamic visual representation of inside the body. Practically, the sound waves are sent to the region to be investigated (region of interest), and the echoes returned are collected to give the physician a 'live' and real-time view of the regions of interest, as shown in Fig. 6.3. The real-time images through ultrasound imaging system can demonstrate the movement and structure of the region, different views, intra-relationship and connectivity among the neighboring parts, blood flowing through the blood vessels, etc. with a reasonable clarity and accuracy. The statistical information that resulted from the reflection of the sound waves is used for producing the images. The inner image processing on the ultrasound

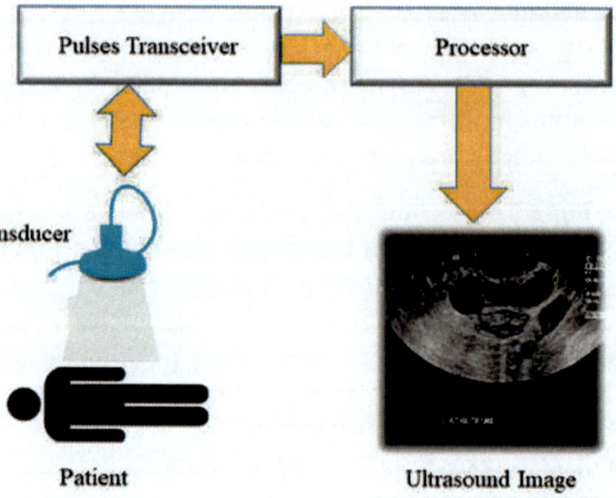

Fig. 6.3 Ultrasound image capturing system

images can provide more subtle information to a physician. Hence, we process the ultrasound data to decipher the inherent unknown issues that are very crucial.

Merits of Ultrasound Imaging

Ultrasound imaging is a widely explored screening tool for medical diagnosis [7]. Because its non-invasive nature (though it is required to use gel on the skin and probe around region from outside), relatively low cost compared to the MRI or CT scanning (though the outputs are different), and the ability to shape real-time images—it is a very beneficial mode of screening. Because of its flexibility, it plays a key role in medical imaging.

- It is based on non-ionizing radiation and hence, no health hazard issues compared to MRI, X-ray or CT scan.
- It is generally painless and does not require special consideration like needles, injections, or incisions.
- It is widely explored in the pregnancy test and to know the growth and development of fetus. Doctors can even use an ultrasound scan to estimate how large a baby is just before the delivery.
- It is valuable in helping to detect potential problems, including some birth defects.

Risks on Human Heath

Though it does not consider any radiation or ionization, it may have slightly negative issues. Ultrasound introduces energy into the body. It may have little impact on skin or tissues underneath, especially, if it is done for a longer period. However, it is usually a safe mode of scanning. The FDA [8] has some recommendations for the healthcare providers to minimize exposure while using ultrasound.

- Ultrasound energy has the ability for biological impacts on the body.
- The waves may heat up the tissues a bit.
- It may generate tiny pockets (e.g., cavitation) of gas in body fluids or tissues.

- However, we do not know any side-effects for long-term usages of ultrasound imaging on a specific region of the body.
- Studies done on mice have shown intestinal bleeding caused by changes in the cells because of ultrasound (similar effects may be in humans).

6.2 Medical Image Enhancement

Image enhancement is a mathematical procedure on a given image aimed at improving its quality for further usages. The resulting image is able to better demonstrate the image features compared to the original image. Based on the adopted physiological experiments, some small shifts in luminance are recognized by the human visual system in continuous grey-tone regions and are not shown at all in any discontinuity regions [9]. Hence, image enhancement may be done to smooth images in more uniform and consistent regions. However, it is worth mentioning that enhancement of certain features (e.g., edges) of the degraded image can simplify the image interpretation both for the human visual system as well as machine recognition.

6.2.1 MRI Image Enhancement

MRI image provides very rich information to the doctors or medical staffs to assist in diagnosis and treatment of various diseases. Based on the idea behind the MRI image capturing system, which are explained in Sect. 6.1, pre-processing steps are required to make the MRI as beneficial and more accurate for the post-processing steps—such as image segmentation. These pre-processing steps of the MRI images may include

- Handling various noise issues and proper filtering methods,
- Image registration,
- Image enhancement,
- Correcting inhomogeneity,
- Removing artifacts,
- Stripping skull (surrounding the brain tissues), if the MRI has to handle this region, etc.

A recent approach is proposed in [5] to enhance the visibility and quantification of the Virchow-Robin space or the Perivascular Space (PVS) by using MRI images. In this approach, they have combined T1-weighted and T2-weighted images to improve the contrast ratio between the Perivascular Space and the tissues around. In [5], the Enhanced Perivascular Space Contrast (PVC) method has filtered the non-structured spatial noise by adaptive filtering mechanism. Figure 6.4 summarizes the workflow of the Enhanced Perivascular space Contrast (EPC) technique.

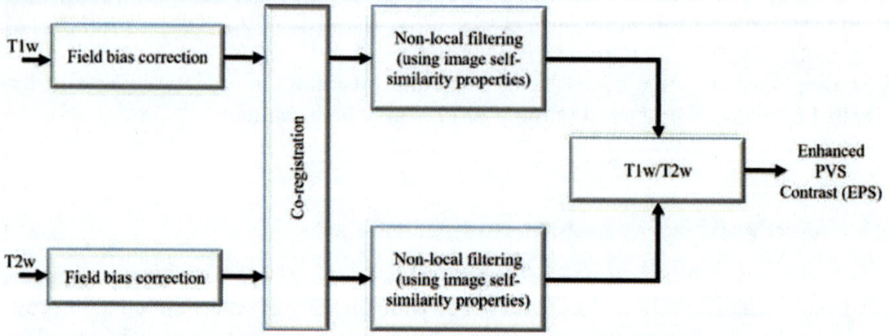

Fig. 6.4 Workflow of the multi-modal approach for the Perivascular space Contrast (EPC) technique. It is based on T1-weighted and T2-weighted images

In [10], a new magnetic resonance imaging technique is proposed for the visualization of molecular changes in the brain. Through this technique, both molecular composition information and water content could be disentangled and decoded the molecular information from the MRI signal. By using Quantitative magnetic resonance imaging (qMRI), aging-related changes of human brains can be explained through some molecular mechanisms. This technique [10] will allow researchers to further understand how the brain works and how it changes with aging or during the onset of neurodegenerative diseases like Parkinson's disease. Moreover, in the future, clinicians may use the brain's 'molecular signature' for early diagnoses, allowing patients to get access to treatment at the early stages of the disease and increasing their likelihood for better outcomes. A new technique is proposed in [11] to produce super resolution slice from MRI images based on convolutional neural networks (CNNs). In particular, a DeepResolve algorithm based on 3D CNN is developed for residual-based transformations for high resolution and low resolution of thin-slice image. For training, 124 Double Echo in Steady-State (DESS) datasets with features 0.7-mm slice thickness are involved. Figure 6.5 shows the overall deep neural network (DNN) structure. In particular, The DeepResolve model is developed to receive the low resolution images as an input and to produce high resolution image.

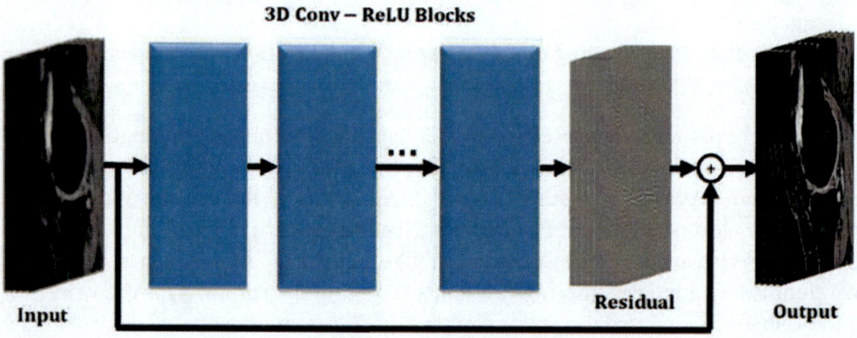

Fig. 6.5 Super resolution deep neural network (DNN) model for MRI image enhancement

6.2.2 X-Ray/CT Image Enhancement

The X-ray images are commonly produced as low intensity noisy gray-scale images with poor contrast, and weak boundary representation [12]. Based on this low-quality image, the feature extraction is quite a challenging task. For efficient feature extraction and segmentation processes, image enhancement techniques can be applied. For instance, a new method in [13] is proposed to automatically enhance the contrast of several X-ray images with high resolution. The morphological operators have been used for contrast enhancement for the best visualization of hard tissues, such as bones and dentin. Contrast enhancement can be accomplished by the joint transforms of the Top-hat and Bottom-hat transform. This concept is also explored in retina vessel segmentation. In this case, the combined approach can enhance the image where the gradient magnitude value is determined for automatic selection of the size of the structuring element.

Experimental evaluation emerges the effectiveness of the method compared to the baselines. Figure 6.6 demonstrates the responses of Top-hat and Bottom-hat transforms' combination. Furthermore, an advanced mammography (digital breast tomosynthesis) X-ray imaging method has been proposed in order to enhance the characterization of breast lesions [15]. In breast tomosynthesis technique, an X-ray tube projects a breast over a short arc of movement [16].

To develop an accurate Computer-Aided Diseases Diagnoses (CADD), the understanding of X-ray scan feature is a critical task. These algorithms are not limited to use in X-ray only, but they can be utilized to understand images for CT-Scan, ECG, ultrasound, and MRI. To design a comprehensive solution for diagnosis analysis and recognition of medical scan, various image processing algorithms have enabled different edge detection techniques. Edge detection algorithms are one of basic strate-

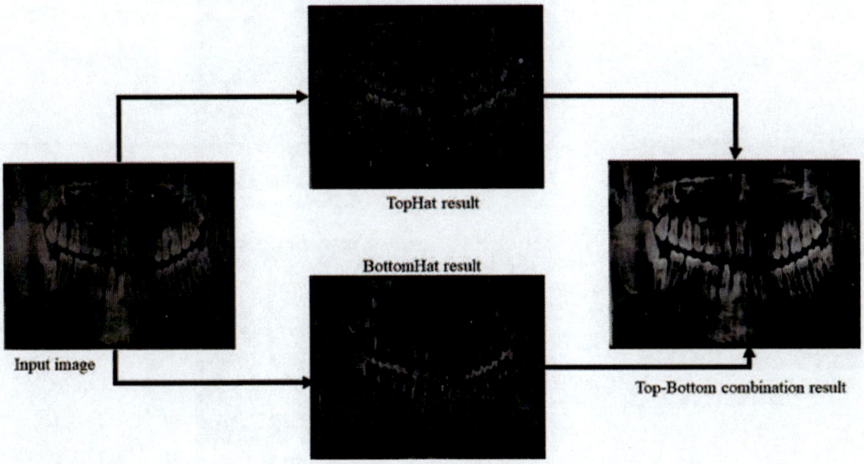

Fig. 6.6 Combination of the top-hat/bottom-hat transforms

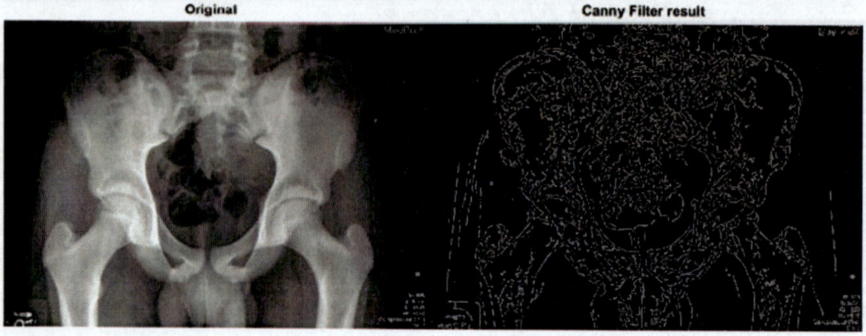

Fig. 6.7 The original X-ray input image (right), the output image after applying the edge detector (left). The original image is taken from the publicly available data on [14]

gies to extract the boundary features of the images of bones and teeth. Practically, the techniques are accomplished by finding the contrast and abrupt brightness changes in image pixels. Figure 6.7 shows the applying of the Canny edge detector, where the right image refers to the input image, and the left image refers to the output after applying the detector.

In a study in [17], an image enhancement algorithm is proposed to solve the medical image blurring problem and to generate an image with more accurate and meaningful features. In particular, the algorithm is developed to deblur the image via Conditional Generative Adversarial Networks (CGAN). The developed convolutional neural network (CNN) is used to reconstruct a sharp CT image as shown in Fig. 6.8. The CNN model is trained as a generator for a sharp CT scan image

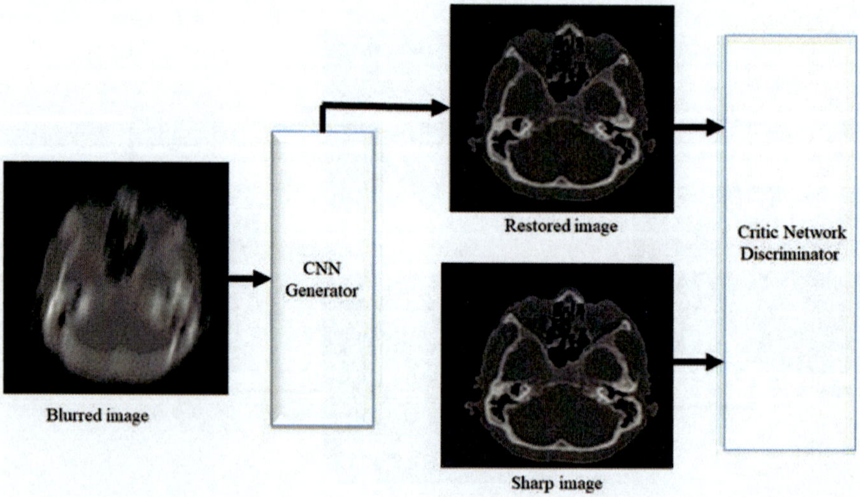

Fig. 6.8 Removal of motion-blind blur for CT images with Wasserstein generative adversarial network (WGAN) model

(output) from a blurred CT scan image (input), so that it can produce a sharp image with accurate features. Meanwhile, to gauge the similarity between the generated restored sharp CT scan image and the sharp CT, a critic network is trained in an adversarial manner, which is worked as the discriminator (see Fig. 6.8). However, The concept of the generator and the discriminator in restoring blurry CT image is introduced by a recent study in [18].

6.2.3 *Ultrasound Image Enhancement*

As ultrasound images are not complete tomographic slices, they are difficult to be processed and reproduced [7]. This is because the ultrasound images are affected by the image processing artifacts, which make the image processing task quite difficult to understand/acquire/extract the quantitative information from ultrasound images in a simple way. Nevertheless, many efforts have been done in order to enable better reading and understanding of ultrasound image information and to make it valuable in healthcare systems. A deep adversarial despeckling approach (DRNN) is developed in [19] to enhance the quality of ultrasound images. In contrast to the existing removal of speckle approaches, the proposed approach ca reduce the speckle extent without altering the structural and qualitative attributes of the ultrasound images. The experimental evaluations demonstrate that the proposed DRNN outperforms the state-of-the-art despeckling approaches in terms of the structural similarity index measure, peak signal to noise ratio, edge preservation index, and speckle region's signal to noise ratio.

A recent study is introduced in [21] to put some light in the construction and release of new experimental databases using an ultrasound device. This study provides a suitable methodology for treatment on experimental data. This study provides an accurate ultrasound identification of the different muscles located within the hindlimb. The major goal is to realize an exploratory analysis of the collected data, representing by,

- the correct range of gain to apply for the ultrasound measurement of muscle structure,
- the structural and functional referent data for a group of healthy mouse muscles, and
- the grayscale index, the texture anisotropy, and the elasticity parameters [21].

The authors argue that with future studies using phantoms (with parameters and geometry similar to mouse muscle), there is an ability for utilizing the technique for monitoring skeletal muscle changes and the response to the treatment over time. Furthermore, an image reconstruction method is proposed in [20] based on generative adversarial network (GAN)-based model to enhance the quality of the ultrasound images. Because of the reliability of the GAN model (see Fig. 6.9) to extract the multi-level nonlinear mapping relationship between the low-quality images and the high-quality images, the imaging quality is expected to be improved in multiple

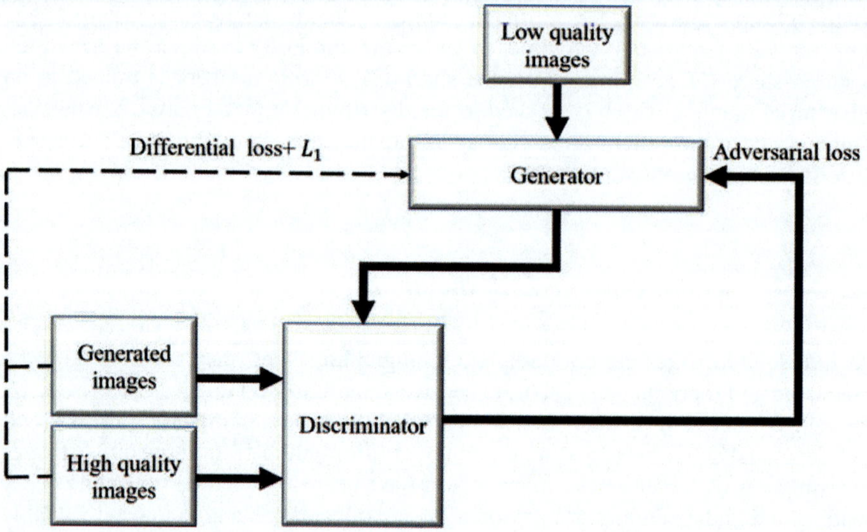

Fig. 6.9 Flowchart of the ultrasound image reconstruction algorithm [20]

aspects. Moreover, the feature extractors has been trained to be applied on the ultrasound images instead of human-designed ones [20], which come with more representative and adaptive to data. On the other hand, the revolution of the information and communication technologies (ICT) enable many opportunities in ultrasound domain. The new generation of ultrasound solution provides automatic measurements for features of streaming frames. Furthermore, the system provides only a few GUI menus for user-interfacing because of the automatic functionality of these solutions, which makes the use of the solution easily than the recent past. Moreover, the revolution of parallel processing has been utilized in these solutions to provide faster processing.

In 2018, Canon Inc. has released an ultrasound solution with 40% fewer GUI buttons to simplify the usage and workflow (the solution is called Aplio i900 CV). Also, Konica Minolta's new Sonimage HS1 provides many algorithms for image optimization that is performed automatically such as frequency, focus, and compounding change automatically proportional to the depth. In the domain of image segmentation/classification, GE Healthcare Logiq$^T M$ E10 provides segmentation and classification of streaming images, i.e., identification of liver lesion, which helps in diagnoses and follow-ups documentation. However, for increased usability of the ultrasound solution, the newest version of the Konica Minolta Sonimage HS1 utilizes speech recognition to perform speech control for the ultrasound devices.

Furthermore, the new revolution of GPU provides parallel processing of the frame rate of multi-dimension images, mostly baud rate of ultrasound systems carried out streaming with 30 frames per second. However, GE Healthcare has released its Imaging Elevated release based on GPU in order to perform real-time image reconstruction for cardiac images with high frame rates, which is named cSound.

Also, the high processing of GPU is utilized to develop an algorithm to recognize and track the blood flow through the heart using fetal ultrasound. This approach helps to evaluate the fetal heart shape features/structure, dimensions, and contractibility within three minutes, i.e., GE Healthcare's fetal HQ.

6.3 Medical Image Compression

As the medial images come from several devices on time, these images are large in resolution and size. Therefore, they need large space for storage and high bandwidth for transferring (i.e., send and receive the images through the Internet). Nowadays, there is massive demand on the remote medication *a.k.a., telemedicine*, wherein the doctor is away from the patient. In many real-world cases, the doctors can not be on-the-fly, even for any urgent situations because of other responsibilities. So, it is better to find such ways for remote diagnosis and treatment. Hence, we need very efficient image compression techniques. However, it is a challenging task due to the expected losses of the medical image content, which may affect the correct diagnostic ability of the doctors. In the following sections, we briefly report the recent medical image compression approaches.

6.3.1 MRI Image Compression

Due to the nature of MRI image acquisition, we may need for both high size and transmission capabilities to serve in telemedicine systems. Therefore, high-quality compression of MRI images is very research-oriented and demanding. Nonetheless, several MRI image compression techniques have been considered so far. In [22], a fast fractal-based compression algorithm for 3D MRI images is proposed. As shown in Fig. 6.10, both the range domain blocks are classified according to the spatio-temporal similarity of 3D objects. As well, a residual compensation mechanism is introduced to achieve high compression/decompression quality of MRI images. The experimental results demonstrate 2–3 times compression improvement, and ten times peak signal-to-noise ration (PSNR) enhancement compared to the baseline [22]. This approach is effective and solves the contradiction between high compression ratio and high quality MRI.

Taking the beneficiaries of the discrete cosine transform (DCT), a new 3D warped DCT is proposed for image compression. The experimental results reveal that the 3D warped DCT-based compression scheme performs better than a similar 3D DCT scheme for 3D datasets at high bit-rates [23]. In [24], a compression method is introduced for real time MRI. The compression process includes decomposing the image using chosen discrete wavelet transform, followed by its encoding through set portioning in the hierarchical tree. For evaluation, the compression performance is quantified in terms of Compression Ratio (CR), PSNR, and Bits per pixel (BPP).

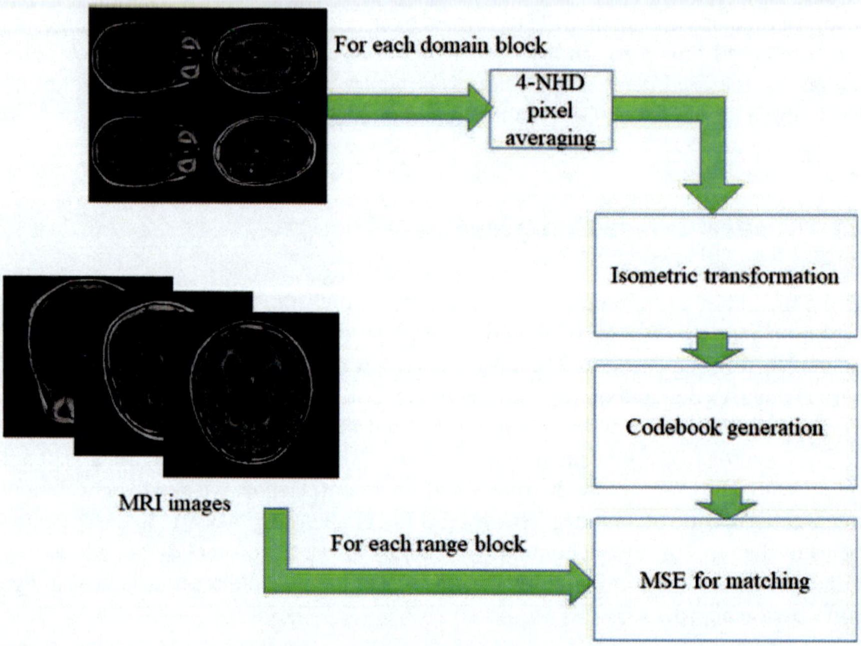

Fig. 6.10 Flowchart of fractal MRI image compression based on sequence of MRI images

Recently, a compression approach is proposed in [3] to exploit the neighbouring pixel redundancy found in MRI images. The authors used asymmetric mother wavelet daubechies (db) combined with the hierarchical embedded bit coding scheme to build a discrete wavelet transform. They also used ten 512 × 512 MRI images dataset to apply a distinct daubechies mother wavelets. This approach has achieved high compression ratio while preserving the MRI image details to great extent.

6.3.2 X-Ray/CT Compression

As an earlier attempts for X-ray image compression, the authors in [25] used the pulmonary tuberculosis X-ray images to investigate the performance of JPEG and wavelet transform based JPEG2000 compression. For qualitative evaluation, the compressed images have been introduced to specialists for assessment. Based on this subjective evaluation, the compressed images had high quality compared to the original images [25]. Relying on the convolutional recurrent neural networks (RNNs), a new model is proposed in [26] for robust X-ray image compression, as shown in Fig. 6.11. The proposed model has trained a set of sub-models at once for a specific dimension of X-ray images to provide variable compression rates during deployment. Afterward, a multi-level pooling scheme is adopted to learn contextualized features. The

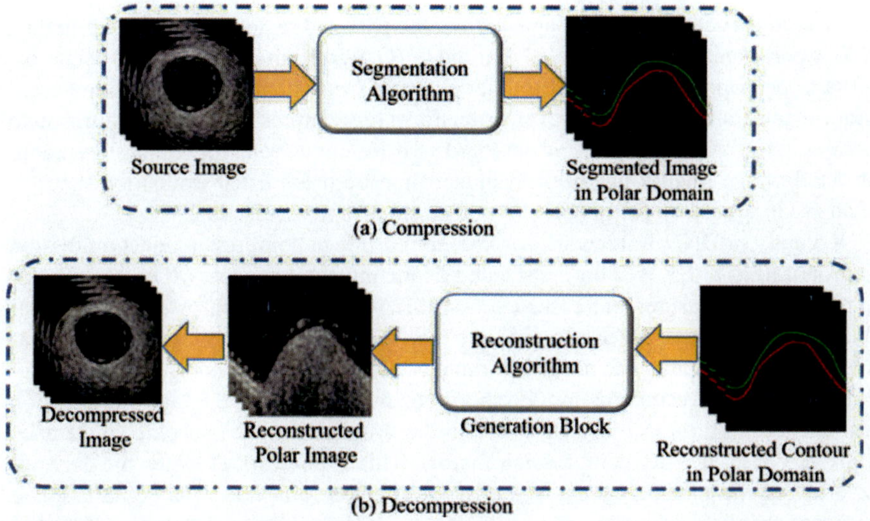

Fig. 6.11 A recurrent neural network (RNN) architecture for X-ray image compression and decompression [26]

experimental results depict the superiority of the model compared to the baselines in terms of structural similarity index and PSNR metrics [26]. The developed convolutional RNN model in [26] has carried out results with high performance compared to the baseline algorithm. Furthermore, a novel compression method is proposed in [27], aiming at excluding the non-valuable medical information from bone X-ray images by eliminating the the background pixels. For that, the histogram dispersion method is used to separate the region of interest (ROI) from the background. However, they have exploited the lossless compression method to preserve medical information of the image.

6.3.3 Ultrasound Image Compression

Due to the massive increasing use and popularity of medical ultrasound images, these are already explored in some remote diagnosis systems. Several attempts have been introduced to find robust ultrasound image compression techniques to handle the storage and transmission challenges while maintaining high diagnostic quality. In [28], a contextual vector quantization method (CVQ) is proposed by defining two regions in the image according to their information content. Those regions are:

- The contextual region, which has the most important information, and
- The background, which has a lower priority.

To reconstruct the output image, both of the encoded regions are merged together. The experimental results revealed that the CVQ algorithm can achieve the state-of-the-art performance compared to other existing methods. Moreover, another technique is introduced based on wavelet transform for compression of breast ultrasound images in [29]. The authors have explored 16 different wavelet functions. The reconstructed image quality has been evaluated into both the usual evaluation metrics, such as Compression Ratio (CR) as well as subjective assessment.

Recently, a DNN framework for ultrasound image compression/decompression is proposed in [30] based on the stacked denoising autoencoders (SDAs). Both linear/nonlinear measurement cases (SDA-L/SDA-NL) have been investigated under the conditions of unlearned compression matrix and the compression is indicated as a layer of the network. The proposed framework has demonstrated its capabilities for compression and reconstruction. Furthermore, a new ultrasound image compression framework is introduced in [31] to retain the originality of the speckle appearance with very high-density compression factors. This framework emerges the generalizability of the method by exploring two variations to develop the compressor. It achieves excellent compression ratio (725:1), while retaining the statistical distribution of the speckles [31].

6.4 Selective Topics of Medical Imaging Innovations

6.4.1 Image Processing for Medical Additive Manufacturing

The additive manufacturing (AM) is a transformative method that enables the creation of lighter, smarter, and stronger systems and structures. AM approach uses any of the data computer-aided-design (CAD) software, or 3D scanners to develop a hardware to engrave material—layer-wise for various geometric models or shapes. Through these steps, we can produce different types of usable products that are usually not feasible to produce easily (or, sometimes, impossible to make) [32]. AM is capable of building complex structures and designs. In the medical industry, it can be utilized to print dental, bones, cardiac stent, etc. The AM machine receives a design of the desired object in the stereolithography (STL) file format [33]. This STL is a format of the CAD program that contains the features of the shape. Afterward, the AM software slices the STL file into G-code to preform a layered concept to add layer by layer. After that, the produced part can be measured via image processing algorithms to validate the product [34, 35].

6.4.1.1 Cardiac 3D Printing

A 3D cardiac printing technique is proposed in [36]. As shown in Fig. 6.12, the steps of cardiac fabrication based on CT images are shown. The basic steps are summarized below:

- In step 1, the dataset is built from many CT scan images of the human heart.
- After that, the segmentation algorithm is applied on the entire dataset to perform the mask filter for all images.
- In step 3, all segmented images will be integrated to reconstruct a 3D mesh. The 3D mesh contains all features data, such as, XYZ-dimensions, resolution, etc.
- In the next step, the 3D mesh file is sliced into multiple layers to perform the G-code for every layer.
- Finally, the G-code will feed to the machine with the required material to produce the desired product (see Fig. 6.12) [36].

In CT image segmentation, all CT datasets should be in Digital Imaging and Communication in Medicine (DICOM) format, while the segmentation process is implemented based on the pixel intensity of the 2D grayscale image. All the pixels with the same intensity values are masked, and the 3D shape will be created. To porting the 3D shape to the AM, the mesh is converted to file format, which can be able to edit by computer aided manufacturing (CAM). For manufacturing purpose, CAM enables to add color to some parts of the 3D object. The challenges are multifarious regarding AM [37], e.g.,

- Less user-friendly equipment,
- Scepticism in the integrity of AM parts,
- Time-consuming,
- A minor flaw in the design may ruin the entire process,
- Closed or restricted architectures of AM machines and their variability, etc.

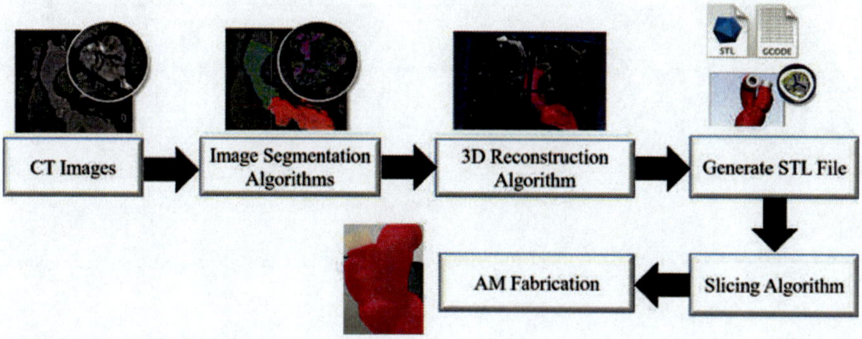

Fig. 6.12 3D printed modeling of a patient-specific anatomy. Various steps are mentioned for additive manufacturing (AM) fabrication

6.4.1.2 3D Bone Printing

3D bone printing is a revolutionary application and it still is an emerging field of research. It has an ample scopes to enrich the field of medicine, surgery, bone replacement, and related treatments. In our daily life, many accidents cause fracture or amputation of bones, apart from bone cancers or other ailments. One of the ways of treatment for these challenges is to implant a bone graft, or explore a donor's bone tissue. Unfortunately, this process needs special considerations for bone graft and plants metal plates. However, if the missing bone limb is large, then it will be difficult for planting and thereby, amputation of the limb deems a very sad but realistic strategy in almost many cases.

Fortunately, most of these aforementioned limitations can be overcome through the 3D printing fashion. Through 3D printing, we are on the verge of more natural, cheaper and more convenient customized solutions for the patients. With 3D printing, there is no need for grafting or donors. Instead, the doctors can simply scan the area of the desired limb and then model the structure of the required structure - as per the requirements of the patient. However, this technology needs more efforts and developments. 3D printers are still not fully-matured as many different designs with highly-varied costs and capabilities are in the market. Most of the designs or companies are sustaining for a longer period. Low-cost printers can not be suitable for bone printing in one hand, and high-cost machines can not be widely-explored all over the World on the other hand. Hence, there is a trade-off and more innovative explorations are needed.

Recently, several 3D printed bone projects have been established to design the implants based on a CT scan of the patient. As shown in Fig. 6.13, the printed bone is able to fit perfectly onto the patient's body part with a very high printing accuracy. It seems that even a complex shape and design can be orchestrated by 3D printer, almost similar to a natural one.

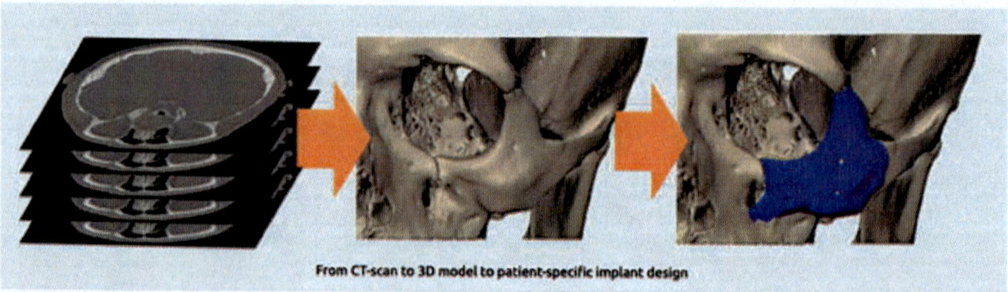

Fig. 6.13 From CT-scan to 3D model to patient-specific implant design. Credit: https://www.xilloc.com/ct-bone/

6.4.2 3D/4D Surgical Visualization and Virtual/Augmented Reality

The revolution in 3D image processing and virtual reality or augmented reality (AR/VR) enables multiple facilities in the domain of orthopaedic surgery. During surgery, doctor needs to be able to visualise the interfacing between the tools and additional parts outside the patient with the bones inside the patient. For instance, the integration between CT scan image and RGB image is introduced with promising results in augmented image/video facilities [38]. To align both images (i.e., the CT-scan and RGB image) with an accurate position, the depth image techniques have been utilized through the usage of depth cameras to preserve the dimensions as shown in Fig. 6.14. Moreover, this framework can track the surgical tool and the affected part of the disease [38]. The virtual/augmented reality has been started with a C-arm solution in [39]. It was the first augmented reality approach that has been utilized for real-time surgeon inside the hospital. The setup of the solution has the RGB/Depth camera placed beside the C-arm source, and the mirror constructed under the X-ray source, provides the alignment of the optical axis. Another augmented C-arm technique is introduced in [40] based on two cameras. The cameras are placed in the side of the X-ray source. Using the RGB data, the video from the X-ray source can be synthesized to visualize the surgeon's operation state.

A new 3D tracking model is developed in [42] for surgeon visualization. This model allows to segment/track the surgical tool. It can track the screw of bone while operate via real-time localization for screw placement from multiple views. It can also perform the alignment between planned trajectory and tracked drill path from multiple views. This facilitation helps the doctors to find the optimal point for surgeon during or before the operation in a short time [42].

A visualization system for pre-clinical evaluation of a prototype of orthopedic interventions in surgeon is introduced in [41]. This approach supports intuitive visualization of the anatomy and can be integrated in the hand-eye coordination for the orthopedic surgeon. Moreover, it enables real-time realization for surgeon and patient in order to provide accurate virtual realty as shown in Fig. 6.15.

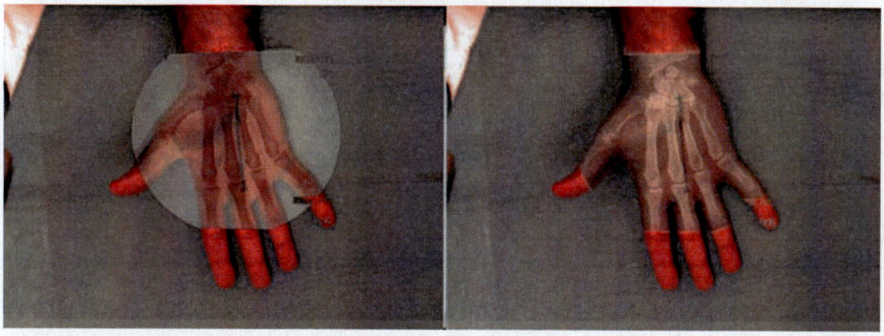

Fig. 6.14 A 3D augmented reality system

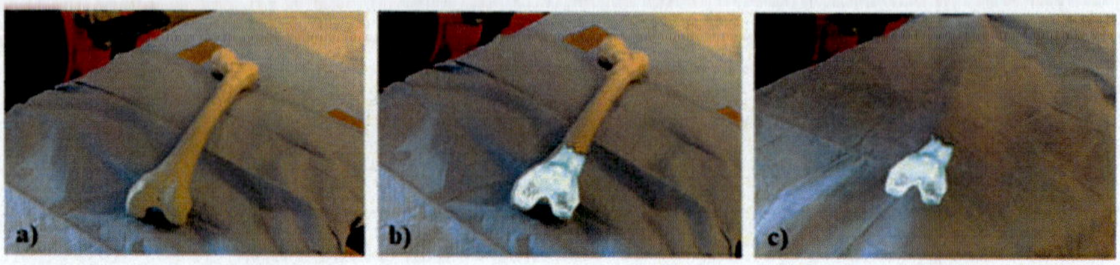

Fig. 6.15 Augmented bone: **a** the natural object, **b** the object overlaid with the rendered volume, and **c** the correct overlay persistence [41]

6.4.3 Smart Phones and IoT Applications

Due to the revolution of the Internet of Things (IoT) technologies and smartphones, it can move the routines of medical checks from the hospital to the patient's home [43–47]. There is a mutual hope to involve the IoT technology and smartphones into medical applications because it allows clinics and medical centers to function more competently and patients to obtain better treatment. Through these technologies, the quality and efficiency of treatments can be improved and accordingly the health of the patients. Furthermore, the smartphone application development based on iOS or Android provides full reports for the health states and analytical for the vital data such as X-ray, CT, laparoscopy images, etc. (see Fig. 6.16).

The expression of IoT in medical applications is being widely used in telemedicine and tele-healthcare systems. The IoT provides many opportunities for the concept/applications of telemedicine. These opportunities enable real-time monitoring for

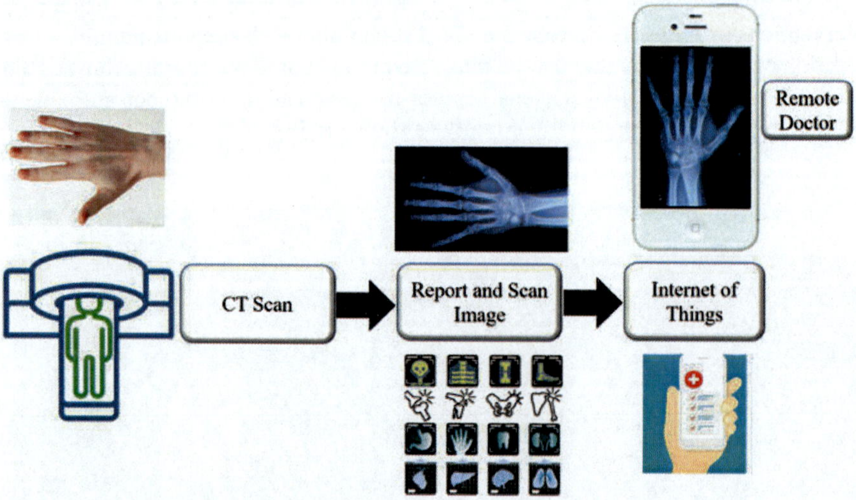

Fig. 6.16 Smart phone-based telemedicine system for CT scan

the patients/elder/kids outside the clinic and hospital. Also, IoT algorithms provide real-time assistance to the doctors to perform remote diagnosis. In [48], an IoT system is introduced for the healthcare system based on non-invasive data acquisition. The developed data acquisition is developed based on convenient image processing algorithms on eulerian video magnification [49]. The image processing algorithm provides real-time computation of heart rate and concatenates this meaningful data in the communication frame via a hybrid architecture. On the other hand, the IoT algorithm is developed based on the integration of LoRa (Long Range-wide area network) modules and the ESP32 module. LoRa has been explored in healthcare facilities [50, 51]. However, the algorithm is restricted to send/visualize the vital data state via IoT without utilization of image processing techniques such as segmentation, analysis, etc. In [52], an image segmentation algorithm for CT medical image is developed to reconstruct segmentation region in a small region to improve the segmentation results. The enhancement accuracy has been increased form 0.978% to 0.981% and the standard deviation improvement from 0.281 to 0.187 compared to the baseline methods.

Because of their small size and usability, smartphones introduce new opportunities in medical applications. It can be utilized for doctor consultation, and for communication with patients [47]. In [47], the authors have reported many smartphones-based medical applications in radiology, i.e., diagnostic reading applications and decision support. IoT-based sensors are very widely explored for many healthcare-related applications [44]. For diagnostic purposes, the FDA in USA has proposed a smartphone-based application to enable displaying CT/X-ray images with a multi-plane reconstructed image. This application is developed to be supported by iOS for iPhones/iPads. Furthermore, this application provides several image processing methods to measure dimensions, display regions of interest and show intensity value [53]. The application works for ultrasonic diagnoses on the smartphone, which is connected through the USB interface with the ultrasonic device or WiFi interface based on socket communication [54]. Furthermore, the IoT has been adopted in tele-ultrasound solution in order to provide real time streaming of vital data from patient to the doctor remotely. Philips' Lumify portable ultrasound has provided this feature with the capabilities to make video/audio call with the doctor and patients,

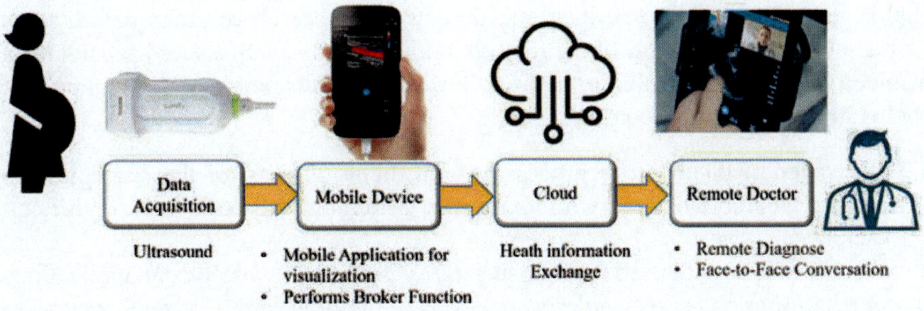

Fig. 6.17 Lumify portable ultrasound system

as shown in Fig. 6.17. The usage of smartphones in medical imaging is not restricted to perform intermediate task, it becomes the core of several medical applications' implementations. This is because the recent advancement of smartphones processing speed as well as the attached high resolution cameras. For instance, an imaging solution for throat visualisation is provided in [55] using the smartphone. The authors argue that the setup of this solution is affordable in order to extract fluorescence image of the throat easily. There are more scopes for applications and advancements in this domain.

6.5 Conclusion

The rapid development of image processing algorithms enables accurate or high quality image acquisition, as well as, enhancement and optimization of the data storage and transfer. This chapter has introduced the recent advancements in medical image enhancement and compression techniques, considering the three main types of medical images: MRI, X-ray/CT, and Ultrasound. Furthermore, we have covered the usage of the traditional image processing techniques, as well as, the usage of the recent deep learning algorithms for medical images processing. With the era of IoT, complex algorithms can be processed and applied in cloud computing based on real-time communication with data acquisition. This end-to-end design may reduce the costs of processing units in the hospital and clinic.

In this chapter, we have reported the recent usage of IoT technology in the medical imaging systems and how it enables exchanges of vital information through medical resources, doctors, nurses, and patients based on the cloud. The ultrasound scans can be compressed and send to the doctor via IoT then, it can be decompressed at the doctor's side to make the desired diagnose. We have also shortly introduced the usage of image processing techniques in the additive manufacturing to assist the modeling of human body parts such as bones, hard tissues, and teeth. We have summarized the integration between augmented reality and additive manufacturing, which could produce an accurate product and help the doctor to use the right way of using the modeled part for surgery. Finally, there are numerous challenges that are face in medical imaging systems and health informatics communities. Many of these challenges still raise several open questions to the research communities to solve partially or generally. Many of the relevant underlying research issues have not been resolved but these are evolving. In the following, we enlist some of these important challenges for the future consideration:

- Low-power medical image processing is difficult as most of the strategies are based on wearable devices with low-power computational costs that are difficult to achieve.
- Wearable sensors are used for human activity monitoring, healthcare applications and rehabilitation centers, elderly support care facilities and related. Now, how to

explore those data, and rationalize with medical records during hospital and after hospital are not studied much. These are important aspects to handle for the future.

- Medical visual diagnosis requires genuine experts and yet, difficult. Therefore, we need to explore on explainable and universal medical visual diagnosis systems and strategies.
- Medical informatics is varied and mostly employable in advanced countries. Moreover, if a hospital wants to deploy an IT-based system that covers medical informatics, it is very expensive.
- Shifting or transformation from one system to another becomes an extremely daunting task due to a lack of clarifying and universality of the existing systems to manage hospitals and hospital data.
- Privacy and security issues are other major concerns. Most of the cases, medical data are not openly available to do research, especially in rare disease cases. Therefore, how to handle the privacy issue or security of the data while opening the core data for researchers is another major challenge. Ethical policies vary from nation to nation.
- 3D computer vision systems/methods in a medical environment are not progressed much till now.
- Real-time applications with more accuracy.
- Microscopy image analysis has many challenging aspects.
- Smart skin image analysis approaches are not available for various skin diseases.
- Medical-based computer vision research and implementations are still not unearthed significantly.

References

1. Ahad, M.A.R., Kobashi, S., Tavares, J.: Advancements of image processing and vision in healthcare. J. Healthcare Eng. **2018** (2018)
2. Daley, B.: 3 types of MRI machines and the difference between an open MTI versus a closed MRI. https://4rai.com/blog/3-types-of-mri-machines (2016)
3. Soni, E., Mahajan, R.: MRI image compression using asymmetric wavelet analysis. In: International Conference on Advanced Informatics for Computing Research, pp. 260–270. Springer (2019)
4. Md Atiqur Rahman Ahad, R.R., Ahmed, M.U.: A study on computer-aided diagnosis of Alzheimer's disease from the ventricular enlargement using s-MRI data. Int. J. Biomed. Soft Comput. Hum. Sci. **24**(2)
5. Sepehrband, F., Barisano, G., Sheikh-Bahaei, N., Cabeen, R.P., Choupan, J., Law, M., Toga, A.W.: Image processing approaches to enhance perivascular space visibility and quantification using MRI, pp. 609–362. BioRxiv (2019)
6. Kak, A.C., Slaney, M., Wang, G.: Principles of computerized tomographic imaging. Med. Phys. **29**(1), 107–107 (2002)
7. Ortiz, S.H.C., Chiu, T., Fox, M.D.: Ultrasound image enhancement: a review. Biomed. Signal Proces. Control **7**(5), 419–428 (2012)
8. Food, U., Administration, D., et al.: Initiative to reduce unnecessary radiation exposure from medical imaging. Center for Devices and Radiological Health (2010)

9. Stockham, T.G.: Image processing in the context of a visual model. Proc. IEEE **60**(7), 828–842 (1972)
10. Filo, S., Shtangel, O., Salamon, N., Kol, A., Weisinger, B., Shifman, S., Mezer, A.A.: Disentangling molecular alterations from water-content changes in the aging human brain using quantitative MRI. Nat. Commun. **10**(1), 1–16 (2019)
11. Chaudhari, A.S., Fang, Z., Kogan, F., Wood, J., Stevens, K.J., Gibbons, E.K., Lee, J.H., Gold, G.E., Hargreaves, B.A.: Super-resolution musculoskeletal MRI using deep learning. Magn. Reson. Med. **80**(5), 2139–2154 (2018)
12. Ramani, R., Vanitha, N.S., Valarmathy, S.: The pre-processing techniques for breast cancer detection in mammography images. Int. J. Image Graph. Signal Process. **5**(5), 47 (2013)
13. Kushol, R., Raihan, M., Salekin, M.S., Rahman, A., et al.: Contrast enhancement of medical X-ray image using morphological operators with optimal structuring element. arXiv:1905.08545 (2019)
14. Applying of canny edge detector. https://medpix.nlm.nih.gov/search?allen=true&allt=true&alli=true&query=fracture, May 2020
15. Helvie, M.A.: Digital mammography imaging: breast tomosynthesis and advanced applications. Radiol. Clin. North Am. **48**(5), 917 (2010)
16. Liu, F., Hernandez-Cabronero, M., Sanchez, V., Marcellin, M.W., Bilgin, A.: The current role of image compression standards in medical imaging. Information **8**(4), 131 (2017)
17. Lyu, Y., Jiang, W., Lin, Y., Voros, L., Zhang, M., Mueller, B., Mychalczak, B., Song, Y.: Motion-blind blur removal for CT images with Wasserstein generative adversarial networks. In: 11th International Congress on Image and Signal Processing, BioMedical Engineering and Informatics (CISP-BMEI), pp. 1–5. IEEE (2018)
18. Kupyn, O., Budzan, V., Mykhailych, M., Mishkin, D., Matas, J.: DeblurGAN: blind motion Deblurring using conditional adversarial networks. arxiv:1711.07064 (2017)
19. Mishra, D., Chaudhury, S., Sarkar, M., Soin, A.S.: Ultrasound image enhancement using structure oriented adversarial network. IEEE Signal Process. Lett. **25**(9), 1349–1353 (2018)
20. Wang, R., Fang, Z., Gu, J., Guo, Y., Zhou, S., Wang, Y., Chang, C., Yu, J.: High-resolution image reconstruction for portable ultrasound imaging devices. EURASIP J. Adv. Sig. Process. **2019**(1), 56 (2019)
21. Ternifi, R., Kammoun, M., Pouletaut, P., Subramaniam, M., Hawse, J.R., Bensamoun, S.F.: Ultrasound image processing to estimate the structural and functional properties of mouse skeletal muscle. Biomed. Signal Process. Control **56**, 101–735 (2020)
22. Liu, S., Bai, W., Zeng, N., Wang, S.: A fast fractal based compression for MRI images. IEEE Access **7**, 62412–62420 (2019)
23. Prabhu, K., Sridhar, K., Mischi, M., Bharath, H.N.: 3-d warped discrete cosine transform for MRI image compression. Biomed. Signal Process. Control **8**(1), 50–58 (2013)
24. Soni, E., Mahajan, R.: Symmetric wavelet analysis toward MRI image compression. In: Soft Computing: Theories and Applications, , pp. 533–547. Springer (2018)
25. Dodig, M. Grgic, S., Dodig, S.: Quality of chest X-ray images compressed using JPEG and JPEG. In: EUROCON 2005—The International Conference on Computer as a Tool, vol. 2, pp. 931–934. IEEE (2005)
26. Sushmit, A.S., Zaman, S.U., Humayun, A.I., Hasan, T.: X-ray image compression using convolutional recurrent neural networks. CoRR, arXiv:1904.12271 (2019)
27. Kazeminia, S., Karimi, N., Soroushmehr, S.R., Samavi, S., Derksen, H., Najarian, K.: Region of interest extraction for lossless compression of bone X-ray images, In: 37th Annual International Conference of the IEEE Engineering in Medicine and Biology Society (EMBC), pp. 3061–3064. IEEE (2015)
28. Hosseini, S.M., Naghsh-Nilchi, A.-R.: Medical ultrasound image compression using contextual vector quantization. Comput. Biol. Med. **42**(7), 743–750 (2012)
29. Shahhoseini, E., Nejad, N.A., Behnam, H., Shahhoseini, A.: A new approach to compression of medical ultrasound images using wavelet transform. In 2010 Third International Conference on Advances in Circuits, Electronics and Microelectronics, pp. 40–44. IEEE (2010)

30. Perdios, D., Besson, A., Arditi, M., Thiran, J.-P.: A deep learning approach to ultrasound image recovery. In: IEEE International Ultrasonics Symposium (IUS), pp. 1–4. IEEE (2017)
31. China, D., Tom, F., Nandamuri, S., Kar, A., Srinivasan, M., Mitra, P., Sheet, D.: Ultracompression: framework for high density compression of ultrasound volumes using physics modeling deep neural networks. In: IEEE 16th International Symposium on Biomedical Imaging (ISBI 2019), pp. 798–801. IEEE (2019)
32. Bertling J., Rommel, S.: A critical view of 3d printing regarding industrial mass customization versus individual desktop fabrication. In: The Decentralized and Networked Future of Value Creation, pp. 75–105. Springer (2016)
33. Charles, A., Elkaseer, A., Thijs, L., Hagenmeyer, V., Scholz, S.: Effect of process parameters on the generated surface roughness of down-facing surfaces in selective laser melting. Appl. Sci. **9**(6), 1256 (2019)
34. Elkaseer, A., Salem, M., Hagenmeyer, V., Scholz, S.: Vision system-based inspection and alignment of laminated polymer films for 3d-integration of microsystems. IFAC-PapersOnLine **52**(15), 13–18 (2019)
35. Elkaseer, A., Salama, M., Ali, H., Scholz, S.: Approaches to a practical implementation of industry 4.0. Resource **3**, 5 (2018)
36. Vukicevic, M., Mosadegh, B., Min, J.K., Little, S.H.: Cardiac 3d printing and its future directions. JACC Cardiovas. Imaging **10**(2), 171–184 (2017)
37. Keicher D.: CAD/CAM Approach to Additive Manufacturing. https://www.osti.gov/servlets/purl/1341361. Accessed 1 Sep 2016
38. Wang, L., Traub, J., Weidert, S., Heining, S.M., Euler, E., Navab, N.: Parallax free long bone X-ray image stitching. In: Yang, G.-Z., Hawkes, D., Rueckert, D., Noble, A., Taylor, C. (eds.) Medical Image Computing and Computer- Assisted Intervention—MICCAI 2009, , pp. 173–180. Springer, Berlin, Heidelberg (2009). ISBN 978-3-642-04268-3
39. Navab, N., Heining, S.-M., Traub, J.: Camera augmented mobile c-arm (CAMC): calibration, accuracy study, and clinical applications. IEEE Trans. Med. Imaging **29**(7), 1412–1423 (2009)
40. Newcombe, R.A., Izadi, S., Hilliges, O., Molyneaux, D., Kim, D., Davison, A.J., Kohli, P., Shotton, J., Hodges, S., Fitzgibbon, A.W.: Kinectfusion: Real-time dense surface mapping and tracking. In: ISMAR, vol. 11, pp. 127–136 (2011)
41. Hajek, J., Unberath, M., Fotouhi, J., Bier, B., Lee, S.C., Osgood, G., Maier, A., Armand, M., Navab, N.: Closing the calibration loop: an inside-out-tracking paradigm for augmented reality in orthopedic surgery. In: International Conference on Medical Image Computing and Computer-Assisted Intervention, pp. 299–306. Springer (2018)
42. Lee, S.C., Fuerst, B., Tateno, K., Johnson, A., Fotouhi, J., Osgood, G., Tombari, F., Navab, N.: Multi-modal imaging, model-based tracking, and mixed reality visualisation for orthopaedic surgery. Healthcare Technol. Lett. **4**(5), 168–173 (2017)
43. Ahmed, M., Das Antar, A., Ahad, M.A.R.: An approach to classify human activities in real-time from smartphone sensor data. In: 2019 Joint 8th International Conference on Informatics, Electronics Vision (ICIEV) and 2019 3rd International Conference on Imaging, Vision Pattern Recognition (icIVPR), pp. 140–145 (2019)
44. Ahad, M.A.R., Antar, A.D., Ahmed, M.: IoT sensor-based activity recognition. In: IoT Sensor-based Activity Recognition. Springer (2020)
45. Ahad, M.A.R., Antar, A.D., Shahid, O.: Vision-based action understanding for assistive healthcare: a short review. In: IEEE CVPR Workshop (2019)
46. Noman, M.T.B., Ahad, M.A.R.: Mobile-based eye-blink detection performance analysis on android platform (2018)
47. Székely, A., Talanow, R., Bágyi, P.: Smartphones, tablets and mobile applications for radiology. Eur. J. Radiol. **82**(5), 829–836 (2013)
48. Salem, M., El-Maddah, I., Youssef, K., Mohamed, H.: Internet of things solution for non-invasive vital data acquisition: a step towards smart healthcare system. In: International Conference on Sustainable Design and Manufacturing, pp. 387–397. Springer (2019)
49. Wu, H.-Y., Rubinstein, M., Shih, E., Guttag, J., Durand, F., Freeman, W.: Eulerian video magnification for revealing subtle changes in the world (2012)

50. Hossain, T., Ahad, M. A. R., Tazin, T., Inoue, S.: Activity recognition by using lorawan sensor. In: Proceedings of the 2018 ACM International Joint Conference and 2018 International Symposium on Pervasive and Ubiquitous Computing and Wearable Computers, pp. 58–61. (2018)
51. Hossain, T., Doi, Y., Tazin, T., Ahad, M. A. R., Inoue, S.: Study of lorawan technology for activity recognition. In: Proceedings of the 2018 ACM International Joint Conference and 2018 International Symposium on Pervasive and Ubiquitous Computing and Wearable Computers, pp. 1449–1453. (2018)
52. Chae, S.-H., Moon, D., Lee, D.G., Pan, S.B.: Medical image segmentation for mobile electronic patient charts using numerical modeling of IoT. J. Appl. Math. **2014** (2014)
53. Kastania, A.N., Moumtzoglou, A.: Quality implications of the medical applications for 4G mobile phones. Int. J. Reliab. Qual. E-Healthcare (IJRQEH) **1**(1), 58–67 (2012)
54. Pianykh, O.S. : Dicom and teleradiology. In: Digital Imaging and Communications in Medicine (DICOM): A Practical Introduction and Survival Guide, pp. 281–317. Springer, Berlin, Heidelberg (2012). https://doi.org/10.1007/978-3-642-10850-1_13. ISBN 978-3-642-10850-1
55. Pratavieira, S., Vollet-Filho, J.D., Carbinatto, F.M., Blanco, K., Inada, N.M., Bagnato, V.S., Kurachi, C.: Adapting smartphones for low-cost optical medical imaging. In: Biophotonics South America. International Society for Optics and Photonics, vol. 9531, p. 95313J (2015)

Chapter 7
Artificial Intelligence, Machine Learning and Reasoning in Health Informatics—An Overview

Mobyen Uddin Ahmed, Shaibal Barua, and Shahina Begum

Abstract As humans are intelligent, to mimic or models of human certain intelligent behavior to a computer or a machine is called Artificial Intelligence (AI). Learning is one of the activities by a human that helps to gain knowledge or skills by studying, practising, being taught, or experiencing something. Machine Learning (ML) is a field of AI that mimics human learning behavior by constructing a set of algorithms that can learn from data, i.e. it is a field of study that gives computers the ability to learn without being explicitly programmed. The reasoning is a set of processes that enable humans to provide a basis for judgment, making decisions, and prediction. Machine Reasoning (MR), is a part of AI evolution towards human-level intelligence or the ability to apply prior knowledge to new situations with adaptation and changes. This book chapter presents some AI, ML and MR techniques and approached those are widely used in health informatics domains. Here, the overview of each technique is discussed to show how they can be applied in the development of a decision support system.

Keywords Artificial Intelligence · Machine learning · Reasoning · Fuzzy logic · Support Vector Machine (SVM) · Random Forest (RF) · Artificial Neural Network (ANN) · K-Nearest Neighbor (k-NN) · K-means clustering · Fuzzy C-means (FCM) Clustering · Case-Based Reasoning (CBR)

7.1 Introduction

In the medical/health informatics domain, the knowledge is today expanding so quickly to the extent that even experts have difficulties in following the latest

M. U. Ahmed (✉) · S. Barua · S. Begum
School of Innovation, Design and Engineering, Mälardalen University, Västerås, Sweden
e-mail: mobyen.ahmed@mdh.se

S. Barua
e-mail: shaibal.barua@mdh.se

S. Begum
e-mail: shahina.begum@mdh.se

M. A. R. Ahad and M. U. Ahmed (eds.), *Signal Processing Techniques for Computational Health Informatics*, Intelligent Systems Reference Library 192,
https://doi.org/10.1007/978-3-030-54932-9_7

new results, changes and treatments. Computers surpass humans in their ability to remember and such property is very valuable for a computer-aided system that enables improvements for both diagnosis and treatment. Decision Support System (DSS) are computer-based systems that can simulate expert human reasoning by understanding the principle of human intelligence, can be served as an assistant to a physician in the medical domain is increasingly important and. They are typically designed for medical knowledge, patient's data/information and an inference engine into assist clinicians in their decision-making tasks namely diagnosis and treatment. In the medical domain diagnostics, classification and treatment are the main tasks for a physician. System development for such a purpose is also a popular area in Artificial Intelligence (AI) research. DSSs that bear similarities with human learning and reasoning have benefits and are often easily accepted by physicians in the medical domain [1–6]. Today many clinical DSSs are developed to be multi-purposed and often combine more than one AI methods and techniques. The multi-faceted and complex nature of the medical domain motivates researchers to design such multi-modal systems [5–7]. Several challenges associated with multi-modal machine learning framework [8] have been addressed, which are:

- Representation: Data processing requires for representing and summarizing heterogeneous data to achieve multiple complementary modalities.
- Translation: Identify and acknowledge the relationship among the multimodal data.
- Alignment: Identify the relations between different health related conditions and the measuring parameters.
- Fusion: Apply data-level and feature-level fusion between two or more modalities to improve system performance.
- Co-learning: Explore the advantages and limitations of each modality and use that knowledge to improve the performances of models trained on a different modality.

This book chapter presents AI technique, such as Fuzzy Logic. Several supervised machine learning e.g. Support Vector Machine (SVM) and Random Forest (RF); unsupervised learning e.g. K-means clustering, Fuzzy C-means (FCM) clustering, Gaussian mixer model and Hierarchical clustering. Also, several machine reasoning algorithms such as Fuzzy Rule-Based Reasoning (RBR), Case-Based Reasoning (CBR) and Textual Case Retrieval.

7.2 Overview of Artificial Intelligence (AI)

Artificial Intelligence (AI) is an area of computer science that is used to develop intelligent machines to think and react like humans. As humans are intelligent, to mimic or models or simulation of humans' certain intelligent behaviour to a computer or a machine is called AI. Even though the concept of AI technology has been changed over time, the fundamental concept of AI is building machines that are capable of thinking (i.e., thought processes and reasoning) and reacting (i.e., behaviour and performance) like humans. Arthur Lee Samuel coined the term "machine learning" in his 1959 paper [9], who was an American pioneer in computer gaming and artificial intelligence. He defined machine learning as the process of programming a digital computer that could behave similarly to the way that human beings or animals learn while doing some task. One of the popular AI algorithms e.g. fuzzy logic has been used in the case studies (discussed in another chapter later) of health informatics domain are presented.

7.2.1 Fuzzy Logic

Information can be incomplete, inconsistent, uncertain, or all of these three and it is often unsuitable for solving a problem. For example, "The temperature of the machine is *really hot,* or Anders is a *very tall* man". Here, it can be seen that most of the time we rely on common sense when we solve problems. To deal with such vague and uncertain information exact mathematical techniques are not sufficient, we need a technique or approach that uses a much closer concept of human thinking. Fuzzy logic is specifically designed to mathematically represent this uncertainty and vagueness. So, fuzzy logic is not a logic that is fuzzy, but a logic that is used to describe fuzziness. It is a theory of fuzzy sets, sets that calibrate vagueness. Moreover, it is a form of multi-valued logic with more than two truth values to deal with reasoning i.e. an approximate value rather than an exact value. Opposite to the binary or crisp logic, it handles the perception of 'Partially Truth' i.e. the values between completely 'true' and completely 'false'. The degree of truth of a statement can range between false (0) and true (1) and considers more than two truth values. Aristotle was the first to realize that logic based on "True" or "False" alone was not satisfactory. Plato left the foundation of a third region beyond the true and false [10]. Multi-valued logic was introduced by a Polish philosopher Jan Lukasiewicz in the 1930s. He presented logic that extended the range of truth values to all real numbers in the interval between 0 and 1 [11, 12]. In 1965, Lotfi Zadeh a professor at the University of California at Berkley, available his famous paper "Fuzzy sets". He prolonged the work on possibility theory into a formal system of mathematical logic and initiated a new concept for applying natural language terms. This new logic for demonstrating and manipulating fuzzy terms was called fuzzy logic [13, 14]. The term "fuzzy logic" derives from the fuzzy set theory or the theory of fuzzy sets. The fuzzy set theory has successfully been applied in controlling uncertainties in various application domains [15] including the medical application areas.

The use of fuzzy logic in medical informatics has begun in the early 1970s. Figure 7.1 illustrated a binary logic with a crisp boundary of 4 different seasons in Sweden; where the X-axis corresponds to dates according to the month of the year and the Y-axis represents the probability between zero and one. In binary logic, the function that relates to the value of a variable with the probability of a judged statement is a 'rectangular' one. The output probability for any input will always be 'one' i.e. only one season and 'zero' for the rest of the seasons. The crisp boundary of

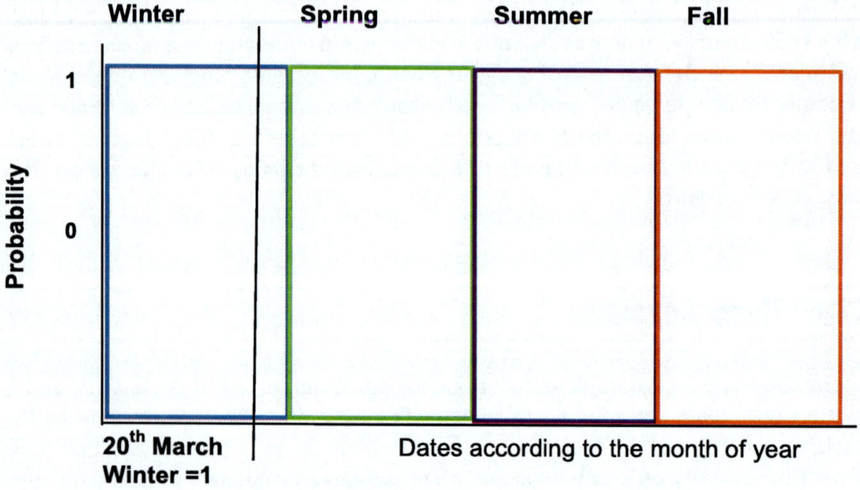

Fig. 7.1 Binary or crisp logic representation for the season statement

the season winter drawn at 31st March and 20th March is winter with the probability of one. In fuzzy logic, the function can take any shape. As the season example illustrated, with the Gaussian curve in Fig. 7.2, here, the X-axis is the universe of discourse which shows the range of all possible days for each month in a year for input. The Y-axis represents the degree of the membership function i.e. the fuzzy set of each season's day values into a corresponding membership degree. In fuzzy logic,

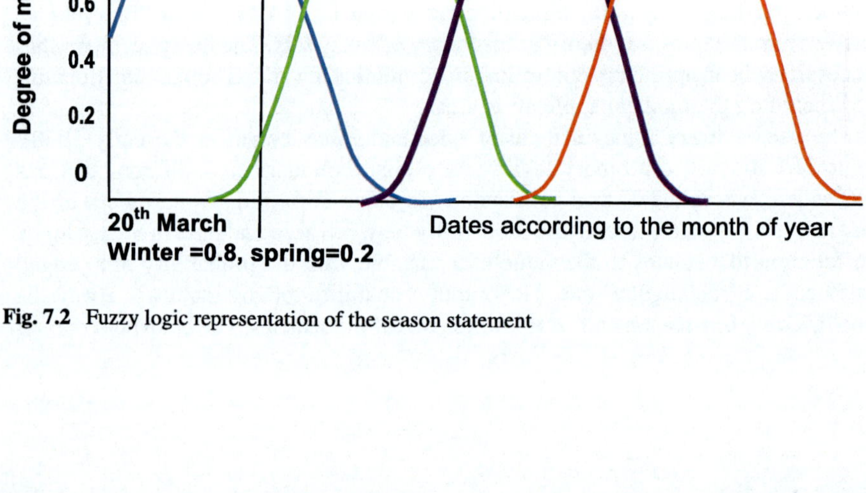

Fig. 7.2 Fuzzy logic representation of the season statement

the truth of any statement becomes a matter of degree. Considering the 20th March as an input in the fuzzy system, it is winter with the degree of truth 0.78 and at the same time spring with the degree of truth 0.22. So according to Zadeh [13], "*Fuzzy logic is determined as a set of mathematical principles for knowledge representation based on degrees of membership rather than on crisp membership of classical binary logic*".

7.3 Overview of Machine Learning (ML)

As stated earlier, simulation of humans' certain intelligent behaviour is AI, there are several ways to do this. For example, it can be a set of 'if-then statements', rules explicitly programmed by a human hand. Machine learning is a subset of AI and thus all machine learning counts as AI. According to –Tom Mitchell, 'a computer program is said to learn from experience E with respect to some class of tasks T and performance measure P if its performance at tasks in T, as measured by P, improves with experience E'. Machine learning provides automated data analysis and automates analytical model building by detecting patterns in the data. Machine learning methods can also predict the patterns of future data and aid in decision making under uncertainty [16]. When there is no analytical solution exists, but data are available in that problem domain then machine learning is useful to build an empirical solution. Arthur Lee Samuel in his experiment was teaching a machine to play the game of checkers, subsequently, machine learning research diverse to many areas where often the focus is to find relationships in data and analysing the processes for extracting such relations [9]. This book chapter focuses on the applications of machine learning, here, both supervised and unsupervised (e.g. clustering) are considered.

7.3.1 Supervised Machine Learning Algorithms

Supervised classification problems involve an input space (i.e., the instances of χ) and an output space (e.g., the labelling of Υ). An unknown target function $f : \chi \rightarrow \Upsilon$ defines the functional relationship between the input space and output space. As mentioned above, a dataset D exists containing input-output pairs $(\chi_1, \Upsilon_1), \ldots\ldots, (\chi_n, \Upsilon_n)$ drawn as an independent and identical distribution (i.i.d) from an unknown underlying distribution $P(\chi, \Upsilon)$. The goal is to find a function $g : \chi \rightarrow \Upsilon$ that can approximate the solution of f with minimum errors. The function $g : \chi \rightarrow \Upsilon$ is called a classifier [17].

7.3.1.1 Support Vector Machine (SVM)

The SVM is a supervised machine learning method first developed by Vapnik [18] and is now commonly used in pattern recognition: it can be used for both classification and regression purposes [19, 20]. An SVM finds the hyperplane that not only minimizes the empirical classification error but also maximizes the geometric margin of the classification [18]. SVM maps the original data points in the input space to a high dimensional feature space, making the classification problem simpler. Hence, SVM is suitable for classification problems with redundant datasets [21]. Consider an n-class classification problem with a training data set $\{\chi_i, \Upsilon_i\}_{i=1}^{n}$, where $\chi_i \in \mathbb{R}^d$ is the input vector, and Υ_i is the corresponding class label. The SVM maps the d-dimensional input vector space to a d_h-dimensional feature space and learns the separating hyperplane $\langle w, \chi \rangle + b = 0, b \in \mathbb{R}$ that maximizes the margin distance $\frac{2}{\|w_2^2\|}$, where w is a weight vector, and b is the bias. The SVM classifier obtains a new label $\hat{\Upsilon}$ for the test vector by evaluating Eq. (7.1):

$$\hat{\Upsilon} = \sum_{i=1}^{N} w_i.K(\chi, \chi_i) + b \tag{7.1}$$

where N is the number of support vectors, w_i are the weights, b is the bias that is maximized during training and K is the kernel function.

The solid line represents the optimal hyperplane, dotted line denotes maximal margin; circles and diamonds on the margin are the support vectors [22]. Here, w is the weight vector and b is the threshold such that $\Upsilon_i(\langle w, \chi_i \rangle + b) > 0 (i = 1, \ldots\ldots, N)$. In this study, the Radial Basis Function (RBF) kernel was used for classification. The RBF can be denoted as $K(\chi, \Upsilon) = exp\left(-\frac{\|\chi - \Upsilon^2\|}{2\sigma^2}\right)$, where σ is the variance of the Gaussian. An SVM with RBF is a weighted linear combination of the kernel function computed between the data points and each of the support vectors. Figure 7.3 depicts an example of binary classification with linear separability.

7.3.1.2 Random Forest (RF)

RF is a standard ensemble algorithm in machine learning that consists of a series of randomizing decision trees [23]. Each decision tree in the random forest is trained using bootstrap data samples, where bootstrapping is the process of creating samples with replacement. During the bootstrapping process, not all data are selected for training; the selected data are referred to as out-of-bag data, and these out-of-bag data are used to find the generalization error or the out-of-bag error. A generic architecture for a random forest classifier is shown in Fig. 7.4.

During the tree-generation process, for the k-th tree, a random vector υ_k is generated, which is drawn from the same data distribution but independent of previous

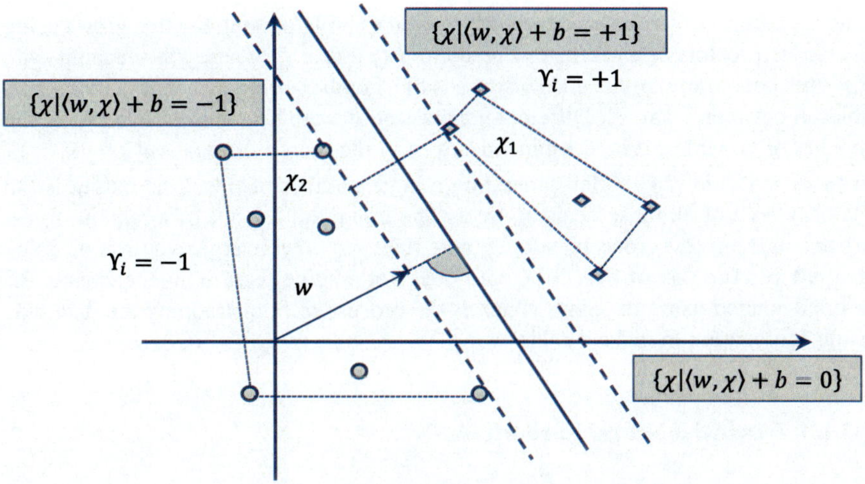

Fig. 7.3 An example of SVM separation of 2-dimensional binary class problem

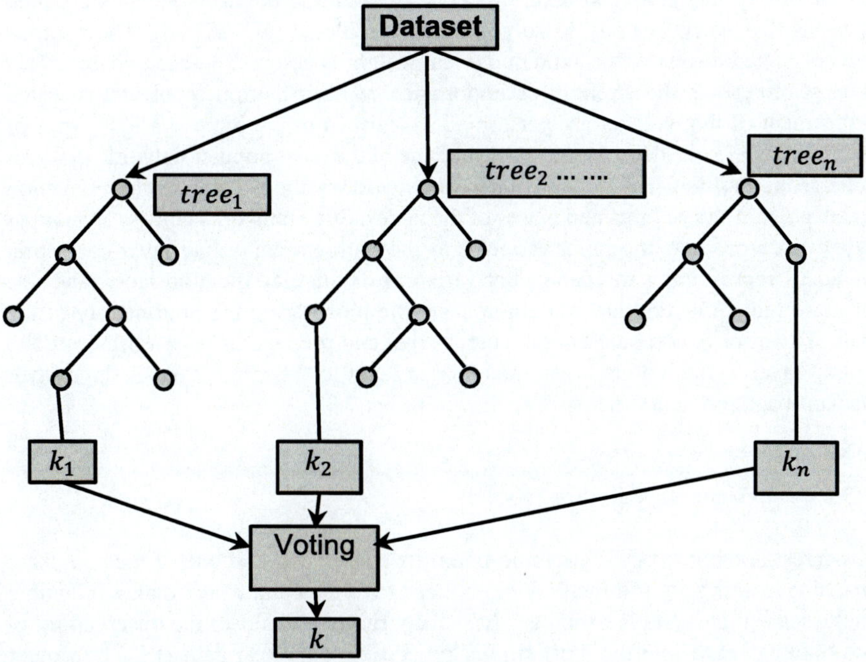

Fig. 7.4 Generic structure of random forest classification

random vectors $\upsilon_1, \ldots\ldots, \upsilon_{k-1}$. For the given training dataset, the tree grows using the random vectors υ_k and creates a predictor $h(\chi, X_k, \upsilon_k)$, where χ is the input data, X_k is the bootstrap sample, and υ_k consists of a number of independent random variables m between 1 and K. Different generalizations can be achieved by varying the number of variables; it is recommended to start the search from $m = \lfloor \log_2 K + 1 \rfloor$ or $m = \sqrt{K}$ [23, 24]. After generating a large number of trees, the output is the majority vote of all these decision trees. The important aspects of a random forest are that as the forest grows by adding more trees, it will converge to a limiting value that reduces the risk of overfitting and does not assume feature independence. RF is implemented using bagging, which is the process of bootstrapping the data plus using aggregation to make a decision.

7.3.1.3 Artificial Neural Network (ANN)

In the artificial intelligence paradigm, one of the most popular learning methods is the Artificial Neural Network (ANN). ANN is a method that is vaguely inspired by the biological nervous system. It is composed of interconnected elements called neurons that work in unity to solve specific problems [20, 25, 26]. The neurons are connected through links, and numerical weight is assigned to each neuron. This weight represents the strength or importance of each neuron input and repeated adjustment of the weights are performed to learn from the input. Various types of neural networks are described in [20], and one of the most popular network architectures is the multilayer feedforward neural network methods using backpropagation to adapt/learn the weights and biases of the nodes. Such networks consist of an input layer that represents the input variables to the problem, an output layer consisting of nodes representing the dependent variables or the classification label, and one or more hidden layers that contain nodes to help capturing the nonlinearity of the data. The error is computed at the output layer and propagates backwards from the output layer to the hidden layer, then hidden layer to the input layer. A three-layer backpropagation neural network is shown in Fig. 7.5.

7.3.1.4 K-Nearest Neighbor (K-NN)

K-nearest neighbor (k-NN) is a non-parametric approach and one of the simplistic machine learning algorithms. It does not need to fit the data, which makes it flexible in the sense that k-NN is a memory-based algorithm which uses the observations in the training set to find the most similar properties of the test dataset [27]. In other words, k-NN classifies an unseen instance using the observations that have closest match similarity (k-number nearest neighbors) to it. In the statistical settings, k-NN does not make any assumptions about the underlying joint probability density, rather uses the data to estimate the density.

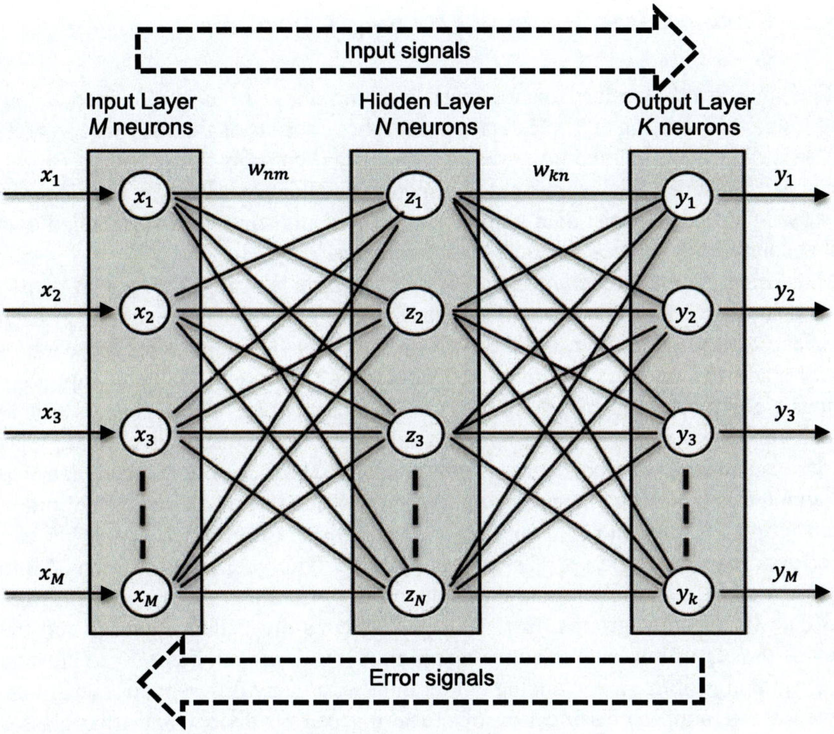

Fig. 7.5 Multi-layer perceptron with backpropagation [58]

In the k-NN algorithm a distance function e.g., the Euclidean distance function is often used to find the k most similar instances. Then methods like majority voting is used on the k-neighbor instaces that indicates most commonly occurring classification to make the final classification. The bias-variance trade-off of k-NN depends of the selection of k, i.e. the number of nearest neighbors to be considered. As the value of k gets larger the estimation smoothed out more. Since k-NN is based on a distance function, it is straightforward to explain the nearest-neighbour model when predicting a new unseen data. However, it may be difficult to explain what inherent knowledge the model has learned. Further, the assumption of closest similarity that is similar data shares similar classification has a drawback in high dimensional feature spaces i.e., similar data may not be close together in the high dimensional spaces. Thus, it requires to ensure that there are enough data that rationalize the dimensionality of the feature space and the data density.

7.3.2 Unsupervised Machine Learning Algorithms

Unlike supervised learning, unsupervised learning does not have a defined output space (e.g., the labelling of Υ). Here, the input space consists of a set of n observations $(\chi_1, \chi_2, \ldots\ldots \chi_n)$ of a random ρ-vector χ that has joint probability density $Pr(\chi)$. The goal of unsupervised learning is to directly infer this probability density i.e., the underlying structure in the data without the help of any supervisor or labelled data Υ that can tell the degree-of-error for each observation [17].

Clustering is an approach of unsupervised machine learning that a set of data is divided into several subsets where the data within one subset are similar to each other and are different from the data of other subsets. The clustering approach or cluster analysis is not an algorithm itself rather it is a task to be solved by applying various algorithms. A formal definition can be presented as "These clusters should reflect some mechanism at work in the domain from which instances or data points are drawn, a mechanism that causes some instances to bear a stronger resemblance to one another than they do to the remaining instances" [28]. A mathematical definition of clustering as stated in [29], which can be express as follows: let $X \in R^{m \times n}$ in a set of data representing a set of m points x_i in R^n. The goal is to partition X into K groups and C_k so that all data that belongs to the same group are more "alike" than data in different groups. Each of the K groups are called a cluster and the result of the algorithm is an injective mapping $X \rightarrow C$ of data items X_i to clusters C_k. Several algorithms are available in literature with many different classifications. However, one simple classification of clustering can be divided into two classes as: (1) parametric and (2) non-parametric clustering. *Parametric* clustering helps to minimize a cost function where the main goal of this kind of algorithm is to solve an optimization problem in a satisfactory level imposed by the model. However, this algorithm requires a better understanding about data distribution and a proper probability distribution. This class can be further divided into two groups: (a) generative or probability-based model and (b) reconstructive models. In the probability-based model, the model relies on a guess that the data comes from a known distribution, but this is not true for many situations. So, this model cannot be usefully applied where the probability distribution is not known and/or the data are not numerical. The Gaussian mixture model is one example of such model. However, a proper probability distribution in data can be achieved using this algorithm. On the other hand, the reconstructive model aims to minimize the cost function. A most common and basic algorithm is K-means as an example of reconstructive models. For *non-parametric* clustering, the hierarchical algorithms or an agglomerative and divisive algorithm is a good example. The algorithm works based on dis-similarities among the current clusters for each iteration. The agglomerative algorithm merges and the divisive algorithm divides the clusters depending on similarities. Both of them also produce dendrograms, which presents clusters in a tree structure as bottom up or top down. A detailed elaboration of parametric and non-parametric clustering can be found in [30] and the difference between parametric and non-parametric clustering can be summarized in Table 7.1.

Table 7.1 Comparison of parametric and non-parametric clustering

Criteria	Parametric	Non-parametric
Algorithm	Optimises a cost function Most costs are NP-hard problem Assumes more detailed knowledge of cluster Assumes K is known Gets harder with larger K Older, more widely used and studied	Density-based method No cost functions Does not depend on initialisation K and outliers selected automatically Requires hyper-parameters
When to use	Shape of clusters is known K not too large or known Clusters of comparable size	Shape of cluster is arbitrary K is large or has many outliers Cluster size in large range Lots of data

A summary of the 4 common and well-known clustering algorithms (1) K-means clustering, (2) Fuzzy C-means clustering, (3) Gaussian mixer model and (4) Hierarchical clustering are presented here.

7.3.2.1 K-Means Clustering

K-means clustering expresses groups in a numeric domain and partitions data samples in disjointed groups. The main objective of the algorithm is to minimize the cost objective function and it requires the number of clusters and its initial centre points. The centre points can be given manually or randomly in the initial stage of the algorithm and later in each iteration the algorithm will automatically adjust in order to minimize the value of the distance matrix. Considering the distance matrix values, each iteration is repeated and as soon as the two distance values (previous and next) become the same, the algorithm stops. The Euclidean distance function is used in this algorithm in most of the cases and performance of the algorithm is strongly depends on the distance value. Although the algorithm is easy to implement and takes less time to compute compared to others, it has a drawback that it can be stuck in a local minimum since the algorithm depends on the provided initial centre point. The procedure starts work by giving a set of initial cluster numbers and the centre points for each cluster. Then the centre points are replaced by the mean point for each cluster. These steps are repeated until the two distances become the same. The algorithm can be illustrated as below [31]:

- Step 1. Choose K initial cluster centres $Z_1, Z_2, \ldots\ldots, Z_k$ randomly from the n points $\{X_1, X_2, \ldots\ldots, X_n\}$.
- Step 2. Assign point $X_i, i = 1, 2, \ldots\ldots, n$ to the cluster $C_j, j \in \{1, 2, \ldots\ldots, K\}$, if

$$\|X_i - z_j\| \leqq \|X_i - z_p\|, p = 1, 2, \ldots\ldots, K \text{ and } j \neq p$$

- Step 3. Calculate new cluster centers:

$$z_i^{new} = \frac{1}{n_i} \sum_{x_i \in C_i} X_j, i = 1, 2, \ldots, K$$

- Step 4. Continue step 2 and 3 and if $\left\| z_i^{new} - z_i \right\| < \varepsilon, i = 1, 2, \ldots\ldots, K$ then stop.

7.3.2.2 Fuzzy C-Means (FCM) Clustering

FCM is also referred to as soft clustering; it is an unsupervised clustering algorithm that has been applied to a wide range of problems involving feature analysis, clustering and classifier designs. It is similar in structure to the K-means algorithm and also behaves in a similar way [32, 33] except that fuzzy behaviour is also considered. It is a clustering algorithm where each data point belongs to a cluster to a degree specified by a membership grade whereas traditional clustering algorithms assign each data point to one and only one cluster. It is a clustering method that allows one piece of data to belong to two or more clusters. It associates each element that represents a set of membership levels. Thus, it creates the concept of fuzzy boundaries which is opposite from the traditional concept of well-defined boundaries. The algorithm is presented in several steps in Fig. 7.6.

Step 1: U=[u$_{ij}$] matrix is initialize, $U^{(0)}$
Step 2: At k-step: calculate the centre vectors $C^{(k)}$=[c$_j$] with $U^{(k)}$
Step 3: Update $U^{(k)}$, $U^{(k+1)}$
Step 4: If $\| U^{(k+1)} - U^{(k)} \| < \delta$ then STOP; otherwise return to the step 2,

where m is any real number greater than 1, u_{ij} is the degree of membership of x_i in the cluster j, x_i is the ith of d-dimensional measured data, c_j is the d-dimension centre of the cluster, and ||*|| is any norm expressing the similarity between any measured data and the centre. The equation of the cluster centres c_j and the updated membership matrix function u_{ij} are given bellow:

$$c_j = \left(\sum_{i=1}^{N} u_{ij}^m . x_i\right) / \sum_{i=1}^{N} u_{ij}^m \quad \text{and} \quad u_{ij} = \frac{1}{\sum_{k=1}^{c} \left(\| x_i - c_j \| / \| x_i - c_k \| \right)^{2/(m-1)}}$$

Fig. 7.6 Steps of the FCM clustering technique are taken from [33]

7.3.2.3 Gaussian Mixer Model

It is an example of a generative model where data are presented by a calculated Gaussian Mixture distribution of data points. Each distribution represents a different cluster and during clustering it computes the expectation maximisation of a data point. It is associated with fitting a set of data and identifies a set of Gaussian distribution that presents the highest probability for the data. The data is fitted using an expected maximisation algorithm that assigns probability to each component based on individual observations. This probability is sometimes also called as membership score or rank. Each data point has a membership score of belonging to each cluster. It appears to solve many problems related to other clustering techniques and has been identifying as yielding a more stable cluster especially when the requested number of clusters changes. The details of the model and the basic algorithm can be found in [30].

7.3.2.4 Hierarchical Clustering

The algorithm clusters data over a variety of scales by creating a hierarchical structure (tree) or dendrogram. The tree is not a single set of clusters, but rather a multilevel hierarchy, where clusters at one level are joined with clusters at the next level [34]. It is then further divided into two categories; bottom up i.e. agglomerative and the top down i.e. divisive clustering. This algorithm does not require any initialisation of centre points. To group the data together, a suitable proximity measure is used that estimates firstly the similarity between points and secondly the similarity between groups of points. It has several advantages, such as it starts with the number of clusters equal to the population of the initial data points then through an iterative process of grouping similar data points it finally ends up with a single cluster containing all the given data points. It makes it easy to catch the distance between clusters. If the agglomeration occurs between clusters at a greater distance than the previous agglomeration, one can decide whether to stop when the clusters are too far apart or when there is a sufficiently small number of clusters. However, it is not very efficient when it comes to dealing with large data. To perform agglomerative hierarchical clustering on a data set the algorithm uses the following procedures:

1. It calculates the distance between every pair of objects in the data set in order to find similarity or dissimilarity.
2. It collects or groups the objects into a binary, hierarchical cluster tree. Here, pairs of objects that are close to each other are linked. Since all the objects are paired into the binary clusters, newly formed clusters are grouped to larger clusters until a hierarchical tree is formed.
3. It determines the cutting position of the hierarchical tree into clusters. Here, it prunes the branches off at the bottom of the hierarchical tree and assigns all the objects below the cutting point to a single cluster.

In the hierarchical algorithm, the distance between pairs of objects is generally calculated using Euclidean distance. However, there are some other distance functions which can be used and available in MATLAB function 'pdist', such as Standardised Euclidean distance, cityblock, cosine, hamming, jaccard etc. Similarly, the linkage function applies 'single' (i.e. shortage distances) as a default parameter which determines the objects in the data set that should be grouped into clusters. However, other linkages can be used and available in MATLAB, such as average, centroid, complete etc. [30]. Finally, a cluster function is applied to group the sample data set into clusters where it specifies the cluster's number.

7.4 Overview of Machine Reasoning (MR)

A program or software in a machine or a computer system that can perform reasoning to generate a conclusion form a knowledgebase using some logic or decision i.e. IF-THEN rules. This is an important area of AI approach to develop decision support systems [35]. According to Léon Bottou, machine reasoning is "A plausible definition of 'reasoning' could be algebraically manipulating previously acquired knowledge in order to answer a new question." [36]. Similarly, Jerry Kaplan, describes the reasoning systems with two basic components including "knowledge base"—a collection of facts, rules and relationships and a "inference engine" that described how to manipulate [37].

7.4.1 Fuzzy Rule-Based Reasoning (RBR)

Fuzzy Rule-Based Reasoning is a combination of the fuzzy logic approach with traditional Rule Based Reasoning (RBR) which is also called Fuzzy Inference Systems (FIS). Fuzzy inference is a computer paradigm based on fuzzy set theory, fuzzy if-then-rules and fuzzy reasoning. A traditional RBR system contains a set of if-then rules in a crisp format. A general form of a rule is "If < antecedent > then < consequence>". An example of such a rule is; "If speed is > 100 then stopping distance is 100 meters". In 1973, Lotfi Zadeh outlined a new approach to analyse complex systems, where human knowledge is captured as fuzzy rules [13, 38]. A fuzzy rule is a linguistic expression of causal dependencies between linguistic variables in the form of if-then conditional statements. If we consider the previous example in a fuzzy format "If *speed* is ***fast,*** then stopping *distance* is ***long***". Here the term '*speed*' and '*distance*' are linguistic variables, while '***fast***' and '***long***' are linguistic values determined by fuzzy sets. Therefore '*speed* is ***fast***' is the antecedent and 'stopping *distance* is ***long***' is the consequence [13, 14].

Fuzzy decision making or inference systems can be defined as a process of mapping a given input to an output with the help of the fuzzy set theory i.e. fuzzification $\rightarrow$ fuzzy reasoning $\rightarrow$ defuzzification [15]. Well known inference systems are

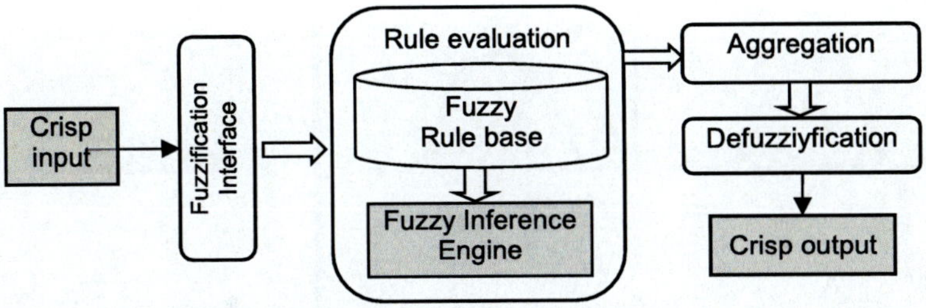

Fig. 7.7 Steps in a Fuzzy Inference System (FIS)

the Mamdani-style and Sugeno-style but both of them perform the 4-step process as described in Fig. 7.7 which illustrates the steps of a fuzzy inference system for the Mamdani-style. Here, the *step1* is the fuzzification of an input variable i.e. crisp input is fuzzified against appropriate fuzzy sets. Given an input in a crisp format, *step1* computes the membership degree with respect to its linguistic terms. Consequently, each input variable is fuzzified over all the Membership Functions (*MF*s) used by the fuzzy rules. In a traditional rule-based system, if the antecedent part of a rule is true then the consequent part is also true. But in a fuzzy system, the rules are met to some extent. If the antecedent is true to some degree of membership, then the consequent is also true to that degree. *Step2* is the rule evaluation where it takes fuzzified inputs and applies them to the antecedent part of the fuzzy rules. So, it compares facts with the antecedents of the fuzzy rules to find degrees of compatibility. The value or firing strength is a single number from each rule represented in the result of the antecedent evaluation. This number is then applied to generate consequent MFs. Aggregation in *step3* is the process that merges all the output MFs for all the rules i.e. all outputs are combined into a single fuzzy set. The last and final phase (*step4*) in the inference process is defuzzification that determines a crisp value from the output membership function as a solution. The input for defuzzification is the aggregate fuzzy set and the output is a single number.

A simple example of fuzzy inference with multiple rules and multiple antecedents is illustrated in Fig. 7.8. The rules and inputs are as follows: *Rule 1*: if x is A_1 and y is B_1 then z is C_1 and *Rule 2*: if x is A_2 and y is B_2 then z is C_2; Inputs: x is A and y is B then z is C (?). First the inputted crisp values (A and B) are converted into the fuzzy sets A' and B'. Then for the rule R_1 and R_2, A' and B' are fuzzified with the fuzzy sets A_1, B_1 and A_2, B_2. The dotted line in Fig. 7.6 presents the clipped area of the membership functions in the antecedent part of the rules. As the rules contain multiple antecedents with AND operators, fuzzy intersection is used to obtain a single number that represents the evaluation result of the antecedents. W_1 and W_2 are the evaluation results applied to the MFs in the consequent part of the rules. Upward and downward diagonal patterns in the fuzzy sets C_1 and C_2 show the firing strengths for the rule's evaluation. After aggregation, the clipped fuzzy set C_1 and C_2, and the new fuzzy set C' are obtained. A defuzzification algorithm could convert this fuzzy

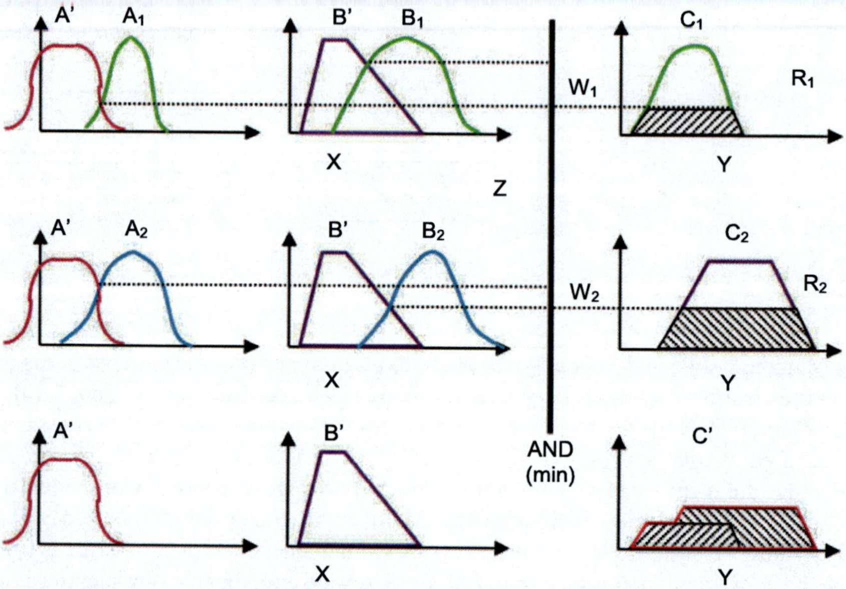

Fig. 7.8 Graphical representation of an example of fuzzy inference

set into a crisp value which is a single number that represents the final output [15, 38].

7.4.2 Case-Based Reasoning (CBR)

Case-Based Reasoning (CBR) is a problem-solving method that gives priority to past experiences for solving current problems (solutions for current problems can be found by reusing or adapting the solutions to problems which have been solved in the past). Riesbeck and Schank presented CBR as, "A case-based reasoner solves new problems by adapting solutions that were used to solve old problems" [39]. The CBR method in a problem solving context can be described as follows: (1) given a particular problem case, the similarity of this problem with the stored problems in a case library (or memory) is calculated (2) one or more most similar matching cases are retrieved according to their similarity values (3) the solution of one of the retrieved problems is suggested for reuse by doing revision or possible adaptation (if needed e.g. due to differences in problem descriptions) (4) finally, the current problem case and its corresponding solution can be retained as a new solved case for further use [40]. The root of CBR can be traced from the work of Schank and his student at Yale University in the early 1980s but Watson presented in [41] that the research of CBR began in 1977. CYRUS [42, 43] developed by Janet Kolodner, is the basic and earliest CBR system. She employed knowledge as cases and used an indexed memory structure. Other early CBR systems such as CASEY [44] and MEDIATOR [45] have been implemented based on CYRUS.

In the medical domain around the 1980s, early CBR systems were developed by Konton [44], and Braeiss [46, 47]. According to Kolodner in [48] a case is a "contextualised piece of knowledge representing experience that teaches a lesson fundamental to achieving the goals of the reasoner". The *problem* part describes the condition of a case and the *solution* part presents advice or a recommendation to solve a problem. A comprehensive case structure has been proposed by Kolodner in [43] as follows: (1) a state with goal, (2) the solution (3) the outcome (4) explanations of results and (5) lessons learned. Further ahead, Bergmann et al. [49] classified case representation in the following three categories: (a) feature vector representations or propositional cases (b) structured representations or relational cases, and (c) textual representations or semi-structure cases [49].

A schematic or lifecycle that presents the key processes involved in the CBR method is shown in Fig. 7.9. Aamodt and Plaza [50] have introduced a four-step model of CBR in a cyclical process comprising the four REs: Retrieve, Reuse, Revise and Retain. Retrieval is essential since it plays a vital role for calculating the similarity of two cases. The similarity value between cases is usually represented as 0 to 1 or 0 to 100, where "0" means no match and "1 or 100" means a perfect match. One of the most common and well-known retrieval methods is the *nearest neighbour* (or kNN) [51] which is based on the matching of a weighted sum of the features. For a feature vector, local similarity is computed by comparing each feature value and a global similarity value is obtained as a weighted calculation of the local similarities. A standard equation for the nearest-neighbour calculation is illustrated in Eq. (7.2):

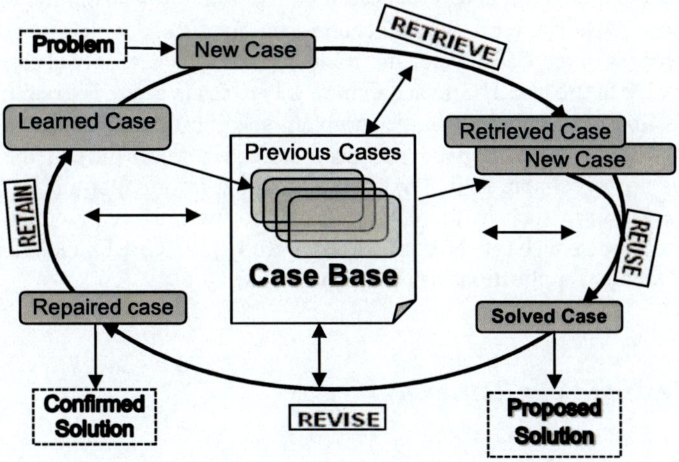

Fig. 7.9 CBR cycle. The figure is introduced by Aamodt and Plaza [50]

$$Similarity(T, S) = \frac{\sum_{i=1}^{n} f(T_i, S_i) \times w_i}{\sum_{i=1}^{n} w_i} \quad (7.2)$$

In Eq. (7.2):

T is the target case
S is the source case
n is the number of attributes in each case
i is an individual attribute from 1 *to n*
f is a similarity function for attribute i in cases T and S
w is the importance for weighing of attribute i.

The weights allocated to each feature/attribute provide them a range of importance. But determining the weight for a feature value is a problem and the easy way is to calibrate this weight by an expert or user in terms of the domain knowledge. However, it may also be determined by an adaptive learning process i.e. learning or optimizing weights from the case library as an information source. The *Reuse* step is reusing one of the retrieved cases from the case library and returning it as the proposed solution for a current case. But in some cases, this phase can become more difficult, especially when there are notorious differences between the current case and the closest one retrieved. An *adaptation* of the obtained solution is required in order to provide a solution for the current problem. For adaptation, it could calculate the differences between the retrieved case and the current case. Then it is possible to apply algorithms or rules that take the differences into account to suggest a solution. This adaptation could be done by an expert/user in the domain. The expert determines if it is a reasonable solution to the problem and they can modify the solution before approval. After that the case is sent to the *Revise* step where the solution is verified and evaluated for the correctness and presented as a confirmed solution to the new problem case [51]. The term *Retain* becomes the final stage which functions as a learning process in the CBR cycle, and it incorporates the new solved case into the case library for future use. The most common way to retain a case is to simply record the information concerning the target problem specification and its final solution (assuming that the solution given was accurate and correct) [40]. If the solution retrieved is not as reliable as it should be, additional information might be stored into the case library such as the changes made to the retrieved solution. So, the information to be saved has to be considered carefully [52]. CBR is applied in a large number of medical applications as presented in [53].

7.4.3 Textual Case Retrieval

Bergmann et al. [49] have proposed that a case could be represented as a textual or semi-structural format. Textual case retrieval could be defined as matching a user query against a bunch of free-text cases. Text retrieval is a branch of Information Retrieval (IR) if the information is stored in the form of text. IR is a science used for searching documents and/or for information within a document or metadata about the document. In this research the knowledge of IR is used to search and retrieve cases with features containing information in a textual format. The idea of this process begins when a query is entered by a user into the system through a user interface. Then the system extracts information from the query. The extracted features may match with several objects (cases) in the collection (case library) with different degree of relevance. The degree of relevance can be computed by the system as a numerical value that shows how well each case is matched with the query. Finally, according to this numerical value, all the cases will be sorted, and the top ranked cases will be presented to the user [54]. There are several ways to find a match between a user query and the stored cases, such as Boolean model, fuzzy retrieval, vector space model, binary retrieval etc. [54]. The Vector Space Model (VSM) [55] is the most common and well-known method that has been used in information retrieval.

VSM or term vector model is an algebraic model that represents textual cases in a vector of terms. It identifies similarity between a query case Q and the stored cases C_i. One of the best-known schemes is the *tf-idf* (term frequency—inverse document frequency) [56] weighting used together with cosine similarity [57] in the vector space model [55] where the word "document" is treated as a case. The *tf-idf* is a traditional weighting algorithm and is often used in information and/or textual retrieval. The similarity/relevancy is measured from the cosine angle between a query case Q and the stored cases C_i inside a vector i.e. a deviation of angles between the case vectors. "$\cos\theta = \frac{Q.C_i}{\|Q\|\|C_i\|}$" is a general equation to calculate the cosine similarity where $Q.C_i$ is the dot product and $\| Q \| \| C_i \|$ is the magnitude of the vectors (a query and the stored case), i is the index of the cases in the case library. The value of the similarity lies in the range of -1 to $+1$, where -1 means no matching and $+1$ means exactly the same. In terms of IR, the cosine similarity of two cases will range from 0 to 1, since the *tf-idf* weights cannot be negative. The final result 1 is a full match and 0 means no words match between Q and C_i. To measure the similarity we need two things, the weight of each term in each case and the cosine similarity between the cases inside a vector space.

The terms are words, keywords, or long phrases in a case and the dimension of the vector is the number or frequency of each term in the vocabulary of cases. If a term occurs in a case the value will be non-zero in the vector. Each word *tf* is the relative frequency of the word in a specific case (document represent as a case) and it presents the importance of the word inside the case. *idf* is the inverse proportion of the word over the whole case corpus which presents the importance of the word over the entire case pool. The weight vector for a case c is $V_c = \left[w_{1,c}, w_{2,c}, \ldots, w_{N,c}\right]^T$ and $w_{t,c} = tf_t . \log \frac{|C|}{|\{t \in c\}|}$ where tf_t is the term frequency or the number of times a term/word t occurs in a case c and is the inverse case frequency. The symbol "$|C|$" is the total number of cases in the case library and $|\{t \in c\}|$ is the number of the cases containing the term t i.e. case frequency.

7.5 Summary and Discussion

This book chapter presents some methods on AI, ML and MR those can be applied in health informatics domain to develop DSS. Here, fuzzy logic can be used to handle uncertainty issues in decision-making tasks, an example of a Parkinson disease application domain with fuzzy logic with rules is presented in the case study chapter. Some well-known machine learning methods both considering supervised and unsupervised are also presented, for example, kNN, SVM, ANN and RF are presented as supervised machine learning algorithms. For unsupervised learning, several clustering approaches are presented, such as K-means, Fuzzy C-means, Gaussian mixer model and Hierarchical. Also, the definition of parametric and non-parametric clustering together with their comparison is presented. Three different approaches to machine reasoning is discussed, such as fuzzy RBR, CBR, and textual case retrieval. Applications of such ML and MR in health informatics domains are presented in the use-case study chapter. It has been observed not a single method is enough to develop a DSS and most common is to combine more than one method as in a hybrid manner. Due to the multi-faceted and complex nature of the health informatics domains, it is necessary to design such hybrid systems that can handle several challenges associated with multi-modal machine learning.

References

1. Begum, S., Ahmed, M.U., Funk, P., Xiong, N., Von Schéele, B.: A case-based decision support system for individual stress diagnosis using fuzzy similarity matching. Comput. Intell. **25**(3), 180–195 (2009). https://doi.org/10.1111/j.1467-8640.2009.00337.x
2. Corchado, J.M., Bajo, J., Abraham, A.: GerAmi: improving healthcare delivery in geriatric residences. IEEE Intell. Syst. **23**(2), 19–25 (2008). https://doi.org/10.1109/MIS.2008.27
3. Marling, C., Whitehouse, P.: Case-based reasoning in the care of Alzheimer's disease patients. Case-Based Reasoning Research and Development, pp. 702–715. Springer, Berlin Heidelberg (2001)
4. Marling, C., Shubrook, J., Schwartz, F.: Case-based decision support for patients with type 1 diabetes on insulin pump therapy. Advances in Case-Based Reasoning, pp. 325–339. Springer, Berlin Heidelberg (2008)
5. Marling, C., Wiley, M., Cooper, T., Bunescu, R., Shubrook, J., Schwartz, F.: The 4 diabetes support system: a case study in CBR research and development. In: Case-Based Reasoning Research and Development, pp 137–150. Springer, Berlin Heidelberg (2011)
6. Montani, S.: Exploring new roles for case-based reasoning in heterogeneous AI systems for medical decision support. Appl. Intell. **28**(3), 275–285 (2008). https://doi.org/10.1007/s10489-007-0046-2
7. Nilsson, M., Funk, P., Olsson, E.M.G., von Schéele, B., Xiong, N.: Clinical decision-support for diagnosing stress-related disorders by applying psychophysiological medical knowledge to an instance-based learning system. Artif. Intell. Med. **36**(2), 159–176 (2006). https://doi.org/10.1016/j.artmed.2005.04.004
8. Baltrušaitis, T., Ahuja, C., Morency, L.-P.: Multimodal machine learning: a survey and taxonomy. IEEE Trans. Pattern Anal. Mach. Intell. (2018)
9. Samuel, A.L.: Some studies in machine learning using the game of checkers. IBM J. Res. Dev. **3**(3), 210–229 (1959). https://doi.org/10.1147/rd.33.0210

10. Salmani, D., Akbari, M.: Fuzzy and research paradigms relationship: a mutual contribution. Acad. Leader. Online J. **6**(2), 7 (2008)
11. Lukasiewicz, J.: Logical foundations of probability theory. Jan Lukasiewicz, Selected Works, pp. 16–63 (1970)
12. Łukasiewicz, J.: A system of modal logic. In: Proceedings of the 11th International Congress of Philosophy vol. 14, pp. 82–87 (1953)
13. Zadeh, L.A.: Fuzzy sets. Inf. Control **8**(3), 338–353 (1965). https://doi.org/10.1016/S0019-9958(65)90241-X
14. Marks-II, R., Zadeh, L.: Fuzzy logic technology and applications. IEEE Technological Activities Board (1994)
15. Jang, J-S.R., Sun, C.-T.: Neuro-Fuzzy and Soft Computing: a Computational Approach to Learning and Machine Intelligence. Prentice-Hall, Inc., (1997)
16. Robert, C.: Machine Learning, a Probabilistic Perspective. Taylor & Francis (2014)
17. Friedman, J., Hastie, T., Tibshirani, R.: The Elements of Statistical Learning, vol 1. vol 10. Springer, New York (2001)
18. Vapnik, V.N.: Principles of risk minimization for learning theory. Adv. Neural. Inf. Process. Syst. **4**, 831–838 (1992). doi.org/citeulike-article-id:431737
19. Jain, A.K., Duin, R.P.W., Jianchang, M.: Statistical pattern recognition: a review. IEEE Trans. Pattern Anal. Mach. Intell. IEEE Trans. **22**(1), 4–37 (2000). https://doi.org/10.1109/34.824819
20. Basheer, I.A., Hajmeer, M.: Artificial neural networks: fundamentals, computing, design, and application. J. Microbiol. Methods **43**(1), 3–31 (2000). https://doi.org/10.1016/S0167-7012(00)00201-3
21. Guyon, I., Weston, J., Barnhill, S., Vapnik, V.: Gene selection for cancer classification using support vector machines. Mach. Learn. **46**(1), 389–422 (2002). https://doi.org/10.1023/a:1012487302797
22. Hearst, M.A., Dumais, S.T., Osuna, E., Platt, J., Scholkopf, B.: Support vector machines. IEEE Intell. Syst. Appl. **13**(4), 18–28 (1998). https://doi.org/10.1109/5254.708428
23. Breiman, L.: Random forests. Mach. Learn. **45**(1), 5–32 (2001)
24. Breiman, L.: Bagging predictors. Mach. Learn. **24**(2), 123–140 (1996). https://doi.org/10.1023/a:1018054314350
25. Drew, P.J., Monson, J.R.T.: Artificial neural networks. Surgery **127**(1), 3–11 (2000). https://doi.org/10.1067/msy.2000.102173
26. Zhang, G.P.: Neural networks for classification: a survey. Syst. Man Cybern. Part C Appl. Rev. IEEE Trans. **30**(4), 451–462 (2000). https://doi.org/10.1109/5326.897072
27. Larose, D.T.: k-nearest neighbor algorithm. In: Discovering Knowledge in Data. Wiley, pp 90–106 (2005). https://doi.org/10.1002/0471687545.ch5
28. Witten, I.H., Frank, E., Hall, M.A., Pal, C.J.: Data Mining: Practical Machine Learning Tools and Techniques. Morgan Kaufmann (2016)
29. Graepel, T.: Statistical physics of clustering algorithms. Technical Re-port 171822 (1998)
30. Fung, G.: A comprehensive overview of basic clustering algorithms (2001)
31. Guldemır, H., Sengur, A.: Comparison of clustering algorithms for analog modulation classification. Expert Syst. Appl. **30**(4), 642–649 (2006)
32. Chuai-Aree, S., Lursinsap, C., Sophasathit, P., Siripant, S.: Fuzzy c-mean: a statistical feature classification of text and image segmentation method. Int. J. Uncertainty Fuzziness Knowl. Based Syst. **9**(06), 661–671 (2001)
33. Velmurugan, T., Santhanam, T.: Performance evaluation of k-means and fuzzy c-means clustering algorithms for statistical distributions of input data points. Eur. J. Sci. Res. **46**(3), 320–330 (2010)
34. Chen, G., Jaradat, S.A., Banerjee, N., Tanaka, T.S., Ko, M.S., Zhang, M.Q.: Evaluation and comparison of clustering algorithms in analyzing ES cell gene expression data. Statistica Sinica 241–262 (2002)
35. Wos, L., Overbeck, R., Lusk, E., Boyle, J.: Automated Reasoning: Introduction and Applications. Prentice Hall Professional Technical Reference (1984)
36. Bottou, L.: From machine learning to machine reasoning. Mach. Learn. **94**(2), 133–149 (2014)

37. Kaplan, J.: Artificial Intelligence: What Everyone Needs to Know. Oxford Univcrsity Prcss, Oxford (2016)
38. Zadeh, L.A.: Outline of a new approach to the analysis of complex systems and decision processes. IEEE Trans. Syst. Man Cybern. SMC **3**(1), 28–44 (1973). https://doi.org/10.1109/tsmc.1973.5408575
39. Riesbeck, C.K., Schank, R.C.: Inside Case-Based Reasoning. L. Erlbaum Associates Inc. (1989)
40. Lopez De Mantaras, R., Mcsherry, D., Bridge, D., Leake, D., Smyth, B., Craw, S., Faltings, B., Maher, M.L., Cox, M.T., Forbus, K., Keane, M., Aamodt, A., Watson, I.: Retrieval, reuse, revision and retention in case-based reasoning. Knowl. Eng. Rev. **20**(03), 215–240 (2005). https://doi.org/10.1017/S0269888906000646
41. Watson, I., Perera, S.: Case-based design: a review and analysis of building design applications. AI EDAM **11**(01), 59–87 (1997). https://doi.org/10.1017/S0890060400001840
42. Kolodner, J.L.: Reconstructive memory: a computer model. Cogn. Sci. **7**(4), 281–328 (1983). https://doi.org/10.1016/S0364-0213(83)80002-0
43. Kolodner, J.: Case-Based Reasoning. Morgan Kaufmann (2014)
44. Koton, P.A.: Using Experience in Learning and Problem Solving. Massachusetts Institute of Technology (1988)
45. Simpson, Jr R.L.: A computer model of case-based reasoning in problem solving: an investigation in the domain of dispute mediation. AIR FORCE INST OF TECH WRIGHT-PATTERSON AFB OH (1985)
46. Bareiss, R.: Exemplar-Based Knowledge Acquisition: A Unified Approach to Concept Representation, Classification, and Learning, vol. 2. Academic Press, London (2014)
47. Bareiss, E.: Protos: a unified approach to concept representation, classification, and learning (1989)
48. Lindgaard, G.: Intelligent decision support in medicine: back to bayes? In: Proceedings of the 14th European conference on Cognitive ergonomics: invent! explore!, ACM, pp 7–8 (2007)
49. Bergmann, R., Kolodner, J., Plaza, E.: Representation in case-based reasoning. Knowl. Eng. Rev. **20**(3), 209–213 (2005). https://doi.org/10.1017/s0269888906000555
50. Aamodt, A., Plaza, E.: Case-based reasoning: foundational issues, methodological variations, and system approaches. AI Commun **7**(1), 39–59 (1994)
51. Watson, I.: Applying Case-Based Reasoning: Techniques for Enterprise Systems. Morgan Kaufmann Publishers Inc. (1998)
52. Ontañón, S., Plaza, E.: Collaborative case retention strategies for CBR agents. In: Paper presented at the Proceedings of the 5th international conference on Case-based reasoning: Research and Development, Trondheim, Norway (2003)
53. Begum, S., Ahmed, M.U., Funk, P., Ning, X., Folke, M.: Case-based reasoning systems in the health sciences: a survey of recent trends and developments. Syst. Man Cybernetics Part C Appl. Rev. IEEE Trans. **41**(4), 421–434 (2011). https://doi.org/10.1109/TSMCC.2010.2071862
54. Singhal, A.: Modern information retrieval: a brief overview. IEEE Data Eng. Bull. **24**(4), 35–43 (2001)
55. Salton, G., Wong, A., Yang, C.S.: A vector space model for automatic indexing. Commun. ACM **18**(11), 613–620 (1975). https://doi.org/10.1145/361219.361220
56. Salton, G., Buckley, C.: Term-weighting approaches in automatic text retrieval. Inf. Process. Manage. **24**(5), 513–523 (1988). https://doi.org/10.1016/0306-4573(88)90021-0
57. Weber, R.O., Ashley, K.D., BrÜNinghaus, S.: Textual case-based reasoning. Knowl. Eng. Rev. **20**(3), 255–260 (2005). https://doi.org/10.1017/S0269888906000713
58. Negnevitsky, M.: Artificial Intelligence: A Guide to Intelligent Systems. Addison-Wesley Longman Publishing Co., Inc., (2001)

Chapter 8
Health Information Retrieval

Md Shajalal and Masaki Aono

Abstract Searching health-related information on the Web has been increasing in the recent past. The methodologies and techniques to access and/or retrieve information related to health using the process of information retrieval are referred to Health Information Retrieval (HIR). In other words, a health information retrieval system produces a ranking of relevant documents that covers users' information needs underlying health-related query. In this chapter, we present the noticeable challenges in health IR, the most prominent existing methods to solve the problems and future directions. The methods and techniques for health information retrieval are generally categorized into (a) general classical retrieval models and (b) advanced re-ranking techniques. This chapter also presents the details of the datasets, evaluation metrics and procedures to validate the performance of any HIR methods.

Keywords Health information retrieval · Query reformulation · Document diversity · Document ranking

8.1 Introduction

The methodologies and techniques to access and/or retrieve information related to the health using the process of information retrieval are referred to health information retrieval (HIR) [1]. As the information in the Web is rapidly increasing, people generally are seeking and accessing required information using the commercial search engines by expressing their search intention through some keywords which

M. Shajalal (✉)
Department of Computer Science and Engineering, Hajee Mohammad Danesh Science and Technology University, Dinajpur 5200, Bangladesh
e-mail: shajalal@hstu.ac.bd

M. Aono
Department of Computer Science and Engineering, Toyohashi University of Technology, Toyohashi, Aichi, Japan
e-mail: aono@tut.jp

M. A. R. Ahad and M. U. Ahmed (eds.), *Signal Processing Techniques for Computational Health Informatics*, Intelligent Systems Reference Library 192,
https://doi.org/10.1007/978-3-030-54932-9_8

are collectively called a query. Along with this, the information related to health is also significantly increased in the recent past [2–4]. As the people are habituated in accessing information from the Web, searching health-related information has been very common to the users. According to a survey, almost 72% of users in Web accessed health-related information in the United States [5]. But one of the major challenges in searching is to express the required information needs to the search engines. Unfortunately, a large number of users fail to access the intended information because of their weakness in preparing the right query. For the same reason, the meaning of the maximum queries might be ambiguous. Hence, the queries have multiple interpretation [6, 7]. These types of queries might lead the search engines toward a different direction that may return irrelevant documents. Thus the users remain unsatisfied. However, searching for health-related information using search engines is more challenging. As we noted that users fail to express their information needs and this problem is more complex in health-related information searching for the following reasons:

- Laypeople express their health information need using non-medical terms
- The expert medical practitioners tend to use advanced medical terms for searching.

Therefore, we need a stable IR system that should tackle these types of query variations. For example, laypeople might search using the query "heart attack," instead of "myocardial infarction" (correct medical terms for symptoms). Users also might search with their native language, for example, Bengali. But generally, the Web is full of information written in English. Thus, we might need to translate the users' native query into English before searching and need to provide the translated documents to the users in their native language. That's why we need a cross-lingual information retrieval system (CLIR) [8]. A cross-lingual IR system can process the query written in any language and returns the search results in users' native language.

The structure of the remainder of this chapter is organized as the following: Section. 8.2 presents the model of an HIR system. We present different query reformulation techniques including query aspect identification and query expansion in Sect. 8.3. The explanation about different classical retrieval models is discussed in Sect. 8.4. We present different measures to estimate relevance in Sect. 8.5. We also present multiple document ranking techniques in the same section. The datasets and evaluation metrics are discussed in Sect. 8.6. Section 8.7 presents some conclusion remarks about health information retrieval.

8.2 Model of a Health Information Retrieval System

An information retrieval system has some common components and functional units. We can consider each functional unit as an individual phase that the performance of one phase is dependent on the previous phase. However, it is a step-by-step process. The major steps of an HIR system are:

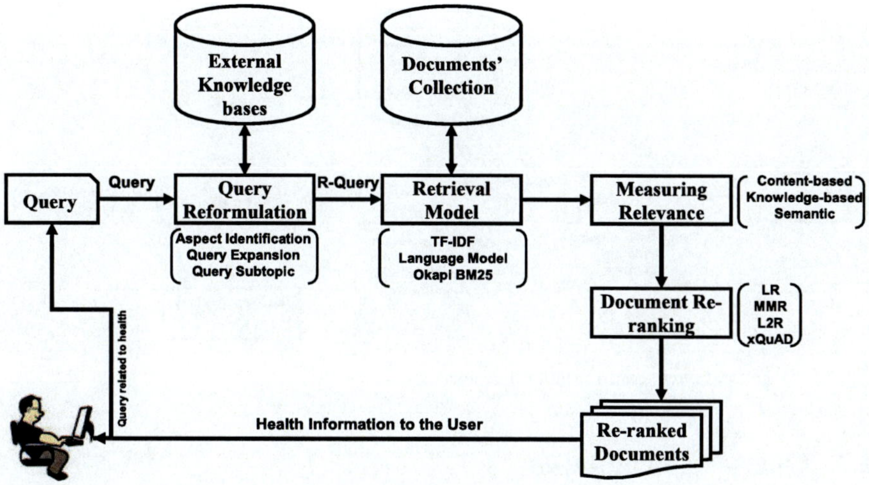

Fig. 8.1 A block-diagram of a health information retrieval system

1. Reformulating under-specified and ambiguous health query
2. Retrieving top documents using a classical retrieval model
3. Measuring relevance between query and documents
4. Producing a ranking balancing documents' relevance and novelty.

A general block diagram of an HIR system considering the above-mentioned steps is illustrated in Fig. 8.1. In summary, an HIR system at first reformulates the users' query to represent their health search intention in an efficient way. As we noted that queries are short, ambiguous and broad, different reformulation techniques including query aspect identification, subtopic mining, query expansion and query suggestion generation can be applied. This step is referred to as query reformulation. Different external resources such as Wikipedia, WordNet, and FreeBase, etc., are commonly used as knowledge-bases for query reformulation. Then the reformulated query is applied to retrieve a list of relevant documents from the index that consists of a vast collection of documents. Generally used retrieval models are Okapi BM25 [9], Language Model [10], TF-IDF etc.

The top retrieved documents are used to produce an efficient diverse ranking after measuring their relevance with the reformulated query. The techniques for measuring the relevance can be classified considering the resources including the content information, different knowledge-bases and semantic information. There are also multiple re-ranking approaches including linear ranking, maximum marginal relevance (MMR) [11], coverage-based diversification [12], learning to rank (L2R) [13] and xQuAD [14]. The remaining contents of this chapter describe the details of the phases of the above-mentioned block diagram.

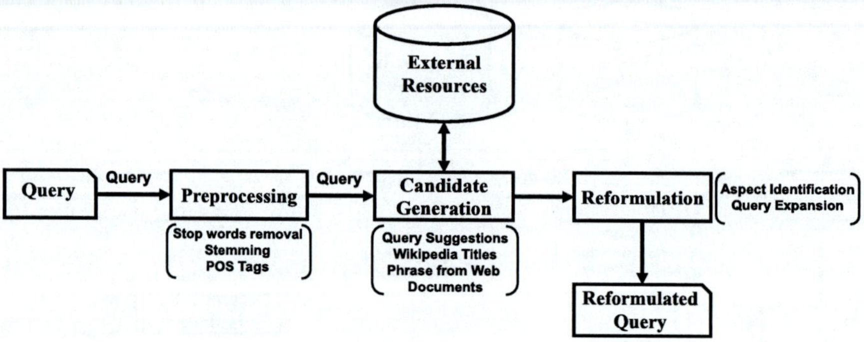

Fig. 8.2 A general query reformulation framework

8.3 Query Reformulation

Users are laconic in describing their search intention. According to the previous study on web queries, the average length of the queries are short and about 2.3 terms long [15]. Moreover, general people may not efficiently express their health queries. They might use terms that are not familiar in the medical area. People may search with queries consisting of non-medical terms. On the other hand, medical practitioners (i.e doctors or individuals related to the medical field) might search with advanced medical terms. Therefore, the HIR system may need to reformulate the query [16]. Different existing efficient techniques are available including query aspects identification [17], subtopic mininig [18] and query expansion [19, 20]. The general query reformulation framework is illustrated in Fig. 8.2.

8.3.1 Preprocessing

In the preprocessing phase, the punctuation marks are filtered out from the query. Then, the query can be converted into lower case. Some words have very little importance and carry less content and semantic information refereed to as stopwords. These words should be removed from the query. There are a standard Indri's[1] stopword list which can be utilized to select and remove stopwords from the queries. The remaining terms can be converted to their original form. The most usable stemmers (that converts each word into its original form, i.e. utilized–>utilize) to convert word into its original form are Porter Stemmer, Krovertz Stemmer and NLTK lemmatizer. It is also useful to make a map to store the corresponding part-of-speech (POS) for each lemmatized word which can be used later. Stanford NLP tool and NLTK POS tagger can be utilized for this purpose.

[1]Indri's Stopwords: http://www.lemurproject.org/stopwords/stoplist.dft .

8.3.2 Candidate Generation

To reformulate a query, the first step is to identify the query type. If the type belongs to short, ambiguous, or under-specified then the query should be reformulated after identifying the query aspects and applying query expansion methods. Query suggestions and completion from the commercial search engine, Wikipedia titles and headings, Google Keyword Generator and titles, headings, phrases and anchor text from web documents are commonly employed as candidates for selecting query aspects. For a given pre-processed query, a list of different candidates related to the query is extracted from these resources.

8.3.3 Query Aspects Identification

Due to the ambiguity and having multiple meanings of a query, the returned results might make the users unsatisfied. Identifying different aspects behind the query can be a plausible solution. For example, *fever treatment* a query and fever might be happened due to *dengue*, *malaria* or *typhoid*. Therefore, finding the query aspects enhances the effectiveness of the health information retrieval system and HIR can react with returning the documents considering the query aspects. Identification of query aspects is also helpful in some other query reformulation techniques such as subtopic mining and query expansion.

Applying prominent clustering methods on the generated candidates is one of the common ways to group similar candidates into clusters. A meaningful representative subject for each cluster is generated using the candidates of the corresponding cluster. The generated subjects are then used as query aspects. Some commonly used clustering methods includes K-nearest neighbor (KNN) [21, 22], Lingo clustering algorithm [23], Affinity propagation [24] etc.

8.3.4 Query Expansion

Usually, search engines process the users' query (health query) as the process of exact matching in the index. Sometime, the queries may not be matched with the index. This situation generally refereed to as *vocabulary mismatch* problem. This problem occurs when users' submitted query's terms do not match with the index. There are two types of words. One is synonymy where multiple words has a common meaning (i.e. "*read*", and "*study*"). On the other hand, some words have multiple meanings (i.e. "*jaguar*" has multiple meanings such as *animal* and *Car brand*). These types of terms also might direct the search engine in retrieving irrelevant documents. One possible way to solve this problem is to select diverse terms related to the query and append those terms at the end of the original query [25]. This technique is widely

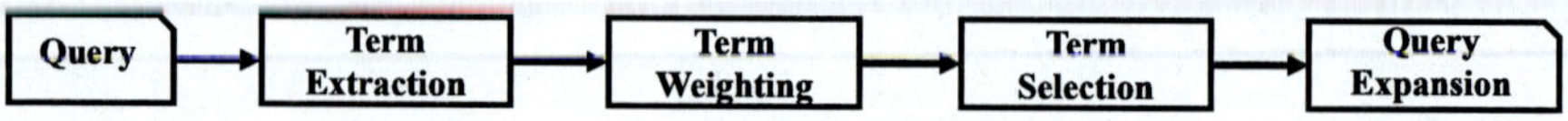

Fig. 8.3 Query expansion process

known as query expansion (QE). There are numerous QE techniques that have been applied to tackle the mismatching problem in HIR [19, 26–29].

Let $Q = \{t_1, t_2, \ldots, t_n\}$ be the preprocessed query except stop words and all terms are in original form. A reformulated query Q_{exp} after query expansion can be defined as following:

$$Q_{exp} = Q \cup T \tag{8.1}$$

where T indicates the set of ranked expansion terms selected from different resources.

The general steps needed to expand a query are depicted in Fig. 8.3. The expansion terms can be extracted from different resources. These resources can be classified into three categories: i. Top retrieved documents, ii. External text collection and iii. External knowledge-bases. For the first one, the QE methods first retrieve top k relevant documents for the users' query. A set of frequently appeared terms similar to the query that share the same subject are extracted from web documents [30–32]. Applying the clustering algorithm is a prominent method to extract terms from top retrieved documents [33]. Two types of clustering are available, term clustering and document clustering [34].

External text collections including Wikipedia, WWW, Query logs, Anchor texts are also very widely used for term extraction [35–37]. There are also numerous types of manual knowledge bases that can be employed to extract expansion terms. WordNet and ConceptNet are two famous knowledge-base for this purpose [38, 39]. However, all extracted terms from different resources have not the same importance and similarity with the query. Therefore, the QE method needs to measure the similarity of the terms with the query. The widely used similarity metrics for estimating the weight of each word are Jaccard similarity [40], Cosine similarity [41], Mutual information, Wu and Pulmar [42], Resnik and semantic similarity [43]. However, considering the approaches and resources, the query expansion methods broadly categorized as (i) Linguistic (ii) Corpus-based (iii) Search query log-based (iv) Web-based (v) Relevance feedback and (vi) Pseudo-relevance feedback.

8.4 Retrieval Model

The most widely used classical models for retrieving documents relevant to the queries are *TF-IDF*, *Okapi BM25* and *Language model* [44]. These classical models can retrieve a number of relevant web documents as a ranking from any particular documents' collection.

8.4.1 TF-IDF

TF-IDF can be used to calculate the degree of importance of a particular word by combining two different statistics, term frequency (TF) and inverse document frequency (IDF). As a retrieval model, TF-IDF can be applied in different setting to estimate the relevancy score of documents with the query. In turn, these scores are employed to generate the ranking. However, TF-IDF can be defined as the following equation:

$$\text{TF-IDF}_{t,d,D} = \text{TF}_{t,d} \cdot \text{IDF}_{t,D} \tag{8.2}$$

where t denotes a particular term in document d in the collection D. The term frequency of t, $\text{TF}_{t,d}$ is the number of occurrence in the document d. Mathematically,

$$\text{TF}_{t,d} = 0.5 + 0.5 \cdot \frac{f_{t,d}}{\max\left\{f_{t',d} : t' \in d\right\}} \tag{8.3}$$

where $f_{t,d}$ indicates the frequency in document d and $\max\left\{f_{t',d} : t' \in d\right\}$ the frequency of a word that appears mostly in the document. The constant is used to control the bias for a longer document. There are also some other variation of TF. On the other hand $\text{IDF}_{t,D}$ decides whether the term t is common in the corpus or not. This can be calculated as the following:

$$\text{IDF}_{t,D} = \log \frac{|D|}{1 + |\{d \in D : t \in d\}|} \tag{8.4}$$

8.4.2 Okapi BM25 Model

Let the document $d \in D$ contains V number of words and d is represented as a vector of the corresponding term frequencies, $\mathbf{d} = \{TF_1, TF_2, TF_3, \ldots, TF_V\}$. BM25 [45] is a ranking approach that can also be utilized in ad-hoc retrieval.

$$W(\mathbf{d}, q, C) = \sum_j \left] \frac{(k_1 + 1) \cdot TF_j}{k_1(1 - b) + b\frac{dl}{avdl}} \log \frac{N - DF_j + 0.5}{DF_j + 0.5} \right[\cdot TF_{q_j} \tag{8.5}$$

where DF_j return the document frequency of j-th term and $avdl$ returns the average document length. k_1 and b be the tuning parameter range in [0,1].

8.4.3 *Language Model*

One of the prominent retrieval models in IR is language model. Let each document is represent by a bag-of-words, a unigram technique. According to the multinomial distribution, the maximum likelihood measure for word w in d can be defined as [10, 46]:

$$P_{ML}(q|d) = \frac{TF_{w,d}}{|d|} \tag{8.6}$$

where the total number of words is denoted by $|d|$. An user query can be represented as a set of words $q = \{q_1, q_2, q_3, \ldots, q_k\}$. Then the query likelihood is estimated by

$$P(q|d) = \prod_{i=1}^{k} P(q_i|d) \tag{8.7}$$

Let cf_w be the frequency of w in whole collection and λ is a parameter for smoothing. Then applying the Jelinek-mercer smoothing approach, it can be computed as following:

$$p(w|d) = \lambda \frac{tf_{w,d}}{|d|} + (1 - \lambda) \frac{cf_w}{|C|} \tag{8.8}$$

8.5 Measuring Relevancy and Document Ranking

The final step to produce the documents' list covering maximum aspects of a health query is to apply a particular ranking approach to the documents retrieved by any retrieval model. Thus the users' satisfaction might increase. Accurately estimating the relevance of the query-document pair is the prior step to build the ranking. A large variety of techniques and ways are available to estimate the relevancy. Some of them used the content information of queries and documents, others might take help from different knowledge-bases and resources. Recently, word-embedding [12, 47, 48], sentence-embedding [49], short-text embedding, etc., are also employed for the same purpose. Several prominent deep learning techniques has been gotten attention in the research community that can capture better similarity/relevancy between texts. The techniques of measuring relevancy between text-pairs can be broadly categorized into three types: (a) Content-based (b) Knowledge-based and (c) Semantic. The content-based measures estimate the relevancy considering the content information of queries and documents. Different kinds of resources including WordNet, ConceptNet, Wikipedia, etc. are exploited in knowledge-based approaches. On the other hand, semantic measures compute the relevance score with the help of the semantic information of terms in a distributed corpus. The Word-embedding technique is an example of this purpose.

However, the re-ranking approaches try to increase the document relevancy which might increase the redundancy too. When more than two different documents in the ranking serve a similar user aspect, then those two documents are redundant to each other. That's why the ultimate goal of any diversified ranking method is to increase the relevancy and decrease the redundancy. Thus we need to think about the novelty of the documents. Decreasing the redundancy of a ranking ensures the novelty. Therefore, the ranking techniques should try the balance the relevance and novelty. Maximum Marginal Relevance (MMR) [11] is one of the most prominent ranking approaches which makes the final rank list balancing the relevancy and novelty. Let D denotes the list of web documents for a given health query q, retrieved by any of the classical retrieval models discussed in Sect. 8.4. MMR is a greedy approach that iteratively selects a document in each iteration and adds it to the tail of the ranking. Let $\mathcal{R}_n$ is the ranking of n documents after n-th iteration. Then $(n+1)$-th selected document according to the maximum marginal relevance can be defined as follows:

$$\mathcal{R}_{n+1} \stackrel{def}{=} \underset{d_i \in D \setminus \mathcal{R}_n}{\text{argmax}}[\rho \, Rel(q, d_i) + (1-\rho) Novelty(d_i)] \tag{8.9}$$

where ρ is a kind of threshold and the value is lies in [0,1]. The relevancy between query and document is denoted as $Rel(q, d_i)$. The relevancy can be estimated by combining all relevance measures. The novelty, $Novelty(d_i)$ of the document d_i can be estimated as follows:

$$novelty(d_i) = -\max_{d_j \in \mathcal{R}_n} Sim(d_i, d_j) \tag{8.10}$$

where the function $Sim(d_i, d_j)$ indicates the degree of similarity for a pair of documents. The similarity is generally estimated using any of the measures such as cosine similarity, Jaccard similarity coefficient, etc. Anyone can also apply there own sophisticated similarity function.

Santos et al. [14] introduced an explicit ranking technique exploiting different query aspects. The technique is widely known as Explicit Query Aspect Diversification and in short *xQuAD*.

$$f_{xQuAD}(q, d, \mathcal{R}) = (1-\gamma)p(d|q) + \gamma p(d, \overline{\mathcal{R}}|q) \tag{8.11}$$

where $p(d|q)$ indicate the probability such that the query appears in d. The function $p(d, \overline{\mathcal{R}}|q)$ returns the similar results as previous but it utilized only the unselected documents in the ranking $\mathcal{R}$. These probability distributions can be defined as computing the relevance and the diversity of document d, respectively. The value of γ lies in between [0,1]

In the recent past, researchers try to rank the documents using the pre-trained distributed representation of words which are known as word embedding [47] as well as *word2vec* [19]. The ranking basically depends on similarity measures based on *word2vec* defined as follows:

$$cosine(q,d) = cosine\left(\frac{1}{|q|}\sum_{t_i \in q} \mathbf{w_{t_i}}, \frac{1}{|d|}\sum_{t_j \in d} \mathbf{w_{t_j}}\right) \tag{8.12}$$

where *word2vec* model represents each term t as a high dimensional vector $\mathbf{w_t}$. The operator $|d|$ indicates the cardinality that returns the number of terms in d.

8.6 Datasets and Evaluation Metrics

8.6.1 Datasets

The performance of any health information retrieval system can be measured by conducting experiments on numerous datasets prepared by CLEF eHealth evaluation lab[2] [50–53] . CLEF has been organizing different research computations on health information retrieval from 2013 to 2018. The datasets contain a set of health queries. Using these queries, the health information retrieval system needs to rank relevant documents from a particular document corpus. ClueWeb09[3] [54] and ClueWeb12[4] [55] are widely used document collection which are built by millions of web documents. Carnegie Mellon University has been prepared these collections. The organizer of the CLEF eHealth task has also built a ground truth for each query. The organizers also provided a list of documents related to the health query that can be used as a gold-standard. The evaluation method utilizes the ranking generated by a specific method and the organizers' ranking. The methods of HIR can be tested using these datasets and can measure the performance using the following evaluation metrics.

8.6.2 Evaluation Metrics

Evaluating the performance of a health information retrieval system is a similar process to any other conventional IR system. However, numerous evaluation measures are being used to test the performance of any HIR system. The measures include normalized discriminating cumulative gain, expected reciprocal rank-intent aware and novelty and rank-biased precision. The metrics try to judge the effectiveness of any particular method in terms of user satisfaction. The satisfaction of a user depends on the underlying health information needs. However, the document relevancy with the users' query is measured by the coverage of the aspects underlying a query. In

[2]http://clef-ehealth.org/.

[3]https://lemurproject.org/clueweb09.php/.

[4]https://lemurproject.org/clueweb12/.

the remainder of this section, we present the most prominent evaluation metrics to test the performance of any health information system.

8.6.2.1 α-nDCG (α-Normalized Discriminating Cumulative Gain)

Given a query q, let $S(q)$ be the set of subtopics or underlying health information needs. The relevancy between any particular subtopic s and the document d_i (analogous for d_j) at the i-th position can be represented as $rel(d, s)$. The discriminating cumulative gain $\alpha - DCG@k$ [56] can be defined as follows:

$$\alpha - DCG@k = \sum_{j=1}^{k} \frac{\sum_{s \in S(q)} rel(d_j, s)(1-\alpha)^{\sum_{i=1}^{j-1} rel(d_i, s)}}{log_2(1+j)}$$

The value of α ranges in [0,1] and this is also used as the user satisfaction threshold. The normalized DCG is estimated as the following equation.

$$\alpha - nDCG@k = \frac{\alpha - DCG@k}{\alpha - DCG'@k}$$

Previously ranked documents are also exploited to evaluate the k ranked document [56]. The value of α can control the coverage of the particular users' aspect behind the query.

8.6.2.2 ERR-IA (Expected Reciprocal Rank—Internet Aware)

Let $ERR(s, D)$ be the expected reciprocal rank of document d for the query aspect s. The importance of any subtopic s for query q can be defined as $p(s|q)$. Then the ERR-IA(q, D) [57] is calculated as:

$$ERR - IA@k = \sum_{s \in S(q)}^{k} p(s|q) \cdot ERR(s, D)$$

8.6.2.3 NRBP (Novelty and Rank-Biased Precision)

The major hypothesis behind this metric is to check whether at least one particular user aspect has been addressed by the ranking or not [58, 59]. Let N be the number of underlying subtopics for a query and the function $J(d, i)$ returns 1 such that the document d satisfies and relevant for the i-th subtopic. Otherwise it returns zero. The NRBP is calculated as:

$$NRBP = \frac{1-(1-\alpha)^{\beta}}{N} \cdot \sum_{k=1}^{\infty} \beta^{k-1} \cdot \sum_{i=1}^{N} J(d_k, i)(1-\alpha)^{C(k,i)}$$

where k indicates the cut-off and $C(k, i)$ returns the number of relevant document related for i-th subtopic. The value of α and β range in [0,1].

8.7 Conclusion and Future Directions

In conclusion, a health information retrieval system produces a ranking of web documents that satisfies the different underlying aspects for given health query. The system also tries to cover as many underlying query aspect as possible which increase the satisfaction level of the user. To build a health information retrieval system, some general steps and different resources are needed. The general steps include query reformulation, retrieval model, relevance measures and re-ranking approaches. The resources can be utilized by any of these steps. In short, query reformulation techniques refine the users' health query by covering underlying aspects. Retrieval model retrieves top documents related to the query and the re-ranking approaches try to build an efficient ranking balancing the relevancy and novelty with the help of different relevance measures. The performance of any HIR method can be measured by several evaluation metrics.

In the future, the HIR system will surely have a significant impact on the medical community. The recent advancement in the computing area such as deep neural networks with its different variants including CNN, LSTM, could be interesting to apply to improve the performance of the health IR system. Moreover, applying vertical search techniques in health information search can also boost the performance and achieve user satisfaction by providing health information needs.

References

1. Goeuriot, L., Jones, G.J., Kelly, L., Müller, H., Zobel, J.: Medical information retrieval: introduction to the special issue. Inf. Retrieval J. **19**(1–2), 1–5 (2016)
2. Wu, S., Huang, C., Li, L., Crestani, F.: Fusion-based methods for result diversification in web search. Inf. Fusion **45**, 16–26 (2019)
3. Jimmy, J., Zuccon, G., Koopman, B., Demartini, G.: Health cards for consumer health search. In: Proceedings of the 42nd International ACM SIGIR Conference on Research and Development in Information Retrieval, pp. 35–44 (2019)
4. Zuccon, G., Koopman, B., Demartini, G.: Health card retrieval for consumer health search: an empirical investigation of methods. In: Proceedings of the 28th ACM International Conference on Information and Knowledge Management, pp. 2405–2408 (2019)

5. Saleh, S., Pecina, P.: Cuni team: Clef ehealth consumer health search task 2018. In: CLEF (Working Notes) (2018)
6. Rodrygo, L.T., Macdonald, C., Ounis, I., et al.: Search result diversification. Found. Trends Inf. Retrieval **9**(1), 1–90 (2015)
7. Shajalal, M., Ullah, M.Z., Chy, A.N., Aono, M.: Query subtopic diversification based on cluster ranking and semantic features. In: 2016 International Conference On Advanced Informatics: Concepts, Theory And Application (ICAICTA), pp. 1–6. IEEE (2016)
8. Vulić, I., Moens, M.-F.: Monolingual and cross-lingual information retrieval models based on (bilingual) word embeddings. In: Proceedings of the 38th international ACM SIGIR conference on research and development in information retrieval, pp. 363–372. ACM (2015)
9. Whissell, J.S., Clarke, C.L.: Improving document clustering using okapi bm25 feature weighting. Inf. Retrieval **14**(5), 466–487 (2011)
10. Metzler, D., Croft, W.B.: Combining the language model and inference network approaches to retrieval. Inf. Process. Manage. **40**(5), 735–750 (2004)
11. Carbonell, J.G., Goldstein, J.: The use of mmr, diversity-based reranking for reordering documents and producing summaries. In: SIGIR, vol. 98, pp. 335–336 (1998)
12. Shajalal, M., Aono, M.: Coverage-based query subtopic diversification leveraging semantic relevance. Knowl. Inf. Syst. (2020)
13. Liu, T.-Y., et al.: Learning to rank for information retrieval. Found. Trends Inf. Retrieval **3**(3), 225–331 (2009)
14. Santos, R.L., Macdonald, C., Ounis, I.: Exploiting query reformulations for web search result diversification. In: Proceedings of the 19th international Conference on World Wide Web, pp. 881–890. ACM (2010)
15. Lau, T., Horvitz, E.: Patterns of search: analyzing and modeling web query refinement. In: UM99 User Modeling. Springer, pp. 119–128 (1999)
16. Zheng, Wei, Wang, Xuanhui, Fang, Hui, Cheng, Hong: Coverage-based search result diversification. Inf. Retrieval **15**(5), 433–457 (2012)
17. Santos, R.L., Macdonald, C., Ounis, I.: Intent-aware search result diversification. In: Proceedings of the 34th International ACM SIGIR Conference on Research and Development in Information Retrieval, pp. 595–604. ACM (2011)
18. Jiang, Z., Wen, J.R., Dou, Z., Zhao, W.X., Nie, J.Y., Yue, M.: Learning to diversify search results via subtopic attention. In: Proceedings of the 40th international ACM SIGIR Conference on Research and Development in Information Retrieval, pp. 545–554. ACM (2017)
19. Oh, H.S., Jung, Y.: Kisti at clef ehealth 2016 task 3: ranking medical documents using word vectors. In: CLEF (Working Notes), pp. 103–108 (2016)
20. Carpineto, C., Romano, G.: A survey of automatic query expansion in information retrieval. Acm Comput. Surv. (CSUR) **44**(1), 1 (2012)
21. Fukunaga, K., Narendra, P.M.: A branch and bound algorithm for computing k-nearest neighbors. IEEE Trans. Comput. **7**, 750–753 (1975)
22. Gou, J., Qiu, W., Yi, Z., Xu, Y., Mao, Q., Zhan, Y.: A local mean representation-based k-nearest neighbor classifier. ACM Trans. Intell. Syst. Technol. (TIST) **10**(3), 1–25 (2019)
23. Osiński, S., Stefanowski, J., Weiss, D.: Lingo: search results clustering algorithm based on singular value decomposition. In: Intelligent Information Processing and Web Mining, pp. 359–368. Springer (2004)
24. Wang, K., Zhang, J., Li, D., Zhang, X., Guo, T.: Adaptive affinity propagation clustering. arXiv preprint arXiv:0805.1096 (2008)
25. Saleh, S., Pecina, P.: Term selection for query expansion in medical cross-lingual information retrieval. In: European Conference on Information Retrieval, pp. 507–522. Springer (2019)
26. Song, Y., He, Y., Liu, H., Wang, Y., Hu, Q., He, L., Luo, G.: Ecnu at 2016 ehealth task 3: patient-centred information retrieval. In: CLEF (Working Notes), pp. 157–161 (2016)
27. Chen, S., Hu, Q.V., Song, Y., He, Y., Wu, H., He, L.: Self-attention based network for medical query expansion. In: 2019 International Joint Conference on Neural Networks (IJCNN), pp. 1–9. IEEE (2019)

28. Zayani, S., Ksentini, N., Tmar, M., Gargouri, F.: Miracl at clef 2018: consumer health search task. In: CLEF (Working Notes) (2018)
29. Diaz-Galiano, M.C., Martin-Valdivia, M.T., Maria, S., Jiménez-Zafra, A.A., López, L.A.U.: Sinai at clef ehealth 2017 task 3. CLEF (2017)
30. Qiu, Y., Frei, H.P.: Concept based query expansion. In: Proceedings of the 16th annual international ACM SIGIR Conference on Research and Development in Information Retrieval, pp. 160–169. ACM (1993)
31. Imran, H., Sharan, A.: Selecting effective expansion terms for better information retrieval (2010)
32. Crouch, C.J., Yang, B.: Experiments in automatic statistical thesaurus construction. In: Proceedings of the 15th Annual International ACM SIGIR Conference on Research and Development in Information Retrieval, pp. 77–88. ACM (1992)
33. Hiteshwar Kumar Azad and Akshay Deepak: Query expansion techniques for information retrieval: a survey. Inf. Process. Manage. **56**(5), 1698–1735 (2019)
34. Willett, P.: Recent trends in hierarchic document clustering: a critical review. Inf. Process. Manage. **24**(5), 577–597 (1988)
35. Kraft, R., Zien, J.: Mining anchor text for query refinement. In: Proceedings of the 13th International Conference on World Wide Web, pp. 666–674. ACM (2004)
36. Dang, V., Croft, B.W.: Query reformulation using anchor text. In: Proceedings of the 3rd ACM International Conference on Web Search and Data Mining, pp. 41–50. ACM (2010)
37. Al-Shboul, B., Myaeng, S.-H.: Wikipedia-based query phrase expansion in patent class search. Inf. Retrieval **17**(5–6), 430–451 (2014)
38. Voorhees, E.M.: Query expansion using lexical-semantic relations. In: SIGIR'94, pp. 61–69. Springer (1994)
39. Hsu, M.H., Tsai, M.F., Chen, H.H.: Combining wordnet and conceptnet for automatic query expansion: a learning approach. In: Asia Information Retrieval Symposium, pp. 213–224. Springer (2008)
40. Jaccard, P.: The distribution of the flora in the alpine zone. 1. New Phytol. **11**(2), 37–50 (1912)
41. Ye, J.: Improved cosine similarity measures of simplified neutrosophic sets for medical diagnoses. Artif. Intell. Med. **63**(3), 171–179 (2015)
42. Wu, Z., Palmer, M.: Verbs semantics and lexical selection. In: Proceedings of the 32nd Annual Meeting on Association for Computational Linguistics, pp. 133–138. Association for Computational Linguistics (1994)
43. Resnik, P.: Using information content to evaluate semantic similarity in a taxonomy. arXiv preprint cmp-lg/9511007. (1995)
44. Shajalal, M., Aono, M., Azim, M.A.: Aspect-based query expansion for search results diversification. In: 2018 Joint 7th International Conference on Informatics, Electronics and Vision (ICIEV) and 2018 2nd International Conference on Imaging, Vision and Pattern Recognition (icIVPR), pp. 147–152. IEEE (2018)
45. Trotman, A., Puurula, A., Burgess, B.: Improvements to bm25 and language models examined. In: Proceedings of the 2014 Australasian Document Computing Symposium, pp. 58. ACM (2014)
46. Lample, G., Conneau, A.: Cross-lingual language model pretraining. arXiv preprint arXiv:1901.07291 (2019)
47. Mikolov, T., Sutskever, I., Chen, K., Corrado, G.S., Dean, J.: Distributed representations of words and phrases and their compositionality. In: Advances in neural information processing systems, pp. 3111–3119 (2013)
48. Klementiev, A., Titov, I., Bhattarai, B.: Inducing crosslingual distributed representations of words. Proc. COLING **2012**, 1459–1474 (2012)
49. Le, Q., Mikolov, T.: Distributed representations of sentences and documents. In: International Conference on Machine Learning, pp. 1188–1196 (2014)
50. Suominen, H., Kelly, L., Goeuriot, L., Névéol, A., Ramadier, L., Robert, A., Kanoulas, E., Spijker, R., Azzopardi, L., Li, D., et al.: Overview of the clef ehealth evaluation lab 2018. In: International Conference of the Cross-Language Evaluation Forum for European Languages, pp. 286–301. Springer (2018)

51. Kelly, L., Goeuriot, L., Suominen, H., Névéol, A., Palotti, J., Zuccon, G.: Overview of the clef ehealth evaluation lab 2016. In: International Conference of the Cross-Language Evaluation Forum for European Languages, pp. 255–266. Springer (2016)
52. Goeuriot, L., Kelly, L., Suominen, H., Névéol, A., Robert, A., Kanoulas, E., Spijker, R., Palotti, J. and Zuccon, G.:. Clef 2017 ehealth evaluation lab overview. In: International Conference of the Cross-Language Evaluation Forum for European Languages, pp. 291–303. Springer (2017)
53. Goeuriot, L., Kelly, L., Suominen, H., Hanlen, L., Névéol, A., Grouin, C., Palotti, J. and Zuccon, G.: Overview of the clef ehealth evaluation lab 2015. In: International Conference of the Cross-Language Evaluation Forum for European Languages, pp. 429–443. Springer (2015)
54. Callan, J., Hoy, M., Yoo, C. and Zhao, L.: Clueweb09 data set (2009)
55. Callan, J.: The lemur project and its clueweb12 dataset. In: Invited talk at the SIGIR 2012 Workshop on Open-Source Information Retrieval (2012)
56. Clarke, C.L.A., Kolla, M., Cormack, G.V., Vechtomova, O., Ashkan, A., Büttcher, S., MacKinnon, I.: Novelty and diversity in information retrieval evaluation. In: Proceedings of the 31st annual international ACM SIGIR Conference on Research and Development in Information Retrieval, pp. 659–666. ACM (2008)
57. Chapelle, O., Ji, S., Liao, C., Velipasaoglu, E., Lai, Larry, Su-Lin, Wu: Intent-based diversification of web search results: metrics and algorithms. Inf. Retrieval **14**(6), 572–592 (2011)
58. Clarke, C.L., Kolla, M., Vechtomova, O.: An effectiveness measure for ambiguous and underspecified queries. In: Conference on the Theory of Information Retrieval, pp. 188–199. Springer (2009)
59. Moffat, A., Zobel, J.: Rank-biased precision for measurement of retrieval effectiveness. ACM Trans. Inf. Syst. (TOIS) **27**(1), 2 (2008)

Chapter 9
Reconfigurable Computing and Hardware Acceleration in Health Informatics

Mehdi Hasan Chowdhury and Ray C. C. Cheung

Abstract Health informatics connects biomedical engineering with information technology to devise a modern eHealth system which often requires precise biosignal processing. This "biosignal" is essentially an electrophysiological signal from a living organism. In practice, these signals are frequently used to assess patients' health and to discover bio-physiological anonymities. However, as most of the biosignal processing units are multichannel systems with extensive datasets, conventional computation techniques often fail to offer immediate execution of data processing. Reconfigurable architecture offers a tangible solution to this problem by utilizing fast parallel computation based on the Field Programmable Gate Array (FPGA). This computation technique ensures "Hardware Acceleration" which essentially means the exclusive utilization of hardware resources to expedite computational tasks. This is the technique of designing application-specific circuits rather than using the general purpose processors to do the signal processing. Because of its low cost and fast computation property, reconfigurable architecture is characteristically suitable for Health Informatics and has become one of the fastest growing research fields of recent years. In literature, several works are found focusing on the efficient use of FPGAs as the biomedical computation units. Some of these researches involve fundamental spatiotemporal signal analysis like Fourier transform, power spectrum density measurement, and identifying significant signal peaks. In other studies, hardware acceleration is used to compress and predict the signal for data storage, processing, and transmission. Some of the works include digital filter designing for denoising the acquired signal, while a few of the advanced research projects incorporated reconfigurable architectures to develop artificial bio-organs and high-level prosthesis as a part of rehabilitation. In this chapter, these works will be briefly reviewed to find out the state-of-the-art research trends in this research field.

M. H. Chowdhury (✉) · R. C. C. Cheung
City University of Hong Kong, Kowloon, Hong Kong
e-mail: chowdhury.ee@my.cityu.edu.hk

R. C. C. Cheung
e-mail: r.cheung@cityu.edu.hk

M. H. Chowdhury
Chittagong University of Engineering and Technology, Chittagong, Bangladesh

M. A. R. Ahad and M. U. Ahmed (eds.), *Signal Processing Techniques for Computational Health Informatics*, Intelligent Systems Reference Library 192,
https://doi.org/10.1007/978-3-030-54932-9_9

Keywords Biosignal · Electrophysiology · Signal processing · FPGA

9.1 Introduction

Modern eHealth scheme and health informatics combine information technology and electronic communication with the biomedical facility to assure efficient health care. In such a system, biosignal processing is often necessary for disease diagnosis and patient rehabilitation. Biosignals are time, space or spatiotemporal recordings of physiological events that often contain significant information about underlying biological phenomena [1]. Some of the most familiar biomedical signals are electrocardiogram (ECG)- the heart signal, electroencephalogram (EEG)- the brain signal, electromyogram (EMG)- the muscle signal etc.

Most of these bioelectric signals are collected using multiple electrodes [2]. For instance, 12 electrodes are employed while recording a clinical standard ECG and up to 512 electrodes can be used in dense-array scalp EEG acquisition. Due to massive amount of simultaneously incoming data, real-time biomedical signal processing often becomes a computation burden if a conventional microprocessor is used. Reconfigurable architecture offers an excellent solution to this technical problem.

Field Programmable Gate Array (FPGA) frames the fundamental fabric of a reconfigurable computation architecture which combines flexible software characteristics with fast parallel computation. In spite of using a general purpose microprocessor, this technique enables application specific processor designing. This custom-made circuit designing scheme ensures dynamic resource utilization to speed up data processing- the "Hardware Acceleration."

FPGAs are Integrated Circuits (ICs) that can be programmed at the circuit level by consumers in the field deployment. Hence, it is called "Field Programmable" and "Reconfigurable." A contemporary FPGA consists of three basic units- Configurable Logic Blocks (CLB), Programmable Interconnections and I/O Blocks [3]. A simplified FPGA assembly is illustrated in Fig. 9.1.

Configurable Logic Blocks are the most fundamental building blocks of an FPGA. These block can be programmed to implement any desired logic gates. A typical CLB is shown in Fig. 9.2, which consists of a 4-input Look-Up-Table (LUT) and a Flip-Flop (FF) with reset (Rst) and clock (Clk) inputs [4]. CLBs are interconnected via programmable connections. As the name suggests, these interconnections are also reconfigurable according to the application requirements. I/O blocks provide a path to communicate FPGA with peripherals using I/O pins.

Modern FPGAs have a large number of logic cells and I/O pins available within it. For example, Xilinx® Virtex®-7 XC7V2000T FPGA device has 1,954,560 logic cells and 1200 I/O pins available for the user [5]. Therefore, FPGAs can be readily programmed for parallel operation exploiting its reconfigurable feature and the extensive number of I/O pins. This salient property makes FPGA the most appropriate tool for biomedical signal processing.

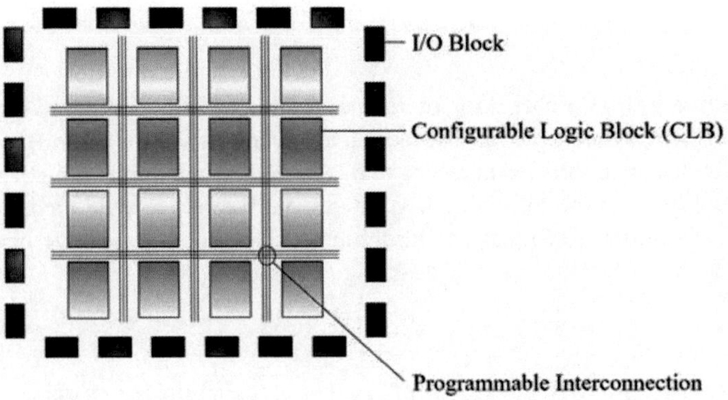

Fig. 9.1 Simplified FPGA assembly

Fig. 9.2 Typical CLB components

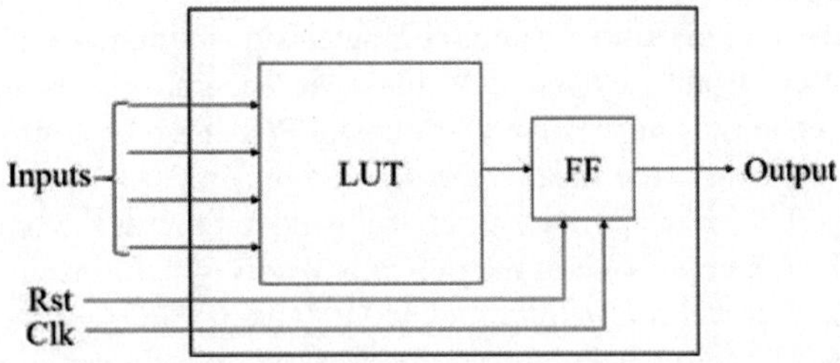

Apart from the parallel computation, the reconfigurable design is also frequently used for Application Specific Integrated Circuit (ASIC) prototyping- the stepping stone for a customized integrated circuit design. FPGA provides a low cost and energy efficient signal processing solution as it only uses a chip (or a development board) instead of complete computer setup like a conventional system. Therefore, reconfigurable computation in biosignal processing is progressively gaining attention from the research community in recent years.

This chapter is divided into four sections for the ease of explaining. Some background information regarding biosignals and reconfigurable computation architecture is discussed in "Introduction". In the next section, recent research trends of FPGA based biosignal processing is reviewed. A classification of reconfigurable computation in the health informatics is given, and several previous works are briefly discussed in the following sub-sections. The subsequent section includes an in-depth systematic analysis of one of the related architectures developed by the authors [6]. The last section contains the conclusions of this chapter and explores some of the future research directions relevant to this field.

9.2 Review of the State-of-Art

Many research groups are working on reconfigurable architecture based biomedical signal processing over the past few decades. However, this section is more focused on the works which are published in recent years. Based on their application these works can be classified into the following five categories: Reconfigurable architecture for i. Medical diagnosis, ii. Signal conditioning, iii. Developing assistive devices, iv. Modeling artificial organs, and v. Designing prosthesis.

9.2.1 Reconfigurable Architecture for Medical Diagnosis

Medical diagnosis or simply "diagnosis" is the process of determining the specific disease, that is causing the patient's medical symptoms or discomfort. As a part of the modern eHealth system, computer-aided automatic disease detection is frequently used to aid physicians to make an accurate decision. Due to the fast computing capability and relatively low cost, FPGA based reconfigurable computation units are often preferred in such medical diagnosis.

Different approaches are followed to process the biosignals for disease detection. For example, one of the previous works took ultrasound imaging as the input signal to detect abnormality of the kidneys using FPGA as the processing unit [7]. Another work is done using ultrasound imaging to estimate arteriovenous fistula stenosis: an end-stage renal disease [8]. There are many FPGA based works done using ECG as the biosignal input to detect cardiac diseases such as arrhythmia [9], myocardial infarction [10], ischemic heart disease [11], and fetal heart abnormalities [12]. Other works include automatic wheezes detection from lung sound [13], differential diagnosis of neuromuscular diseases [14], statistical epistasis detection in GWAS [15], etc. Discussing all of these is beyond the scope of this report and mostly redundant in the technical sense. Here, two of the aforementioned research works will be briefly discussed to demonstrate the working principle and find out the advantages and limitations of FPGA based processing systems.

Krishna et al. [7] have demonstrated an FPGA based kidney abnormality detection scheme which uses an ultrasound imaging scheme- a noninvasive imaging system that uses ultra-high frequency sound waves to generate pictures of organs inside the body. For this detection scheme, firstly the ultrasound image is denoised, and region of interest, i.e. the kidney is identified. After feature extraction, FPGA is employed for two-stage diagnosis. The first stage involves a Look Up Table (LUT) based approach to differentiate between normal and abnormal kidneys. If an unusual kidney is detected, the second stage uses Support Vector Machine (SVM) to detect the presence of cysts or stones in the kidney. The operating flowchart is shown in Fig. 9.3. This scheme can detect the abnormal kidney condition with an accuracy of 86% to 100% depending on the parameter length of the LUT algorithm. However,

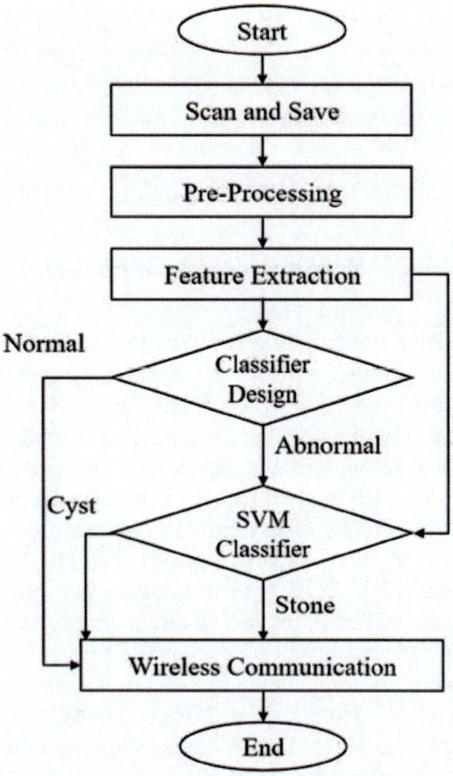

Fig. 9.3 Flowchart of the kidney abnormality detection algorithm [7]

cyst/stone detection demonstrates an accuracy of 41% to 98% using different kernels in SCM classifier.

Wienbrandt et al. [15] have presented a research work to detect statistical epistasis in GWAS which used FPGA to facilitate hardware acceleration. Epistasis is a genotype-by-genotype interaction between genetic markers which is believed to be the source of unexplained genetic variation that causes many complex genetic diseases. However, computing epistasis in Genome Wide Association Studies (GWAS) is mostly overlooked due to its computation complexity. For example, a moderate size dataset requires about 125 billion partwise interactions to be calculated during one stage of simulation. If this processing is performed in a conventional computation system using CPUs or GPUs, it will take a massive amount of time. In their research, Wienbrandt et al. exploited the parallel computation capability of FPGA to reduce the processing time drastically. RIVYERA S6-LX150- an FPGA based reconfigurable computing system is used in this experiment as the processing unit. In this research, the runtime is reduced from 120 h to 4 min by utilizing the parallelism of the reconfigurable architecture. A comparison between the energy consumption and execution run-time of different systems is summarized in Table 9.1.

Table 9.1 Energy and runtime comparison of the different epistasis detection scheme [15]

Architecture	Type	Energy (kWh)	Time	Speed (M tests/sec)
RIVYERA S6-LX150	FPGA	00.05	004 m	520.83
2x Intel Xeon quad-core @ 2.4 GHz	CPU	04.94	019 h	001.83
nVidia GeForce GTX Titan	GPU	25.50	102 h	000.34

9.2.2 *Reconfigurable Architecture for Signal Conditioning*

Signal conditioning is the method of converting a signal to a form which is more compatible for further processing. Reconfigurable architecture is suitable for digital signal conditioning, especially for noise filtering and compression algorithm. There are several works found in the literature which have used FPGAs for filtering biosignals. Reconfigurable architecture can be devised for FIR [16] or wavelet filters [17]. It can also be used to design advanced adaptive filers for neuroprosthetic use [18]. Additionally, reconfigurable architectures are often used for physiological signal compression- either for generic use [19, 20] or for compressing specific biosignal like ECG [21, 22]. In this subsection, one FPGA based filtering scheme and one biosignal compression system is briefly explored.

Dwivedi et al. [16] presented a hybrid Finite Impulse Response (FIR) filter design which is implemented in FPGA for low power application. In this research, the Hybrid Artificial Bee Colony (HABC) algorithm is used to reduce the dynamic power consumption in the reconfigurable filter module by decreasing transitions in the filter coefficient. From the experiment, the maximum dynamic power reduction was found to be 66.67%, which was attainable due to the efficient hardware resource allocation in FPGA design.

Compression of biosignal is often required for telediagnosis and electronic recordings. Lai et al. [21] used a reconfigurable architecture-based hardware acceleration for ECG compression. This complete system comprises a front end signal accusation subsystem with A/D conversion and an FPGA based signal compression subsystem. A simplified system architecture is shown in Fig. 9.4. The compression algorithm is based on the Discrete Cosine Transform of type 4 (DCT-IV), and it demonstrates a high value of compression ratio (5.267) with a low percentage of root-mean-square deviation (0.187).

9.2.3 *Reconfigurable Architecture for Developing Assistive Devices*

Assistive devices are primarily rehabilitative devices which support individuals with physical disabilities. Smart assistive devices use biosignals to actuate distinct functions. Reconfigurable computation is often used to process these physiological signals

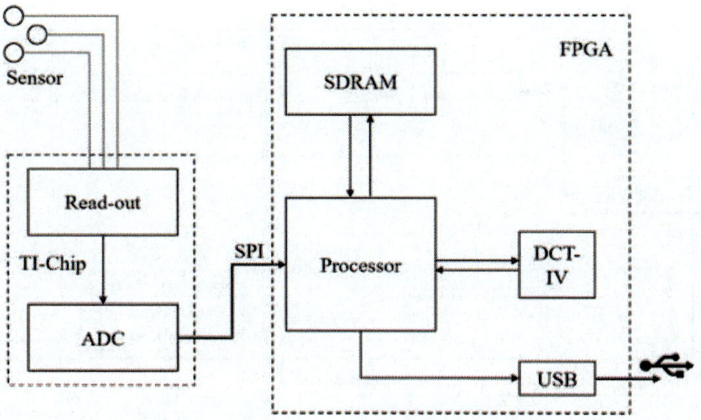

Fig. 9.4 System architecture for the DCT-IV based ECG compression [21]

due to its compact and energy efficient design. For example, a collaborative work between General Motors and NASA was published in 2014 [23] which utilized FPGA to develop the 'RoboGlove'- an assistive device which augments human strength. Some of the other works in this field include the development of assistive robotics [24], exoskeleton devices [25, 26], and assistive technologies for visually impaired people [27].

One of these works is reviewed here to demonstrate the significance of FPGA based signal processing in the evolution of assistive devices. In 2017, Wohrle et al. [26] published their research on an FPGA-based hybrid movement prediction system for exoskeleton development. This work presents an improved movement prediction by combining both EEG and EMG as the actuators.

The reconfigurable architecture is used to process the multiple streams of incoming physiological data in real-time, and it offers the flexibility to choose a suitable combination of predictions for any particular application. The hybrid parallel system architecture is illustrated in Fig. 9.5. The implemented system is smaller in size and consumes lower power, and it can process the biosignals faster than a standard computer which is necessary for the real-time system implementation.

9.2.4 Reconfigurable Architecture for Modeling Artificial Organs

Modeling artificial organs helps to mimic natural organ systems that can be used to either replace a damaged one or provide an in vitro simulation system for biomedical research. As stated earlier, reconfigurable architecture offers a fast and compact biosignal processing solution. Therefore, several previous research works

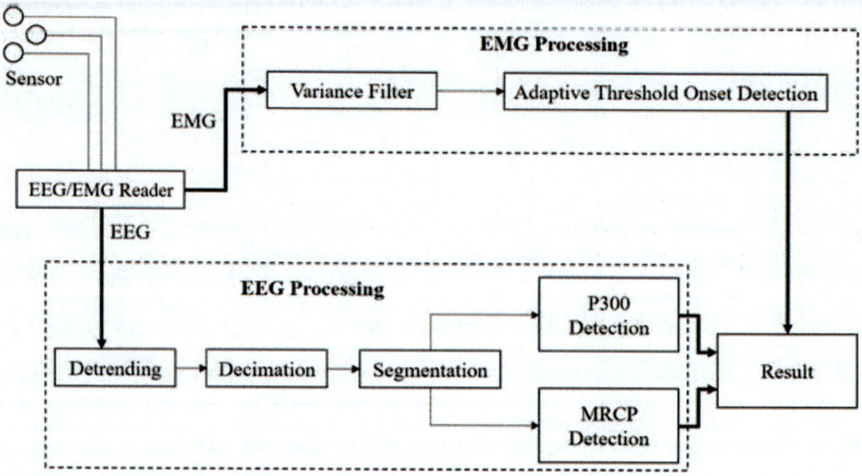

Fig. 9.5 Parallel processing of EMG and EEG for movement prediction [26]

have utilized FPGA to model artificial organs. These works include modeling artificial muscles [28], pancreas [29, 30], and biological neurons [31]. A reconfigurable architecture based Artificial Pancreas System (APS) is briefly described below.

The development of an APS is especially important to assist patients with Type 1 Diabetes mellitus to maintain their glucose level within an acceptable range. This APS system primarily comprises three subsystems- i. a glucose monitor ii. a control unit to estimate the insulin dose iii. an insulin infusion device. Despite several attempts over more than 50 years, a clinically acceptable closed-loop glucose regulator is still not available. Though Cobelli's glucose-insulin model (Fig. 9.6) is a Food and Drug Administration (FDA) approved computer simulator of glucose-insulin interactions, this model was considered difficult to implement on a compact hardware platform as it contains multiple differential equations which requires rigorous computation. To solve this technical problem, Li et al. [29] have published an FPGA based implementation of an artificial pancreas prototype in 2016. The implemented system adopted a simplified Cobelli's glucose-insulin model for computation. Using FPGA as the signal processor, this prototype can provide fast and reliable glucose-insulin estimation, which assists in the further development of extra-corporal portable glucose regulator.

9.2.5 Reconfigurable Architecture for Designing Prosthesis

An artificial device which can replace a missing body part is called prosthesis or prosthetic implant. Over the past few decades, prosthetic technology has become more responsive due to its significant incorporation with biosignals, as it gives a provision

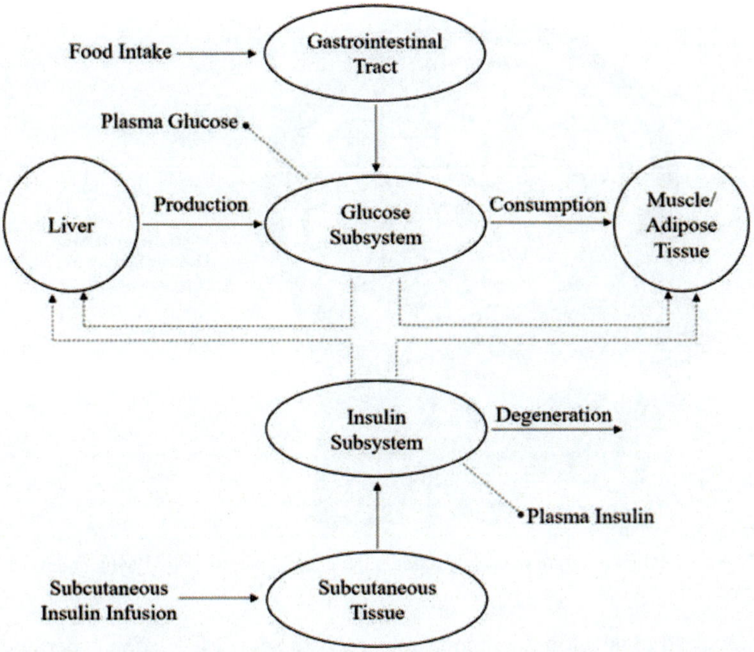

Fig. 9.6 Glucose–insulin interaction scheme. Solid lines denote the real transfer paths and dashed lines symbolize the mutual effect of different parts [29]

of added natural control over the device. There are several prosthesis research works which have utilized the advantage of reconfigurable architecture based biosignal processing because of its fast and customizable computation property. These works include FPGA based neuromuscular control for prosthetic limbs [32, 33], development of retinal prosthesis [34, 35] and modeling hippocampus region for the neural prosthesis [36–38]. Among these research works, the development of FPGA based neural prosthesis is explained here.

Hippocampus is the brain area accountable for the creation of new long-term memories. It processes the upstream neural signal from the CA3 brain region and delivers the downstream signal to region CA1. Thus long-term memories are formed in the neocortices. If this hippocampus region gets damaged due to some injuries or disease, the formation of new long term memory will stop. The development of hippocampus prosthesis is primarily focused on solving this problem. A conceptual diagram of an implanted hippocampal prosthesis is shown in Fig. 9.7. It is designed to mimic the input-output signal transformation of the hippocampal brain region. If this signal processing can be done without any system lag, this neural prosthesis could be used to bypass the damaged region.

It should be noted that the signal processing mentioned here is indeed a Multi-Input Multi-Output (MIMO) system. Therefore, a compact MIMO signal processing

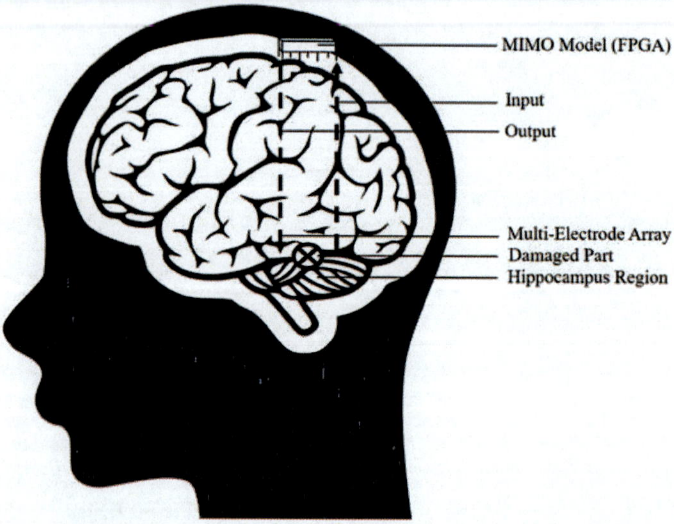

Fig. 9.7 A conceptual diagram of an implanted hippocampal prosthesis (MIMO model) [39]

unit is required to develop the hippocampus prosthesis. FPGA offers a perfect solution to this problem because of its parallel computation capability. Li et al. have published several articles [36–38] to describe the development of the reconfigurable architecture for hippocampal signal processing. Figure 9.8 shows the model for the FPGA implementation of this MIMO system. In this work, the input-output hippocampal transformation is processed using the Generalized Laguerre-Volterra Model (GLVM). However, this research is still limited to the modeling of animal brains due to the extreme complexity of the human neural system. Further research is needed to design a human compatible hippocampal prosthesis that can be used for in vitro and in vivo experimentation.

9.3 Detailed Example: A Reconfigurable Architecture for ECG Compression [6]

Electrocardiogram or ECG is the measurement of the heart's electrical signal. This is one of the most popular cardiovascular diagnostic tools across the world due to its low-cost and non-invasive nature. As a part of the modern eHealth and health informatics, ECG is often required to be compressed for electronic data records and telediagnosis. Reconfigurable computation offers an excellent signal processor for this compression because of its fast parallel computation and compact scalable property.

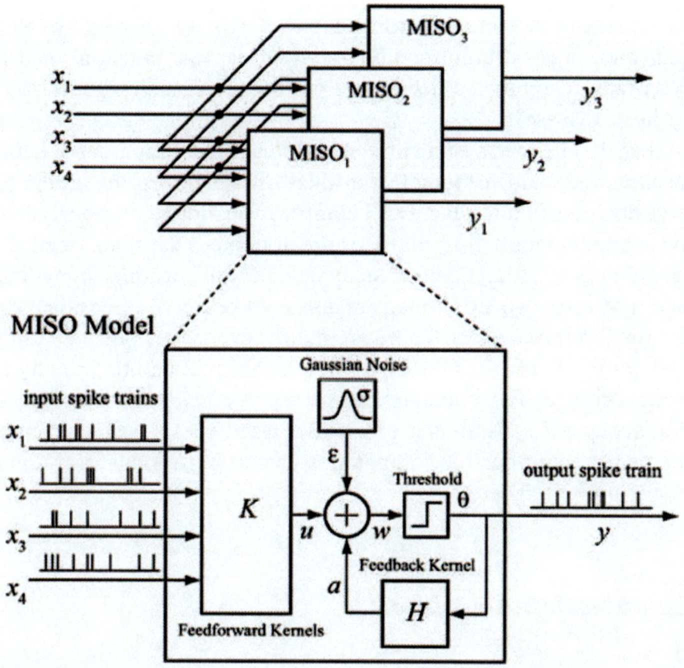

Fig. 9.8 Several MISO (Multi-Input Single-Output) models are combined to create the MIMO (Multi-Input Multi-Output) model in FPGA for the hippocampal prosthesis [36]

9.3.1 Background

ECG is the record of the electrical activities in cardiac muscles over a specified time and measured by placing several electrodes on specific points of the chest [40]. It has been used for more than 70 years as one of the primary tools to assess cardiac health [41]. Clinical standard electrocardiography requires a 12-lead ECG system to evaluate heart condition [42]. As shown in Fig. 9.9, a standard ECG cycle has three characteristic features: i. P wave, ii. QRS complex, and iii. T wave. Each of

Fig. 9.9 A characteristic ECG cycle

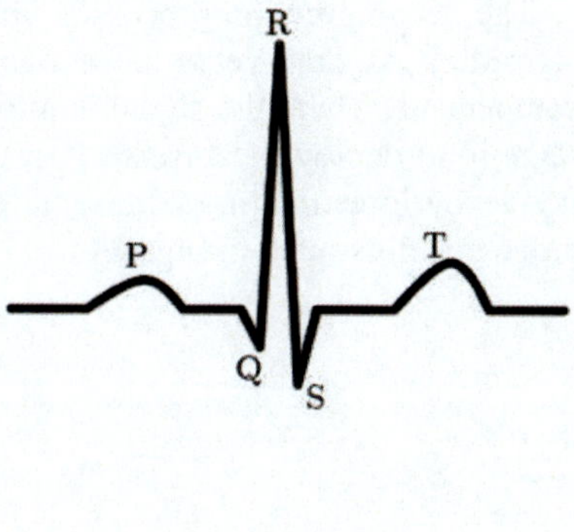

these traits represents a specific cardiac activity. The 12 channels of the clinical ECG system measures different combinations of cardiac potential, and if any of them demonstrates a significant deviation from the reference range, it may indicate a particular heart disease.

Nonetheless, this 12-lead system produces a considerable amount of data for electronic recordings and real-time remote transmission. Therefore, the necessity of ECG data compression comes into play. ECG compression aids to minimize the required bandwidth for telediagnosis [43]. Furthermore, it reduces the space needed for ECG data storage. However, as data compression degrades the original signal quality, the prime concern of effective ECG compression is to preserve the critical diagnostic information for further analysis. There are many approaches presented in the literature for this purpose. The ECG compression techniques can be broadly classified into four categories: i. Time-domain compression scheme, ii. Transform-domain compression scheme, iii. Parameter extraction based compression scheme, and iv. Hybrid scheme. A reconfigurable computation prototype for transform-domain ECG compression is presented here.

9.3.2 Compression Algorithm

Fast Fourier Transform (FFT) is an optimized Discrete Fourier Transform (DFT) technique which takes time sampled data and computes its frequency domain components [44]. When FFT is applied to a time-domain "real" signal, it produces a symmetric "complex" signal with both real and imaginary parts [45]. ECG is recorded in time-domain and is indeed a "real" signal. The compression algorithm of the implemented system is designed exploiting the symmetric property of FFT. At first, the ECG signal is transformed into the frequency domain using FFT. Then, the symmetric frequency domain components of the ECG signal are discarded, as they can be restored from the rest of the signal by simple mirroring. The next step of compression is based on a distinct property of ECG- it is dominant in the lower frequency range (< 30 Hz). Therefore, higher frequency components from the FFT output can be dropped without any significant signal quality distortion. This step is the final stage of the implemented ECG signal compression scheme. Figure 9.10 shows this compression using a standard ECG signal as input.

The decompression process is virtually a reverse procedure of the compression algorithm. At first, zeros are assigned in the places of discarded high-frequency components. Then, the signal is mirrored to recover the symmetric data. The final stage is to deploy the Inverse Fast Fourier Transform (IFFT), which converts the frequency domain signal to the required time domain ECG signal. The decompression process is illustrated in Fig. 9.11.

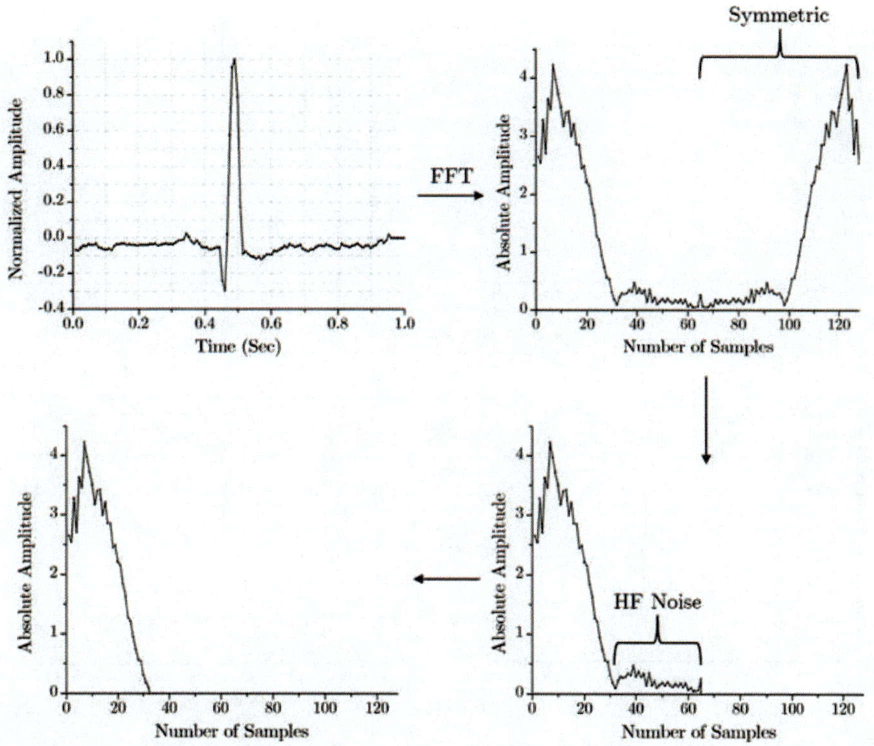

Fig. 9.10 ECG signal compression process

9.3.3 *FPGA Implementation*

Because of the parallel processing capability, the compression algorithm of the previous section is hardware-implemented using the FPGA. Here, 12 channels of the ECG can be designed as 12 structurally identical processing units (core units of Fig. 9.12). The complete multichannel setup is a composition of the core units, as illustrated in Fig. 9.13. Without any significant system delay, this system can process the 12 channel incoming ECG data simultaneously.

System Generator™ is one of the design tools for the implementation of signal processing algorithms in Xilinx® FPGA devices. It works as a toolbox for Simulink®, a graphical programming environment of Matlab®. This tool facilitates the program designers to utilize the rich simulation and verification capabilities of Matlab® [46]. Additionally, it considerably minimizes the time needed to convert the algorithm into Hardware Description Language (HDL) [47], which is the first requirement to program an FPGA. The required design flow for hardware design is presented in Fig. 9.14.

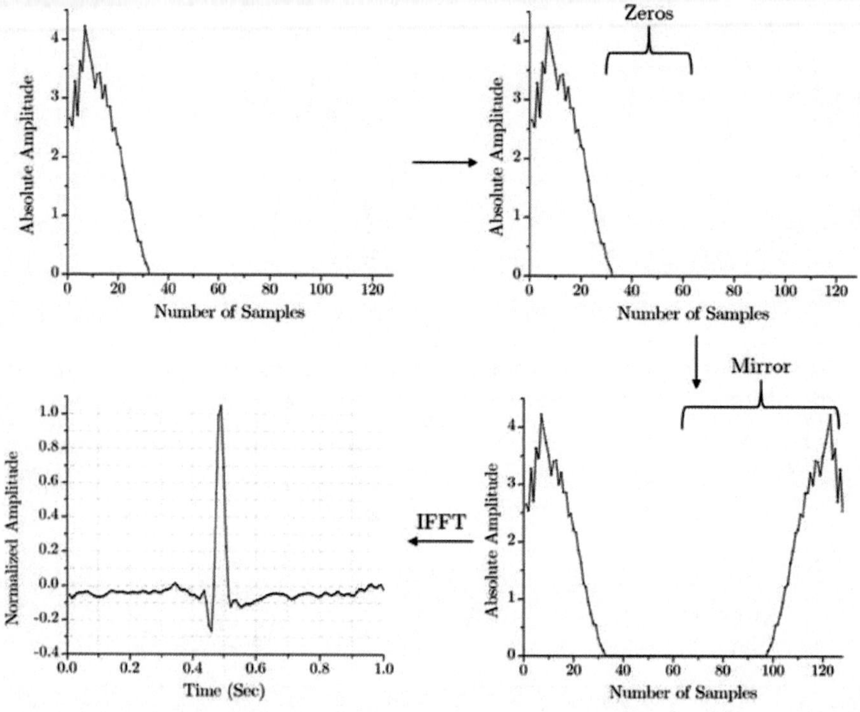

Fig. 9.11 ECG signal decompression process

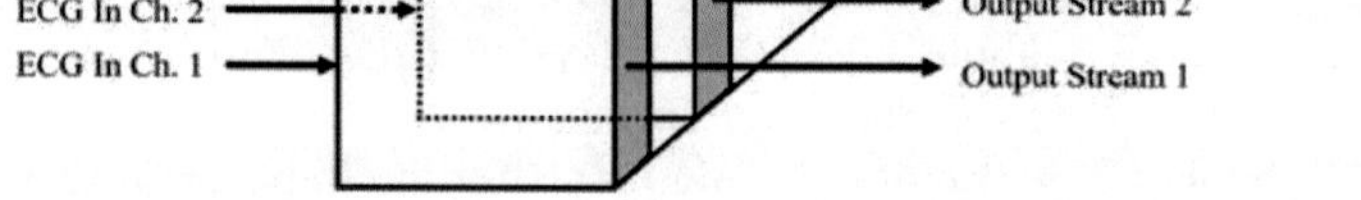

Fig. 9.12 Core units

At first, the System Generator tool is used to design the signal processing unit under the Simulink work environment. After required simulations and design verifications, HDL netlist is generated and passed to Vivado- an HDL Design Suite developed by Xilinx. Vivado runs the synthesis and implementation process to generate the bitstream. Finally, this bitstream is loaded to program the FPGA. For the first

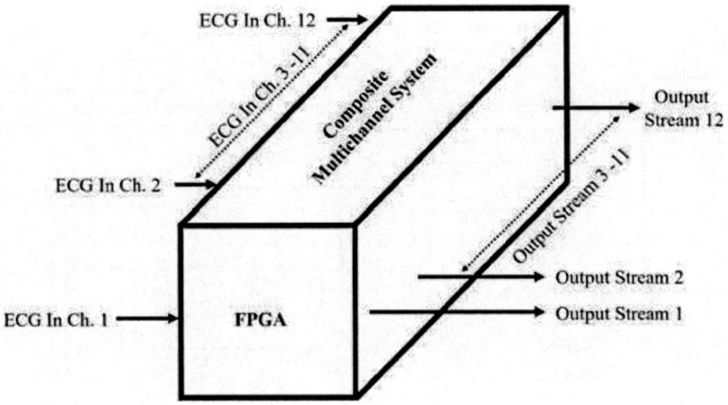

Fig. 9.13 Composite system architecture

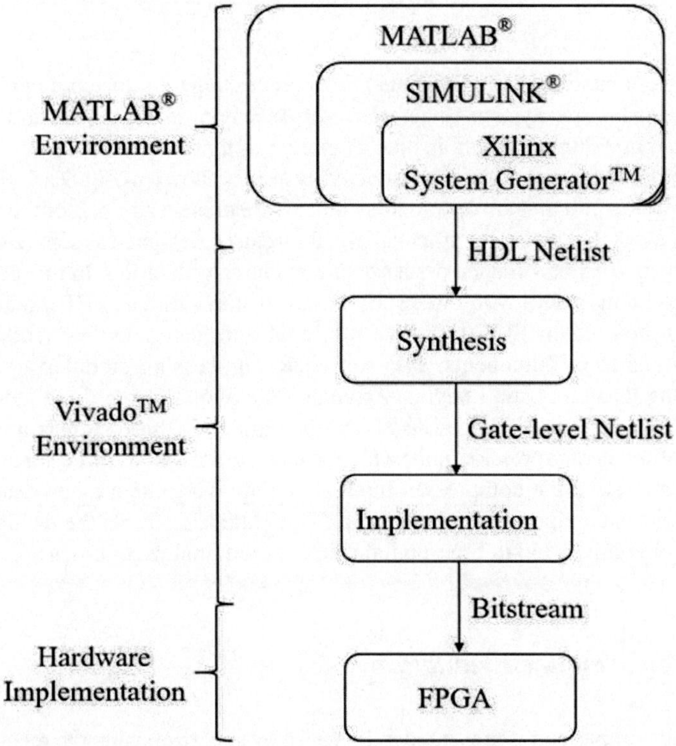

Fig. 9.14 System design flow

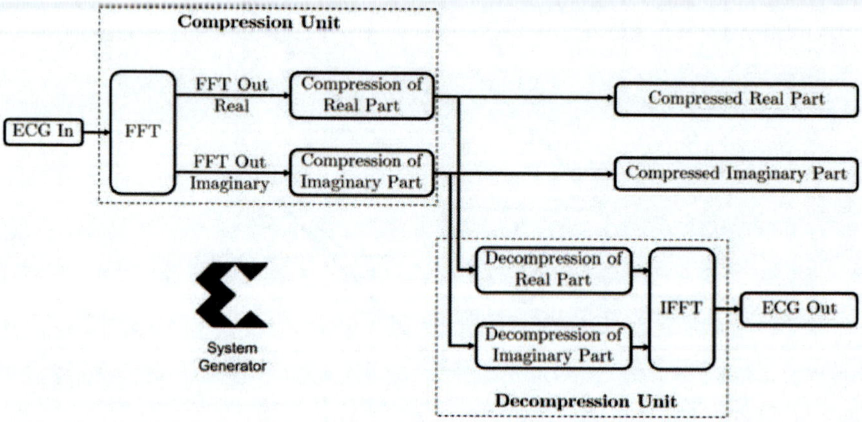

Fig. 9.15 ECG compression and decompression unit design using the System Generator

step of implementation, a single channel ECG processing unit (the core FPGA block) is designed using the System Generator tool. As shown in Figs. 9.12 and 9.13, the complete architecture is a combination of twelve of these core blocks.

A simplified diagram of the implemented system is shown in Fig. 9.15. Here, both the compression unit and the decompression unit are present as a part of the complete signal processor. However, for practical use, they can be designed as separate systems which will significantly reduce the hardware resource utilization. In this design, the compression unit is built with three subsystems. It starts with an FFT module which takes the time-domain ECG signal as the input and generates frequency domain real and imaginary components. Two subsequent processing modules are used for compressing these real and imaginary signals. The outputs from these modules are the required compressed signal. As shown in Fig. 9.15, these signals are used as the input of the decompression unit, which is also comprised of three subunits. First two of them restore the compressed input signal applying the method described in the decompression algorithm. Then, an IFFT module transforms the decompressed frequency-domain signal to time-domain ECG as the final requirement.

9.3.4 *Performance Evaluation*

A graphical comparison is presented in Fig. 9.16 by superimposing the reconstructed ECG signal (output) over the original signal (input). From a thorough visual inspection, it can be recognized that the input and output signals of Fig. 9.16 are virtually identical.

Still, two parameters are needed to be examined for analyzing the performance of a compression algorithm for biosignals to find out how much data compression is done and what is its effect over the signal quality.

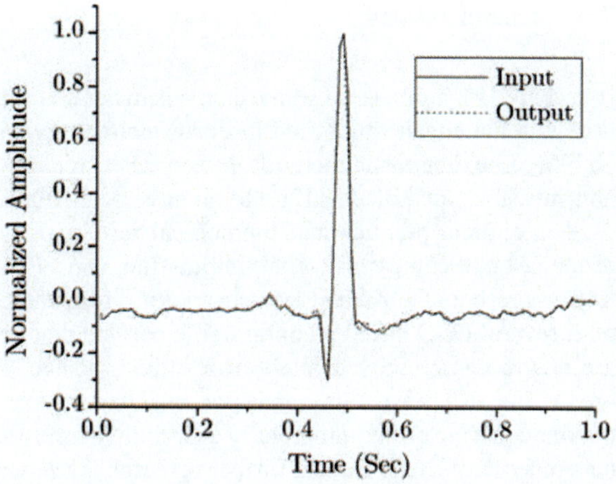

Fig. 9.16 Input and output ECG traces for graphical comparison

Compression Ratio (also known as, the Data-volume Saving in some literature) measures how much the processed signal is compressed compared to the original signal. Percentage of compression ratio (CR%) can be defined [48] by:

$$\mathrm{CR\%} = \left(1 - \frac{size\,of\,the\,output\,stream}{size\,of\,the\,input\,stream}\right) \times 100$$

Normalized Percentage of Root-mean-square Difference (PRDN) is recognized as the most accurate measure for assessing the decompressed signal quality and defined [48] by:

$$\mathrm{PRDN\%} = \sqrt{\frac{\sum_{n=1}^{N}\left[x(n) - \check{x}(n)\right]^2}{\sum_{n=1}^{N}\left[x(n) - \bar{x}(n)\right]^2}} \times 100$$

Here, $x(n)$ is the input signal, $\check{x}(n)$ is the decompressed signal and $\bar{x}(n)$ is the mean value of the input signal. It is important to note that the value of PRDN should be less than 9% for clinical use [48–50].

Following a data analysis, which employs several ECG datasets from the PhysioBank-PhysioNet repository [51], it is found that the implemented system can achieve up to 90% compression ratio with 8.8% PRDN. Because of the high compression rate and superior signal quality, this implemented system is highly suitable for practical applications in an eHealth scheme.

9.4 Conclusions

In recent days, biomedical signal analysis in health informatics is gaining more attention with the advancement in biosensor technology and signal processing research. Unlike some diagnostic methods, biosignal acquisition is mostly low-cost, generally non-invasive, and presents little to no adverse health effect. Hence, it is now widely used in clinical practice and biomedical research. Real-time biosignal processing needs fast and energy efficient computation, and FPGA based reconfigurable architecture presents the perfect low-cost solution for multichannel biosignals. In literature, several ECG based reconfigurable cardiac diagnostic systems are found which are now commercially available for clinical usage. FPGA based EEG and EMG processing also present immense potential to detect several neuromuscular diseases, but there is a lack of commercially available diagnostic units which employs biosignals other than ECG. Hence, further research is needed to ensure the clinical acceptance of this sort of medical tools. As a reconfigurable architecture, the same FPGA chip can be programmed for multiple signal processing tasks. Hence, the development of a unified biosignal processing system for the eHealth system can be a future research direction. The development of artificial organs and prosthesis is also an ongoing research direction which is frequently using FPGAs for hardware acceleration. For example, a neural prosthesis for human brain is still under development and needs further modeling and experimentation for the ultimate validation. Because of its enormous possibilities, many research groups are continuously working on the development of reconfigurable biosignal processing system. The state-of-the-art researches are explored in this chapter to endorse future advancement in this field.

References

1. Escabí, M.A.: Biosignal processing. In: Enderle, J.D., Blanchard, S.M., Bronzino, J.D. (eds.) Introduction to Biomedical Engineering, 2 edn, pp. 549–625. Academic Press, Boston (2005)
2. Rangayyan, R.M., Rangayyan, R.M.: Biomedical Signal Analysis, 2nd edn. Wiley, Hoboken, New Jersey (2015)
3. Ünsalan, C., Tar, B.: Digital System Design with FPGA: Implementation Using Verilog and VHDL. McGraw-Hill Education, New York, NY (2017)
4. Woods, R., Mcallister, J., Turner, R., Yi, Y., Lightbody, G.: FPGA-Based Implementation of Signal and Data Processing Systems. Wiley, New York (2017)
5. Iles, G., Jones, J., Rose, A.: Experience powering Xilinx Virtex-7 FPGAs. J. Instrum. **8**(12), C12037 (2013)
6. Chowdhury, M.H., Cheung, R.C.C.: Reconfgurable architecture for multi-lead ECG signal compression with high-frequency noise reduction. Sci. Rep. **9** (2019)
7. Divya Krishna, K., et al.: Computer aided abnormality detection for kidney on FPGA based IoT enabled portable ultrasound imaging system. Innov. Res. Biomed. Eng. **37**(4), 189–197 (2016)
8. Wu, J.X., Lin, C.H., Du, Y.C., Chen, P.J., Shih, C.C., Chen, T.: Estimation of arteriovenous fistula stenosis by FPGA based Doppler flow imaging system. In: International Ultrasonics Symposium, pp. 1–4 (2015)

9. Kumari, L.V.R., Sai, Y.P., Balaji, N., Viswada, K.: FPGA based arrhythmia detection. Proc. Comput. Sci. **57**, 970–979 (2015)
10. de Carvalho, H.H., Moreno, R.L., Pimenta, T.C., Crepaldi, P.C., Cintra, E.: A heart disease recognition embedded system with fuzzy cluster algorithm. Comput. Methods Programs Biomed. **110**(3), 447–454 (2013)
11. Chatterjee, H.K., Gupta, R., Mitra, M.: Real time P and T wave detection from ECG using Fpga. Proc. Technol. **4**, 840–844 (2012)
12. Rasu, R., Sundaram, P.S., Santhiyakumari, N.: FPGA based non-invasive heart rate monitoring system for detecting abnormalities in Fetal. In: International Conference on Signal Processing and Communication Engineering Systems, pp. 375–379 (2015)
13. Boujelben, O., Bahoura, M.: FPGA implementation of an automatic wheezes detector based on MFCC and SVM. In: International Conference on Advanced Technologies for Signal and Image Processing, ATSIP, pp. 647–650 (2016)
14. Chowdhury, M.H., Cheung, R.C.C.: Point-of-care EMG processor for the differential diagnosis of neuropathy and myopathy. In: IEEE EMB Special Topic Conference on Healthcare Innovations and Point-of-Care Technologies (2019)
15. Wienbrandt, L., Kässens, J.C., González-Domínguez, J., Schmidt, B., Ellinghaus, D., Schimmler, M.: FPGA-based acceleration of detecting statistical epistasis in GWAS. Proc. Comput. Sci. **29**, 220–230 (2014)
16. Dwivedi, A., Ghosh, S., Londhe, N.: Low-power FIR filter design using hybrid artificial bee colony algorithm with experimental validation over FPGA. Circuits Syst. Signal Process. **36**(1), 156–180 (2017)
17. Eminaga, Y., Coskun, A., Kale, I.: Multiplier free implementation of 8-tap daubechies wavelet filters for biomedical applications. In: New Generation of CAS, NGCAS, pp. 129–132 (2017)
18. Xin, Y., Li, W., Zhang, Z., Cheung, R., Song, D., Berger, T.: An Application Specific Instruction Set Processor (ASIP) for Adaptive Filters in Neural Prosthetics. IEEE/ACM Trans. Comput. Biol. Bioinforma. **12**(5), 1034–1047 (2015)
19. Liu, B., Zhang, Z., Fan. H., Fu, Q.: Compression via compressive sensing: a low-power framework for the telemonitoring of multi-channel physiological signals. In: IEEE International Conference on Bioinformatics and Biomedicine, pp. 9–12 (2013)
20. Kim, D.S., Kwon, J.S.: A lossless multichannel bio-signal compression based on low-complexity joint coding scheme for portable medical devices. Sensors **14**(9), 17516–17529 (2014)
21. Lai, S.C., Chien, W.C., Lan, C.S., Lee, M.K., Luo, C.H., Lei, S.F.: An efficient DCT-IV-based ECG compression algorithm and its hardware accelerator design. In: IEEE International Symposium on Circuits and Systems, vol. 101, pp. 1296–1299 (2013)
22. Luo, C.-H., et al.: An ECG acquisition system prototype design with flexible PDMS dry electrodes and variable transform length DCT-IV based compression algorithm. IEEE Sens. J. **16**(23), 8244–8254 (2016)
23. Diftler, M.A., et al.: RoboGlove—a robonaut derived multipurpose assistive device. In: International Conference on Robotics and Automation (2014)
24. Oballe-Peinado, O., Hidalgo-Lopez, J.A., Sanchez-Duran, J.A., Castellanos-Ramos, J., Vidal-Verdu, F.: Architecture of a tactile sensor suite for artificial hands based on FPGAs. In: IEEE RAS and EMBS International Conference on Biomedical Robotics and Biomechatronics, pp. 112–117 (2012)
25. Kumar, J., Kumar, N., Pankaj, D., Kumar, A.: Implementation of real time control algorithm for gait assistive exoskeleton devices for stroke survivors. In: International Conference on Electronic Systems, Signal Processing, and Computing Technologies, pp. 271–275 (2014)
26. Wöhrle, H., Tabie, M., Kim, S.K., Kirchner, F., Kirchner, E.A.: A hybrid FPGA-based system for EEG- and EMG-based online movement prediction. Sensors **17**(7), 1–41 (2017)
27. Ang, L.-M., Seng, K.P., Heng, T.Z.: Information communication assistive technologies for visually impaired people. Int. J. Ambient Comput. Intell. **7**(1), 45–68 (2016)
28. Kim, R.H., Kang, C.H., Bae, J.H., Kang, B.S.: Development of a continuum robot using pneumatic artificial muscles. Int. Conf. Control. Autom. Syst. **Iccas**, 1401–1403 (2014)

29. Li, P., Yu, L., Fang, Q., Lee, S.-Y.: A simplification of Cobelli's glucose insulin model for type 1 diabetes mellitus and its FPGA implementation. Med. Biol. Eng. Comput. **54**(10), 1563–1577 (2016)
30. Vavouras, M., Duarte, R.P., Armato, A., Bouganis, C.S.: A hybrid ASIC/FPGA fault-tolerant artificial pancreas. In: International Conference on Embedded Computer Systems: Architectures, Modeling and Simulation, pp. 261–267 (2017)
31. Slepova, L.O., Zhilenkov, A.A.: Synthesis of model of hardware realization of LIF-model of biological neuron on the basis of FPGA. In: IEEE Conference of Russian Young Researchers in Electrical and Electronic Engineering, vol. 2018, pp. 992–996 (2018)
32. Zhang, G., Tao, H., Shao, J., Lei, S.C., Liang, F.: Low-power programmable linear-phase filter designed for fully balanced bio-signal recording application. Ieice Electron. Express **9**(17), 1402–1407 (2012)
33. Boschmann, A., Agne, A., Witschen, L., Thombansen, G., Kraus, F., Platzner, M.: FPGA-based acceleration of high density myoelectric signal processing. In: International Conference on ReConFigurable Computing and FPGAs, ReConFig, pp. 1–8 (2016)
34. Srivastava, N.R., Troyk, P.R., Bradley, D.: FPGA based visual prosthesis device for testing visual perception on non human primates. In: EEE International Conference on Electro/Information Technology, pp. 21–25 (2007)
35. Al-Yaman, M., Al-Atabany, W., Bystrov, A., Degenaar, P.: FPGA design for dual-spectrum visual scene preparation in retinal prosthesis. In: Annual International Conference of the IEEE Engineering in Medicine and Biology Society, vol. 2014, pp. 4691–4694 (2014)
36. Li, W.X.Y., Chan, R.H.M., Zhang, W., Cheung, R.C.C., Song, D., Berger, T.W.: High-performance and scalable system architecture for the real-time estimation of generalized laguerre-volterra MIMO model from neural population spiking activity. IEEE J. Emerg. Sel. Top. Circuits Syst. **1**(4), 489–501 (2011)
37. Li, W.X.Y., Chan, R.H.M., Berger, T.W., Song, D., Cheung, R.C.C.: A dual mode FPGA design for the hippocampal prosthesis. In: Annual International Conference of the IEEE Engineering in Medicine and Biology Society (EMBC), pp. 4579–4582 (2012)
38. Li, W.X.Y., Cheung, R.C.C., Chan, R.H.M., Song, D., Berger, T.W.: Real-time prediction of neuronal population spiking activity using FPGA. Biomed. Circuits Syst. IEEE Trans. **7**(4), 489–498 (2013)
39. Song, D., Robinson, B.S., Hampson, R.E., Marmarelis, V.Z., Deadwyler, S.A., Berger, T.W.: Sparse large-scale nonlinear dynamical modeling of human hippocampus for memory prostheses. IEEE Trans. Neural Syst. Rehabil. Eng. **26**(2), 272–280 (2018)
40. Chowdhury, M.H., Hossain, Q.D.: Development of two wireless ECG monitoring systems and their performance assessment. In: International Conference on Informatics, Electronics Vision, pp. 459–464 (2018)
41. Shouleice, R.B., Bass, G.: From bench to bedside-developments in electrocardiology. Eng. Journal, Inst. Eng. Irel. **56**(4), 47–49 (2002)
42. Chowdhury, M.H., Hossain, Q.D., Saha, P., Rahaman, M.M.: Design, fabrication and performance evaluation of a three electrode ECG recorder. In: International Conference on Innovations in Science, Engineering and Technology (2016)
43. Chowdhury, M.H., Hossain, Q.D., Hossain, M.A., Cheung, R.C.C.: Single feed circularly polarized crescent-cut and extended corner square microstrip antennas for wireless biotelemetry. Int. J. Electr. Comput. Eng. **9**(3), 1902–1909 (2019)
44. Proakis, J.G., Manolakis, D.G.: *Digital signal processing*, 4th editio. Pearson/Prentice Hall, Upper Saddle River, NJ (2007)
45. Rabiner, L.: On the use of symmetry in FFT computation. IEEE Trans. Acoust. **27**(3), 233–239 (1979)
46. Olivas, J.Á., Sepúlveda, R., Montiel, O., Castillo, O.: Methodology to test and validate a VHDL inference engine through the Xilinx system generator. Soft Computing for Hybrid Intelligent Systems, pp. 325–331. Springer, Cham (2008)
47. Moreo, A.T., Lorente, P.N., Valles, F.S., Muro, J.S., Andres, C.F.: Experiences on developing computer vision hardware algorithms using Xilinx system generator. Microprocess. Microsyst. **29**(8–9), 411–419 (2005)

48. Němcová, A., Smíšek, R., Maršánová, L., Smital, L., Vítek, M.: A comparative analysis of methods for evaluation of ECG signal quality after compression. Biomed Res. Int. **2018** (2018)
49. Zigel, Y., Cohen, A., Katz, A.: The weighted diagnostic distortion (WDD) measure for ECG signal compression. IEEE Trans. Biomed. Eng. **47**(11), 1422–1430 (2000)
50. Blanco-Velasco, M., Cruz-Roldan, F., Godino-Llorente, J.I., Barner, K.E.: ECG compression with retrieved quality guaranteed. Electron. Lett. **40**(23), 1466–1467 (2004)
51. Goldberger, A.L., et al.: PhysioBank, PhysioToolkit, and PhysioNet: components of a new research resource for complex physiologic signals. Circulation **101**(23), e215–e220 (2000)

Chapter 10
Health Informatics: Challenges and Opportunities

Mehedi Hasan Raju, Mosabber Uddin Ahmed, and Md Atiqur Rahman Ahad

Abstract Health Informatics (HI) imposes informatics concepts, theories, and practices to real-life circumstances to attain improved health outcomes, which incorporate not only collection and accumulation of data but also data analysis and presentation. A plethora of research activities has been going on in the field of HI due to the widespread of its probable applications. This chapter presents a comprehensive treatise on HI, its potential challenges, opportunities and some recommendations as the future directions for HI. All the pertinent aspects are discussed in this chapter with a view to relating their significance in HI and its applications. On the whole, the chapter ensures the fundamental information one needs to step into the world of HI.

Keywords Health informatics · Health IT · EHR

10.1 Introduction

Informatics is an extended type of information science and information engineering branch. In this field, information processing and information systems engineering are addressed. This field relates to the human-information relationship as well as the integration of boundaries, connections, experiences, emerging technologies, and controlled networks. This led to the appraisal of informatics with computational, statistical, natural, subjective and social perspectives, including the investigation of technology's social effect. Hence, the field of informatics is exceedingly wide and includes numerous subareas, including data science, information systems, and statistics.

M. H. Raju (✉)
Department of ICT, Bangladesh University of Professionals, Dhaka, Bangladesh
e-mail: 0.mehedihasanraju@gmail.com

M. U. Ahmed · M. A. R. Ahad
Department of Electrical and Electronic Engineering, University of Dhaka, Dhaka, Bangladesh

M. A. R. Ahad
Department of Media Intelligent, Osaka University, Osaka, Japan

M. A. R. Ahad and M. U. Ahmed (eds.), *Signal Processing Techniques for Computational Health Informatics*, Intelligent Systems Reference Library 192,
https://doi.org/10.1007/978-3-030-54932-9_10

In the medicinal sector, the use of computer is not new and it is developing at a very high rate. Healthcare system utilizes innovative technologies to improve medicinal services. Health Informatics (HI) has grown as an advanced science with the extension of electronic health records (EHRs) and health data analytics systems. It has additionally developed with the establishment of health data exchange standards, such as HL7 (Health Level 7) and FHIR (Fast Health Interoperability Resources) [1]. Nowadays, healthcare system organizes, analyzes, and deals with health records by using information technology. It manages the assets, devices, and strategies to use attainment, storage, recovery, and utilization of data in health and medication. It affords to grant access to medical records for patients, specialist doctors, nurses, hospital administrators, caregivers, and the stakeholder related to the system. For that reason, HI is also called the health information system, or biomedical informatics.

It should be mentioned and noted that HI focuses on information related to health, not technology. In HI, health data has been collected, processed, used, analyzed, shared, and stored (Fig. 10.1).

To abridge, HI is an evolving specialization aspect of informatics that connects information technology, communications and healthcare to improve the quality and safety of patient care and ensures higher quality, higher efficiency, lower cost, greater availability, and new opportunities to the existing health care system. It incorporates a set of methodologies for the management of information in the health sector [2, 3].

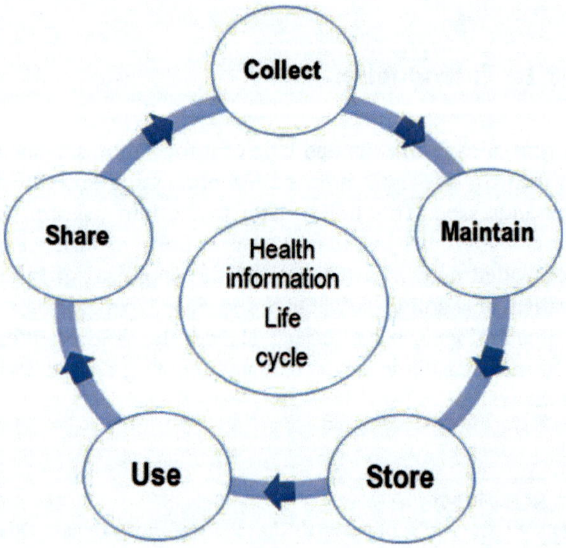

Fig. 10.1 Health information lifecycle

10.2 Aspects of Health Informatics

HI brings state-of-the-art technology in healthcare sectors. Both patients and clinicians are depending on new electronic technology and information system. Several ways of keeping the patient engaged and then being allowed to treat by more informed and prepared clinicians are addressed below:

(1) **Electronic Health Records (EHR)**

Patients visit several doctors because of their several health-related issues. Paper-based records were a matter of hassle for the patients. Similarly, doctors also failed to learn about the patient's health history properly. Electronic Health Records (EHR) makes this situation easier. Patients no longer have to sum up their personal history in case of emergencies. When they consider moving to other clinicians – patients and their families no longer need to worry about forgotten pediatric names or lost records of medicines. Instead, the medical staff will have much of the information available for review in the EHR.

(2) **Decision making support to improve patient care**

For a patient, proper assessment/diagnostic and treatment is the most important of all. HI ameliorates the standard of treatment to patients by healthcare sector. HI helps data to be processed and recovered easily and effectively, but can also be a resource of decision-making. Computerized protocols offer advantages that help make better decisions for physicians and clients. With this, it is possible to maintain high quality care.

(3) **Reduce treatment costs**

Due to medical errors, every year a huge amount of money has been wasted. HI can reduce that cost at a larger amount. Because using Electronic Health Records, patient's information is in safe and reliable hands. EHR not only minimize such mistakes but also work to take most productivity-intensive tasks out of the preoccupied hands of medical personnel. Such procedures are streamlined to save extreme expenses for the health sector and consumers.

(4) **Standards**

HI's involvements in healthcare sector are changing the traditional way of researching on public health and ailment, and are providing better treatment [4]. HI is transforming the standards of thinking and clinician's activities. Doctors are now using different wearable and contactless technologies for patient monitoring as well as remote treatment [5].

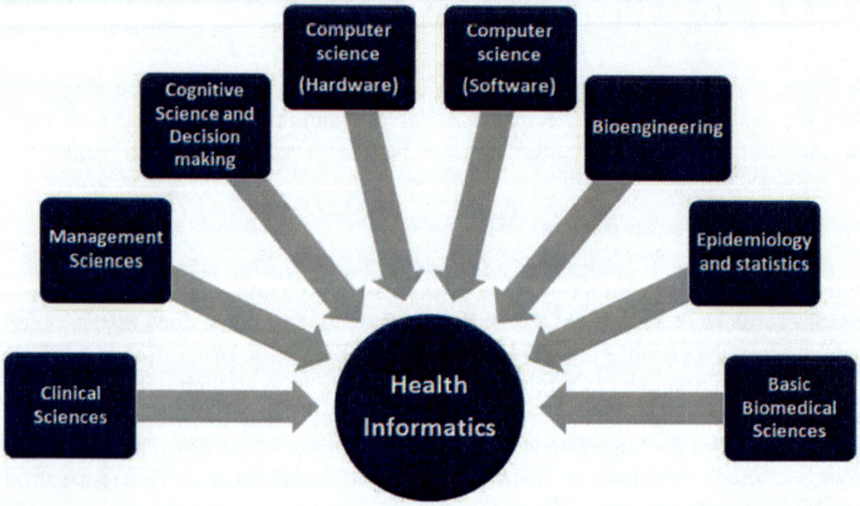

Fig. 10.2 Health informatics with other disciplines

10.2.1 Interdisciplinary Nature of Health Informatics

HI is a multidisciplinary study in identifying, implementing, incorporating and integrating information and technology-based advancements in the distribution, administration, and preparation of public health and health care (Fig. 10.2). It has attachments with clinical science because of clinical research works, cognitive science and decision making. These aid to evaluate the situation based on the statistics. Similarly, the multidisciplinary nature of HI brings together different aspects of biomedical science, bioengineering, computer science, management science, etc.

10.2.2 Health Information Technology (HIT) Versus Health Informatics (HI)

In spite of the fact that the idea of Health Information Technology (HIT) incorporates the utilization of technology in healthcare, HI is not synonymous with HIT. There exists a fine line of difference between these two domains. While the two fields are related, there are distinct differences between health information technology and HI. Health information are exchanged and shared with HIT. This field implements the process that generates electronic health records and electronic prescribing, ensures data security and privacy and interoperates the records across multiple organizations.

On the other hand, HI utilizes the available data to secure, organize and evaluate data related to patient care. HI does so with the help of HIT directly. HI deals with electronic health records in an interdisciplinary approach to create new solutions

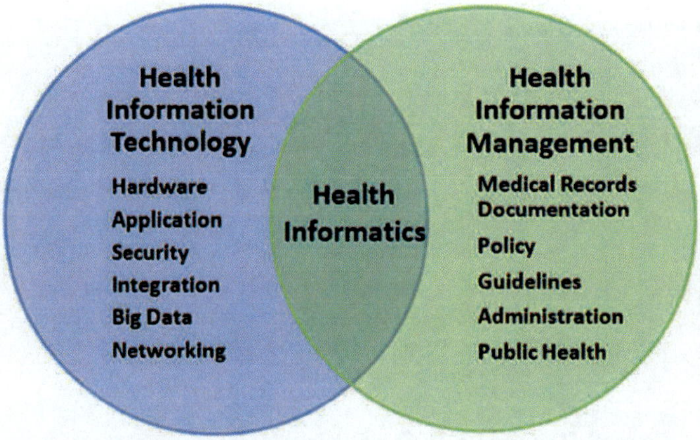

Fig. 10.3 Relation between HIT and HI

intended to improve the delivery of public and private healthcare services. It designs patient data systems, manages information database and analyzes patient data using health information technology. Figure 10.3 demonstrates a relationship between HIT, health information management and HI.

10.3 Application of Health Informatics

10.3.1 Translational Bioinformatics (TBI)

Bioinformatics functional related to human health and disease is termed as Translational Bioinformatics (TBI). It utilizes and expands the ideas and techniques from bioinformatics to support the act of translational medicine, for example, the interpretation of natural disclosures into real effect on clinical consideration and human health. TBI links up the gap between bioinformatics and HI. Translational bioinformatics includes the advancement and utilization of computational techniques that can reason over the tremendous measures of life science information being gathered and put away to make new instruments for medicine [6]. Translational bioinformatics can be defined as "the development of storage, analytic, and interpretive methods to optimize the transformation of increasingly voluminous biomedical data, and genomic data into proactive, predictive, preventive, and participatory health" [2] (Fig. 10.4).

American Medical Informatics Association (AMIA) considers the translational bioinformatics as one of its three major fields of informatics. It is a sub-domain of HI, which integrates molecular and clinical data to facilitate a new translational propositions between the field of biology and medicine [7, 8].

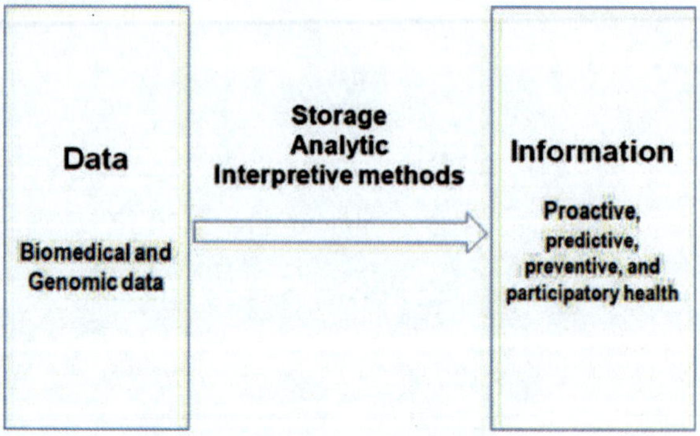

Fig. 10.4 Translational bioinformatics

10.3.2 Clinical Research Informatics (CRI)

An energetic and emergent sub-discipline of informatics has risen at the convergence of biomedical informatics and clinical research, which we will allude to as Clinical Research Informatics (CRI). CRI has added to upgrade the quality, proficiency, and convenience of clinical research. It is associated with developing, analyzing and applying computer theory, processes and applications to amend the scope and conduct of biomedical research and to distribute the acquired information [2]. Clinical research is a science that promotes the assessment of the efficacy and safety of medicines and devices, surgical techniques and differential diagnoses. Therefore, clinical research informatics is a branch of the informatics that advocates all these research activities, especially information gathering, procurement and evaluation for diverse types of claims [9, 10]. The United States describes clinical research as "The range of studies and trials in human subjects that fall into three subcategories: Patient-oriented research, Epidemiologic and behavioral studies, Health services research" [11].

10.3.3 Clinical Informatics

Clinical informatics is the utilization of HI and IT to convey medical services to mass people. It is often alluded to as applied clinical informatics and operational informatics. Clinical informatics offers a wide range of subjects involving medical decision guidance to visual information; from patient records to prescription management systems, and from management to execution and acceptance concerns [12]. When used for health care, American Medical Informatics Association (AMIA) assumes informatics to be practically the same regardless of the community of health professionals' involved. Clinical informatics examines, develops, incorporates and reviews systems information to improve quality of life for the mass people, ameliorate patient care, and reinforce the relationship between doctor and patient. Due to the practice of clinical informatics, electronic health records are being used to carry out medicinal research, public healthcare services, etc. and it is increasing day by day. Moreover, clinical informatics is raising the standards among consumers about how the computer tools communicate [11–13].

10.3.4 Consumer Health Informatics

Considerable growth has been visualized in the consumer health informatics sector for the last 25 years. Consumer health informatics services can promote quality care and can integrate care for patients, modify medical behavior, maintain information and make decisions [14]. It is a subdivision of the health informatics that scrutinizes the needs of users; researches and executes processes of rendering information widely available; and models and strengthens the connection among specialists and patients [15]. Wireless as well as wearable devices have influenced the evolution of consumer health informatics at an early age [16]. Consumer health informatics remains at the intersection of different fields, for example, nursing informatics, healthcare advancement, proper health training, etc. Probably, it is the most tested and quickly extended field in medicinal informatics. Consumer health research helps individuals with non-communicable diseases to manage the complex healthcare environment with real-time tracking, new devices, and quick access to substantial guidance to endorse risk management [17]. Patients face many problems while seeking health services. Consumer health informatics could guide the care seeker for getting proper treatment and run the system from the patient's perspective [18].

10.3.5 Public Health Informatics

Public health services have implemented health information systems and information technology as a potentially transformative tool for developing processes of real-time reporting, coordination, and knowledge sharing through different institutions. Public health informatics is assigned to protect and enhance community health by delivering efficient and productive training, sound ways of life, just as an anticipation of ailment and damage [19]. The effective and reliable assortment of data and knowledge on quality public health is complex. It is the cornerstone of the roles of public health, such as inspection, analysis for public health, and evaluation [20]. When personal data gathering and processing is rapidly being used, there is an overemphasis on information management systems [21].

It factors in the need for public health teams to be able to design and execute these programs of Public Health Informatics (PHI) specialists. PHI professionals refer to the principles of information technology to support technological advances that enhance the quality and efficiency and dissemination of information used only

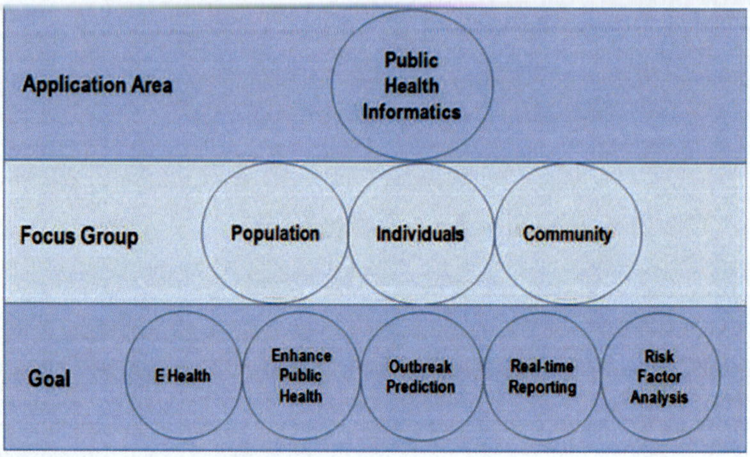

Fig. 10.5 Various aspects of public health informatics

to ameliorate public health and its services [22, 23]. In creating and sharing electronic data, both medical care services and public health organizations are increasingly using public health informatics. Such initiatives reflect substantial growth in a variety of health-centric exchanges of information and insights [24]. Figure 10.5 depicts various aspects of PHI, covering the focused group and goals. PHI focuses on the individuals as well as the whole community with the objective of E-health, improvement of medical facilities, and preparing the community for any kind of pandemic/outbreaks.

10.4 Privacy Issues and Challenges for Health Informatics

Research on health informatics has several interesting challenges to face [25]. Important challenging aspects are highlighted below:

(i) **Conventional healthcare environment**

Embracing new models of reliable information epoch might be a troublesome adventure given the present timetables from production to execution and use. The existing administrative condition encompassing conventional medical devices implies so. Trusted and reliable connections among a range of devices are critical aspects that are required to excel in HI. The expanding connectedness and the reduction of authoritative limits however present data security concerns.

(ii) **Infrastructure issue**

HI brings new security problems and challenges. The issue of dynamic versus static network, with no fixed end focuses implies that a considerable amount of the existent communication mechanism for moving messages safely may not work properly. This implies that there are critical difficulties in the security and administration of this information, just as its assurance and security. At present, these associations are profoundly dependent on trust. If the medical device engineer does not consider cyber-attack threats while designing the devices, it can be termed as technical debt [26]. The faulty devices showed unpredictable and unusual behaviors in their functionalities. The significant concern is the effect of misuse as opposed to the abuse itself.

(iii) **Device diversity, interoperability and vulnerability**

Different types of medical wearable devices have been used in the health informatics system. So, interoperability between those devices is a big concern. It has to be an interoperable system where data need to be transferred both one-to-one and one-to-many connections, including information exchange across multiple interfaces where the devices need to be compatible with one another. It is mandatory to consider that in any communication between multiple systems, the combination of interfaces is almost double. There is no collection of information regarding the capability of the devices. Device registry requires indexes of devices functionality, conventions, phrasings and standards. The system's interoperability made the system invulnerable to different threats.

(iv) **Data integrity and consistency**

Data integrity is a matter of concern for HI. Data integrity means preserving the original data even in the case of any alterations. Ensuring integrity in a HI system guarantees the correctness of data which leads to minimizing errors and improving the safety of patients. As of now, approved clients are also making mistakes because of their inadequate knowledge about the system. Everyone is using the different features of the system without proper knowledge which makes the system inconsistent. Dealing with huge number of data is a challenge for HI [27]. Moreover, for every information exchanging system, heterogeneous data is another issue to face [28].

(v) **Privacy concern**

The utility of information is expanded when a significant number of people in the area use it. A few information or datasets are openly accessible, while numerous different sorts of information have various degrees of privacy concerns. Medical information is considered the most private sorts of information and access to this information is profoundly sensitive and must be approved to be accessed by assigned experts [29]. Privacy in the healthcare sector may make different results to the patients including the refusal of the administration to death. For specialist co-ops, privacy breaches can prompt legitimate authorizations, financial loss, or loss of goodwill [30]. Besides, health data must be audited in regular intervals [31].

(vi) **Data access control**

Information access to information control is considered as topmost constraints for ensuring privacy and security to any data. For HI, it is mandatory to control access over the whole system. The whole system supposed to have different access segmentation. While guaranteeing CIA triads, protecting patients' vital pieces of information from unauthorized divulgence is fundamental under any conditions. All in all, the patient is characterized as the maker of the data. Building up the responsibility for data is essential for securing the system from unauthorized access and manipulating the patient's health-related information. Other than patients, staff who are taking care of the patients can be termed as the supervisor of the health information of the patients [32]. Authorization is mainly carried out by a security mechanism called access control. Medical data are stored in the cloud which is distributed covering a larger area. Sometimes it makes a challenge for the system.

(vii) **Human factors**

Human being becomes a crucial factor while using a system like HI as we have a huge role to play. Staff training is a prerequisite for developing a technology-based health system. Because, as per the research conducted by KTH University, a human factor is considered as the ultimate challenge in 76% of the time [33]. So, a usability study is required before developing and adopting a whole new system of HI.

(viii) **Laws and ethics**

Laws and ethics sometimes become the reason of privacy breach. Hospitals and governments provide records about the patient and his/her diseases to the research agencies so that research agencies could help, in case of a disease outbreak. The government supposed to ensure that the research agencies dealt with that information in the best way without causing any misuse of it.

(ix) **Data authenticity**

Authenticity is simply the validness of the data. Authenticity depicts the accuracy, truthfulness, and specifications related to data. It establishes or confirms that all the claims are true and authentic. Due to the lack of authentication of information, attacks like man-in-the-middle (MITM) could take place. To prevent this kind of attack, endpoint authentication is required in the cryptographic protocol.

(x) **Confidentiality and availability**

Confidentiality includes a lot of rules so that the private information could not be accessed by general mass. The facility to protect the information in the HI system so that it can only be accessed by authorized subjects is called confidentiality. Authorized subjects receive access based on their working role. Thus, nothing about the patient's health record should be shared without their consent.

The system ought to have the option to be accessed whenever required by approved ones, for instance, on account of any crisis circumstance a particular doctor needs access to the patient's record to complete analysis and favor prescription to a patient. The system ought not to be obliged to a particular time generally; a patient may require a doctor's support any time. Thus, the system needs to be available 24/7.

(xi) **Site recruitment**

Different difficulties, for example, issues with site recruitment, are critical to talk about, yet cannot be resolved legitimately through HI alone. Community health centers engage themselves in a network and showed interest in an active collaborative network in order to have a mutually beneficial relationship with other sites and users of the network. The whole process is termed as site recruitment [34].

(xii) **4 V's**

There are 4 V's which are challenging for HI [35]. Those are volume, variety, velocity and veracity. Here volume means lots of medical data, which due to variety of sources with high velocity to process creates complexity because of veracity. It is difficult and daunting to deal with large quantities of healthcare data, coming from varied data sources. Moreover, it varies in its eminence and intricacy and also it is difficult to generate and process such amount data [36]. Health care sector dealt with data that are often biased, full of clatter and anomalies that create a potential threat to proper decision-making processes and treatments for the patients.

10.5 Opportunities and Future Goal of Health Informatics

If we could overcome the challenges mentioned above, there are a lot of opportunities for the HI sector. Let's have a look at those opportunities.

Personalized treatment: Within a very short time, HI will be able to provide personalized treatment to everyone. It will improve the standard of treatment; patients will receive the best practice form the specialists, while doctors will be able to detect any diseases before a patient shows any symptoms. In HI, the recommender system will be used, which realizes a few chances to the healthcare sector in particular in personalized healthcare as they give significant data to the patients [37].

Public health service standards: Through using information science in the healthcare sector, a large number of general people can be benefitted. With the help of a nationwide database for patient's health records, contagious diseases and outbreaks can be prevented easily, consequently benefiting the whole population [38]. Health equity can be achieved through HI [39]. For example, vision-based action analysis like monitoring, rehabilitation treatments are the outcome of improvement of public health standard as well as healthcare sector [40, 41].

Remote monitoring: Caregivers do not require sitting the whole day by the side of patients to monitor his/her health status. HI will allow the clinicians to monitor the patients remotely and observe multiple patients at a time.

Telemedicine: Telemedicine is providing health services from remote distance through electronic signal [42]. HI is a part of telemedicine umbrella that covers distance healthcare service [43]. More specifically, telemedicine can extends its dimension through HI as the use of computerized database, records, information access as well as decision making based on medical data can revolutionize the healthcare sector [44].

Heredity analysis: Heredity analysis is a hot opportunity for HI. HI can incorporate genome analysis in the conventional decision-making methods of health care by designing innovative and reliable tools for gene sequencing. This will create a whole new way of public health treatment. The genomic advancements are capable of facilitating inference, treating especially inherited infections and multi-faceted diseases [45].

10.6 Some Representative HI Service Providers

Eclinicalworks, LLC [46] is a pioneer in healthcare IT, giving thorough EHR and Practice Management (PM) arrangements utilized by more than 850,000 medical professionals in 20 nations. Their service includes telehealth, EHR, population health management, patient management, etc. It offers unified and integrated healthcare IT solutions for medical professionals.

NextGen healthcare [47] is a leading EHR and healthcare practice management software solutions for ambulatory care providers. Their service includes care coordination, EHR, electronic data interchange, health information exchange, population health, patient management, tele solution, etc.

McKesson Corporation [48] is a multifaceted company distributing pharmaceuticals and providing health information technology, medical supplies, and care management tools to the users. Through their services, McKesson ensures improvement in healthcare sector. However, there are other partners and in this chapter, we are not enlisting them. These three examples are mentioned to provide an overview of the few HI service providers.

10.7 Recommendations for Advanced Health Informatics

HI is extremely important in improving quality and minimizing health care costs. Thus, efforts to protect the privacy of patients will focus on finding ways to protect confidential digital medical information in an electronic world. Some recommendations are made for advanced health informatics for the future:

- While considering the improvement of the safety and security of HI, healthcare organizations need to take a more active strategy. HI is lagging due to a lack of active managerial incentives. Strong management and trained manpower/staff will help the system to adopt strong approaches [49].
- The main concerns about patient data privacy emerge from the open exchange of information across the healthcare sector and the dysfunctional central and provincial regulatory system for the careful security of health information. The regulatory sector needs to be more effective and careful regarding the patient's information [29, 50].
- Different countries of the world are getting HI services through many companies. However, it is a matter of concern that the developing/underdeveloped countries are lagging behind. So, there is a lot to develop in this sector in a cost-effective way so that developing/underdeveloped countries could be a beneficiary of HI.
- Government institutions like the ministry of health or other non-profitable health organizations should work actively with the objective of proper health informatics development [24]. The policymakers should develop a sustainable economic model for the healthcare sector incorporating health informatics and initiate infrastructure for HI.
- Health insurance companies should have decisive coordination with health informatics service providers to improve individual health conditions and healthcare care sectors as well.
- Unauthorized access to information should be monitored. The healthcare organization itself should take initiatives to control and design the system as per privileges. Last but not the least, when resolving privacy and security issues, physicians, as well as patients, have vital roles to play.
- Telemedicine has a vital role to play in this modern life; specifically, COVID-19 pandemic makes it clear for us. Integrating HI in telemedicine will add a new dimension to the healthcare sector.
- System and device compatibility are recommended for HI advancement. Transition from conventional to advanced HI cannot be achieved overnight. Ensuring compatibility will make the process smoother.
- Adequate learning opportunities for doctors as well as medical staffs are recommended for developing a new system and for the improvement of the sector as a whole [49, 51].
- There are lots of signal processing techniques for HI. However, all techniques have some flaws or some restrictions to work on [52]. So for advancement of healthcare, advancement in processing techniques is mandatory.

10.8 Conclusion

HI focuses on real-life circumstances, informatics principles, hypotheses, and procedures to produce better health benefits. It collects data, compiles them and does the proper analysis. Because of its possibility of extensive uses, a multitude of research practices has been taking place in the area of HI. In this chapter, the basic concepts of HI have been discussed. Its difference from HIT and other fields of informatics has been stated clearly here. This chapter depicts the widespread activities of the sub-branches of HI and the potentiality of HI as a whole. Challenges and privacy issues are a concern for HI. We stated those issues and provide some potential recommendations for improving the situations. Health informatics with the current ground-breaking improvements has the prospect to further improve the healthcare system in the future.

References

1. Bender, D., Sartipi, K.: HL7 FHIR: an Agile and RESTful approach to healthcare information exchange. In: Proceedings of the 26th IEEE International Symposium on Computer-Based Medical Systems, pp. 326–331 (2013)
2. Shortliffe, E.H., Cimino, J.J.: Computer Applications in Health Care and Biomedicine. Springer, Heidelberg (2006)
3. Collen, M.F.: The origins of informatics. J. Am. Med. Inform. Assoc. **1**(2), 91–107 (1994)
4. Ohno-Machado, L.: Health information technology and patient safety. J. Am. Med. Inform. Assoc. **24**(2), 243 (2017). https://doi.org/10.1093/jamia/ocx008
5. Kobashi, S., Ahad, M.A.R., Kim, N., Tong, Y., Yagi, N.: Special issue on soft computing in medical informatics. Int. J. Innovative Comput. Inf. Control **12**(4), 2 (2016)
6. Butte, A.J.: Translational bioinformatics: coming of age. J. Am. Med. Inform. Assoc. **15**(6), 709–714 (2008). https://doi.org/10.1197/jamia.M2824
7. Sarkar, I.N., Payne, P.R.O.: The joint summits on translational science: crossing the translational chasm. J. Biomed. Inform. **44**, S1–S2 (2011). https://doi.org/10.1016/j.jbi.2011.11.011
8. Dudley, J.T., Pouliot, Y., Chen, R., Morgan, A.A., Butte, A.J.: Translational bioinformatics in the cloud: an affordable alternative. Genome. Med. **2**(8), 51 (2010). https://doi.org/10.1186/gm172
9. Richesson, R.L., Horvath, M.M., Rusincovitch, S.A.: Clinical research informatics and electronic health record data. Yearb. Med. Inf. **23**(01), 215–223 (2014). https://doi.org/10.15265/IY-2014-0009
10. Richesson, R.L., Andrews, J.E., Hollis, K.F.: Introduction to clinical research informatics. In: Clinical research informatics, pp. 3–15, Springer, Cham (2019)
11. Embi, P.J., Payne, P.R.O.: Clinical research informatics: challenges, opportunities and definition for an emerging domain. J. Am. Med. Inform. Assoc. **16**(3), 316–327 (2009). https://doi.org/10.1197/jamia.M3005
12. Singh, S.: Big dreams with big data! use of clinical informatics to inform biomarker discovery. Clin. Transl. Gastroenter. **10**(3), e00018 (2019). https://doi.org/10.14309/ctg.0000000000000018
13. Silverman, H.D., Steen, E.B., Carpenito, J.N., Ondrula, C.J., Williamson, J.J., Fridsma, D.B.: Domains, tasks, and knowledge for clinical informatics subspecialty practice: results of a practice analysis. J. Am. Med. Inform. Assoc. **26**(7), 586–593 (2019). https://doi.org/10.1093/jamia/ocz051
14. Demiris, G.: Consumer health informatics: past, present, and future of a rapidly evolving domain. Yearb. Med. Inform. **25**(S 01), S42–S47 (2016). https://doi.org/10.15265/iys-2016-s005
15. Eysenbach, G.: Recent advances: consumer health informatics. BMJ **320**(7251), 1713–1716 (2000). https://doi.org/10.1136/bmj.320.7251.1713

16. Gibbons, M.C., Shaikh, Y.: Introduction to consumer health informatics and digital inclusion. In: Edmunds, M., Hass, C., Holve, E. (eds.) Consumer Informatics and Digital Health, pp. 25–41. Springer, Cham (2019)
17. Faiola, A., Holden, R.J.: Consumer health informatics: empowering healthy-living-seekers through mhealth. Prog. Cardiovasc. Dis. **59**(5), 479–486 (2017). https://doi.org/10.1016/j.pcad.2016.12.006
18. Featherall, J., Lapin, B., Chaitoff, A., Havele, S.A., Thompson, N., Katzan, I.: Characterization of patient interest in provider-based consumer health information technology: survey study. J. Med. Internet Res. **20**(4), e128 (2018). https://doi.org/10.2196/jmir.7766
19. Williams, F., Oke, A., Zachary, I.: Public health delivery in the information age: the role of informatics and technology. Perspect Pub. Health **139**(5), 236–254 (2019). https://doi.org/10.1177/1757913918802308
20. Wholey, D.R., LaVenture, M., Rajamani, S., Kreiger, R., Hedberg, C., Kenyon, C.: Developing workforce capacity in public health informatics: core competencies and curriculum design. Front. Public Health **6**, 124 (2018). https://doi.org/10.3389/fpubh.2018.00124
21. Freed, J., Kyffin, R., Rashbass, J., Organ, S., Boseley, P., Haworth, A., Brice, A., Schmidt, J., Flowers, J., Sinclair, D., Hughes, A., Kessel, A., Coates, E., Davis, A., Baughan, S., Chappel, D., Mauchline, M., Roberts, N., Kemp, R., Hill, A., Carrigan, C.: Knowledge strategy: harnessing the power of information to improve the public's health. Public Health England, pp. 1–41 (2014)
22. Thiébaut, R., Thiessard, F.: Public health and epidemiology informatics. Yearb. Med. Inf. **26**(01), 248–251 (2017). https://doi.org/10.15265/IY-2017-036
23. McFarlane, T.D., Dixon, B.E., Grannis, S.J., Gibson, P.J.: Public health informatics in local and state health agencies: an update from the public health workforce interests and needs survey. J. Pub. Health Manage. Prac. **25**, S67–S77 (2019). https://doi.org/10.1097/PHH.0000000000000918
24. Gamache, R., Kharrazi, H., Weiner, J.: Public and population health informatics: the bridging of big data to benefit communities. Yearb. Med. Inf. **27**(01), 199–206 (2018). https://doi.org/10.1055/s-0038-1667081
25. Coiera, E., Ammenwerth, E., Georgiou, A., Magrabi, F.: Does health informatics have a replication crisis? J. Am. Med. Inform. Assoc. **25**(8), 963–968 (2018)
26. Williams, P.A.H., McCauley, V.: Always connected: the security challenges of the healthcare Internet of Things. In: 2016 IEEE 3rd World Forum on Internet of Things (WF-IoT), Reston, VA, USA, pp. 30–35. https://doi.org/10.1109/wf-iot.2016.7845455 (2016)
27. Pang, Z., Yang, G., Khedri, R., Zhang, Y.-T.: Introduction to the special section: convergence of automation technology, biomedical engineering, and health informatics toward the healthcare 4.0. IEEE Rev. Biomed. Eng. **11**, 249–259 (2018)
28. Raju, M.H., Ahmed, M.U., Ahad, M.A.R.: Security analysis and a potential layer to layer security solution of medical cyber-physical systems. In: Balas, V.E., Solanki, V.K., Kumar, R., Ahad, M.A.R. (eds.) A Handbook of Internet of Things in Biomedical and Cyber Physical System, vol. 165, pp. 61–86. Springer, Cham (2020)
29. Al-Muhtadi, J., Shahzad, B., Saleem, K., Jameel, W., Orgun, M.A.: Cybersecurity and privacy issues for socially integrated mobile healthcare applications operating in a multi-cloud environment. Health Inf. J **25**(2), 315–329 (2019). https://doi.org/10.1177/1460458217706184
30. Anwar, M., Joshi, J., Tan, J.: Anytime, anywhere access to secure, privacy-aware healthcare services: issues, approaches and challenges. Health Policy Technol **4**(4), 299–311 (2015). https://doi.org/10.1016/j.hlpt.2015.08.007
31. Azeez, N.A., der Vyver, C.V.: Security and privacy issues in e-health cloud-based system: a comprehensive content analysis. Egypt. Inf. J. **20**(2), 97–108 (2019). https://doi.org/10.1016/j.eij.2018.12.001
32. Zhang, R., Liu, L.: Security models and requirements for healthcare application clouds. In: 2010 IEEE 3rd International Conference on Cloud Computing, Miami, FL, USA, pp. 268–275. https://doi.org/10.1109/cloud.2010.62 (2010)

33. Kubbo, M., Jayabalan, M., Rana, M.E.: Privacy and security challenges in cloud based electronic health record: towards access control model. p. 9 (2016)
34. Harris, D.R., Harper, T.J., Henderson, D.W., Henry, K.W., Talbert, J.C.: Informatics-based challenges of building collaborative healthcare research and analysis networks from rural community health centers. In: 2016 IEEE-EMBS International Conference on Biomedical and Health Informatics (BHI), Las Vegas, NV, USA, pp. 513–516. https://doi.org/10.1109/bhi.2016.7455947 (2016)
35. Fang, R., Pouyanfar, S., Yang, Y., Chen, S.-C., Iyengar, S.S.: Computational Health informatics in the big data age: a survey. ACM Comput. Surv. **49**(1), 1–36 (2016). https://doi.org/10.1145/2932707
36. Feldman, B., Martin, E.M., Skotnes, T.: Big data in healthcare hype and hope. Dr. Bonnie **360**, 122–125 (2012)
37. Saha, J., Chowdhury, C., Biswas, S.: Review of machine learning and deep learning based recommender systems for health informatics. In: Deep Learning Techniques for Biomedical and Health Informatics, Springer, pp. 101–126 (2020)
38. Raghupathi, W., Raghupathi, V.: Big data analytics in healthcare: promise and potential. Health Inf Sci Syst **2**(1), 3 (2014). https://doi.org/10.1186/2047-2501-2-3
39. Brewer, L.C., et al.: Back to the future: achieving health equity through health informatics and digital health. JMIR mHealth uHealth **8**(1), e14512 (2020)
40. Ahad, M.A.R.: Activity recognition for health-care and related works. In: Proceedings of the 2018 ACM International Joint Conference and 2018 International Symposium on Pervasive and Ubiquitous Computing and Wearable Computers—UbiComp '18, Singapore, pp. 1765–1766. https://doi.org/10.1145/3267305.3277813 (2018)
41. Ahad, M.A.R., Antar, A.D., Shahid, O.: Vision-based action understanding for assistive healthcare: a short review. In: Proceedings of the IEEE Conference on Computer Vision and Pattern Recognition Workshops 2019, USA, pp. 1–11 (2019)
42. Perednia, D.A.: Telemedicine technology and clinical applications. JAMA J. Am. Med. Assoc. **273**(6), 483–488 (1995). https://doi.org/10.1001/jama.273.6.483
43. Wootton, R.: Recent advances: telemedicine. BMJ **323**(7312), 557–560 (2001). https://doi.org/10.1136/bmj.323.7312.557
44. Clemmer, T.P.: The role of medical informatics in telemedicine. J. Med. Syst. **19**(1), 47–58 (1995). https://doi.org/10.1007/BF02257190
45. Parihar, J., Kansal, P., Singh, K., Dhiman, H.: Assessment of bioinformatics and healthcare informatics. In: 2019 Amity International Conference on Artificial Intelligence (AICAI), pp. 465–467 (2019)
46. eClinicalWorks, eClinicalWorks. https://www.eclinicalworks.com/. Accessed 11 Apr 2020
47. EHR/EMR, RCM Software for Ambulatory Practice, NextGen Healthcare. https://www.nextgen.com. Accessed 11 Apr 2020
48. McKesson | Medical Supplies, Pharmaceuticals and Healthcare Solutions. https://www.mckesson.com/. Accessed 7 Apr 2020
49. Sujan, M.A.: Managing the patient safety risks of bottom-up health information technology innovations: recommendations for healthcare providers. BMJ Health Care Inf. **25**(1), 7–13 (2018). https://doi.org/10.14236/jhi.v25i1.952
50. Xu, Z.: An empirical study of patients' privacy concerns for health informatics as a service. Technol. Forecast. Soc. Chang. **143**, 297–306 (2019)
51. Fridsma, D.B.: Health informatics: a required skill for 21st century clinicians. Br. Med. J. Publ. Group (2018)
52. Ahad, M.A.R., Kobashi, S., Tavares, J.M.R.S.: Advancements of image processing and vision in healthcare. J. Healthc. Eng. **2018**, 1–3 (2018). https://doi.org/10.1155/2018/8458024

Chapter 11
Mental Health and Sensing

Abdul Kawsar Tushar, Muhammad Ashad Kabir, and Syed Ishtiaque Ahmed

Abstract Mental health is a global epidemic, affecting close to half a billion people worldwide. Chronic shortage of resources hamper detection and recovery of affected people. Effective sensing technologies can help fight the epidemic through early detection, prediction, and resulting proper treatment. Existing and novel technologies for sensing mental health state could address the aforementioned concerns by activating granular tracking of physiological, behavioral, and social signals pertaining to problems in mental health. Our paper focuses on the available methods of sensing mental health problems through direct and indirect measures. We see how active and passive sensing by technologies as well as reporting from relevant sources can contribute toward these detection methods. We also see available methods of therapeutic treatment available through digital means. We highlight a few key intervention technologies that are being developed by researchers to fight against mental illness issues.

Keywords Mental health · Wearables · Sensing

11.1 Introduction

Mental health can be termed as a concern that is plaguing the entire earth. There is a worrying number of 450 million around the globe that have been diagnosed with some form of mental or neurodevelopmental illnesses [1] and they often lead to various levels of disability [2]. Mental and neurodevelopmental illnesses give rise to

A. K. Tushar · S. I. Ahmed (✉)
Department of Computer Science, University of Toronto, Toronto, ON, Canada
e-mail: ishtiaque@cs.toronto.edu

A. K. Tushar
e-mail: tushar.kawsar@gmail.com

M. A. Kabir
Charles Sturt University, Bathurst, NSW, Australia
e-mail: akabir@csu.edu.au

M. A. R. Ahad and M. U. Ahmed (eds.), *Signal Processing Techniques for Computational Health Informatics*, Intelligent Systems Reference Library 192,
https://doi.org/10.1007/978-3-030-54932-9_11

a mortality rate that has been compared at a level more than double that of the general population, leading to approximately 8 million deaths [3]. Another impact of such sheer numbers related to these conditions is the financial burden, which generate from expenditure for care as well as the loss in productivity. The numbers related to economic loss has been estimated at more than $400 billion dollars, that only in the United States of America for a year [4].

Well-being of patients suffering from serious mental illness for a sustainable period can be ensured through treatment, management, and care and this can be achieved through granular symptom monitoring [5]. However, existing clinical tools and resources are limited in terms of accessibility and scalability [6]. Mobile health, often termed as mHealth for brevity, is where mobile (or electronic) devices converge with medical professionals and public health administration [7] and has been a well-researched area for exploring the scope of involving qualitative research methods with a view to providing accessible treatment, participant monitoring and retention, and progress of treatment. The growth in the number of mobile devices has also been a significant factor in lending more weight to this type of solutions, since close to 4 billion people around the world own at least one phone(the number is scheduled to double by 2022) [8]. This is remarkable when we consider the fact that studies found more than 70% people suffering from serious mental illness have mobile phones [9]. In addition, an increase of sensors embedded in mobile phones is giving birth to novel possibilities of utilizing these devices into mental health care based on digital evidence, such as quantitative functional and behavioral labels efficiently and without obstacles [10, 11].

What is holding an widespread adoption of sensors in mental health care and management is the scattered and restricted state of evidence that proves the connection between, on one hand, sensor data obtained using wearables and ubiquitous smartphones and, on the other hand, the prevalence and status of mental illnesses [6, 12]. In this paper, we show how technology can help in detection and sensing of mental health problems around the around. Specifically, we focus on the major mental illnesses that are tormenting billions of people across various countries. We see how active and passive sensing by technologies as well as reporting from relevant sources can contribute toward these detection methods. We also see available methods of therapeutic treatment available through digital means. We highlight a few key intervention technologies that are being developed by researchers to fight against mental illness issues.

11.2 Mental Health Problems

In this section, we do not aim to classify mental health disorders as that is not our target for this paper. Instead, our discussion would revolve around the prevalence of these disorder to provide a sense of their different presentations. Characteristics of major mental disorders include a permutation of irregular and atypical belief, concepts, attitude, and expression especially with people in the surrounding. Top

Table 11.1 Major mental health disorders and victims of each of them in the world

Mental health problem	Severity in the world
Depression	264 million
Bipolar disorder	45 million
Schizophrenia	20 million
Dementia	50 million
Autism spectrum disorder	50 million

mental disorders are schizophrenia, bipolar conditions (BP), depression and sadness, and developmental disorders together with autism [13]. Table 11.1 shows the number of people affected by these disorders in the world.

Prevalence: We use the World Health Organization fact sheet [13] to know the prevalence of these illnesses. Depression is a common psychiatric disorder that is a major concern responsible for various forms of disability. Around the world, a population of more than 200 million are affected by depression, majority of whom are women. Schizophrenia can make it difficult for people affected to work or study normally. More tan 40 million humans are affected by BP, which comprises of both manic and depressive periods mingled with regular behavior and mood states. Schizophrenia is another crippling psychiatric disorder that disables around 15 million. Schizophrenia and other psychoses can distort the ability to think, perceive, and express. Another concerning illness that affects more than 50 million worldwide is dementia, which is characterized by a deterioration in cognitive function that exacerbates the regular effects of aging on memory. Lastly, developmental disorders comprise various terms such as intellectual disability and pervasive developmental disorders including autism. 1 in 160 children in the world are estimated to be affected by autism [13].

11.3 Existing Detection Techniques

In this section, we discuss some of the widely popular methods that are used to detect the prevalence and existence of mental health problems in a person. We first discuss how the wide use of mobile phone technology is helping the revolution of mental health sensing methods. Then we discuss the currently available sensing technologies by dividing these technologies in three categories: biological or physiological sensing, behavioral or soft sensing, and social or proximity sensing methods.

11.3.1 Usage of Mobile Phones

The wide availability of mobile and sensor technology has enabled the opportunity for personalized data collection efficiently and without obstacles.

Real-world behavior sensing: A popular technique of estimating the status of one's mental health is to use smartphones sensors to capture behavioral data of humans. We can use a plethora of sensors available in today's smartphones. The aforementioned sensors can be used in different permutations to capture a wide range of human behavior, including mental and physical. A predecessor to this approach was used along with various sensors to capture and classify data of physical activity [14]. Another similar study was utilized to predict social isolation in older adults using sensors and body microphone [15].

Technology-mediated behavior: More and more work is exploring and analyzing online behavior to predict and care for mental health. For instance, a recent study by de Choudhury et al. demonstrated using information from social media to predict the early signs of depression [16].

11.3.2 Physiological Signals

1. **Facial expression**: Facial expressions and associated emotions can convey a person's emotional states and could be useful in diagnosing psychiatric illnesses [17]. Tron et al. tracked facial Action Units using 3D cameras in people with schizophrenia to differentiate patients from control participants [18]. Another study used a similar range of technology to detect the onset of suicidal thoughts in a person [19]. There are other similar studies [20, 21]. These ideas can be paired with the widespread use of mobile phones to diagnose mental illness.
2. **Heart rate variability**: People affected with psychiatric conditions suffer from a high chance of facing cardiovascular morbidity compared to the general population [22–24]. A recent research argued that the reduction in heart rate variability (HRV) could be behind the connection between this heightened cardiac mortality and psychiatric illness [25]. If that is indeed true, then there is a link between HRV and depression and this could be detected through sensing. The same relationship is reported for people with post-traumatic stress disorder [26], anxiety disorders [27], and bipolar disorder and schizophrenia [28]. Traditional HRV measurement devices are heavy; therefore, smart devices can be an apt replacement. Some devices are already in place for this purpose [29].
3. **Eye movement**: Data captured from fine changes in the movement of eyes can be used to draw conclusion and inferences about mental illness, as shown in research on schizophrenia [30] and depression [31, 32]. A technology called EOG glasses (Electrooculography in Wearable form as in glasses) can be used for detecting the movement of eyes and well as the frequency and pattern of

blinking [33]. Additionally, web cameras can also be used for similar purposes to detect the beginning of dementia [34].

4. **Electrodermal activity**: Electrodermal activity (or EDA for short) can be gauged from measuring changes in electrical properties in human skin [35]. Various research has utilized this technique in mental health detection setting to utilize the proposed relationship between heightened EDA and mental illness [36]. For instance, regarding BP, EDA signals can classify various mood states and subsequent swings [37, 38]. EDA can also be used to determine suicidal tendencies [39, 40].

11.3.3 Behavioral/Soft Signals

1. **Mobility and location**: Patterns in our location can be used to predict social activities, which can provide a peek into a person's mental status. A research tried to link lethargic lifestyle with depression [41], while another linked phone location data to depression severity [42]. There are various such other researches (see [43, 44]).
2. **Speech patterns**: Characteristics of speech could be used to judge mental health. There is an established relation between depression and human voice [45], as well as speech monotone [46]. A recent research found that jitters in voice is important to establish a pattern that can identify patients having suicidal thoughts [47]. Three other research has done significant work in developing frameworks to collect audio data for similar purposes [48–50].
3. **Technology use**: The patterns demonstrated in our day-to-day technology usage contain meaningful data and this can be leveraged in the fight against mental illnesses. For instance, patterns of phone use have been linked with people's behaviors related to sleeping and waking up, something that has been explored in relation to screen lock information of modern smartphone devices [51]. These features were discovered to be significantly correlated with mood in BP [52]. Other features pertaining to the pattern of usage of smartphone by a person have been found helpful. Two very recent papers explored the connection between change of technology usage and different mood states of BP patients [53, 54]. Schizophrenia patients also found to display similar connection [44], as did patients of depression [43].
4. **Activity**: While the connection between physical activity and mental state may not seem obvious, research has actually established a strong link between them. For instance, in BP, mania and depression are strongly related with overactivity and under-activity, respectively [55]. This information can be utilized to detect and predict the onset, existence, and duration of either of these mood states in a person. Studies earlier used *actigraph* to determine level of activity in a person [56, 57]. However, different smartphone sensors could be utilized in order to monitor an user activity level on a continuous basis [58]. Studies in recent years

have looked at data of numerous physical activities to connect them with mental disorders line BP [59, 60], depression [42], and schizophrenia [44].

11.3.4 Social/Proximity Signals

1. **Social interaction**: Sensing technologies that can capture data from nearby access points as well as other sensing devices are helpful in obtaining information about social interactions without much obstructions. Although not as accurate as user-filled data, these social proximity data can be used as a replacement which can serve to indicate the level of social interactions of a person with the help of a good algorithm [61, 62].
2. **Communication patterns**: A person's level of social engagement can be indicated by their communication technology usage data. Communication patterns of humans have been used to identify various mental illnesses such as BP [17] and schizophrenia [44, 63]. They found that symptoms are associated with a change of frequency and duration in outgoing SMS or phone calls.
3. **Social media**: Since many individuals are comfortable in sharing their daily life stories on different social media channels, these channels can be a rich source of data to determine social engagement, social network characteristics, mood, and emotion that are related to one's overall well-being. Recent research has worked with Twitter data to predict depression and PTSD [16, 64]. Images and videos in social media posts can be used to collect useful signals about a person. For example, mood [65] and depression [66] can be predicted from sentiment visible in social media photos. This idea has the potential to be scalable in this age of vast social media user engagement.

11.4 Design Interventions

In this section, we explore some of the available intervention techniques that are associated with digital sensing of mental health problems. There are various methods that are used to assist people in judging and caring for their mental health conditions. These technologies can range from using machine learning methods to detect mental illness to providing customized and personalized feedback or treatment routine. In the end, we discuss two popular methods that seamlessly integrate the sensing, inference, and partial treatment procedures.

If we want to a scientific model of how humans behave from the data that we capture from various wearable and mobile sensing devices, we need to develop one or more algorithms that will serve as a bridge between what we know and what we want to predict. This is useful for medical doctors as well as public health administrators alike to have useful insights about the spread and depth of mental illnesses. While statistical modeling can be used as for this purpose, they may not capture the high level of complexity present in human behavioral data [67]. For this reason, researchers have been opting for machine learning methods [68]. For instance, depression [42, 43] and social rhythm metric [69] has been inferred using smartphone data that was passively acquired. Specifically, deep learning has shown success in determining or predicting about the onset of mental illness [70].

11.4.1 Summary and Suggestion Display

Usually, there are two approaches for presenting the captured data using wearable and mobile sensors to the user for useful insights and feedback in the mHealth domain. First, we can summarize the collected data into short bursts of information or visual statistics or both (e.g., UbiFit [71] and BeWell [68]). Second, based on the collected data, we can predict a set of present and future states and based on this prediction, we can provide recommendations to the user. While the first method usually allows for the user to set their goal based on the presented statistics, the second method would often set a goal for the user and provide recommendation to reach that goal with minimum effort and maximum efficiency. The issue is that it is difficult to make maximum or even desired use of the complexity present in the capture data. Hence, the feedback or recommendation presented to people are only partially useful and even sometimes partially correct. Even more, because of the lack of insight into the data, the recommendations can even be dangerous sometimes. The good news is that researchers have been exploring different frameworks that would formalize the process of providing feedback and recommendation that would streamline the process and minimize risks. Additionally, researchers have explore variation in feedback in the forms of data change, augmentation, or subtraction to perceive the resulting change in user behavior [72]. Below, we discuss two such frameworks.

11.4.2 Frameworks for Extracting Useful Information into Recommendations and Feedback

A hierarchical framework extracts data from sensors and extract useful features in two sequential steps. This framework is depicted in Fig. 11.1. The first level at the bottom (in green) has the raw inputs to the sensor device which is often a mobile phone. This data needs to be processed to extract any useful information. The second level (in yellow) is where the system merges statistical algorithms—expert in finding patterns in data—with human intelligence via brainstorming and relevant domain expertise to construct low-level features. The boxes at the top (in blue) combine the middle-level features into behavioral markers by using machine learning and deep learning.

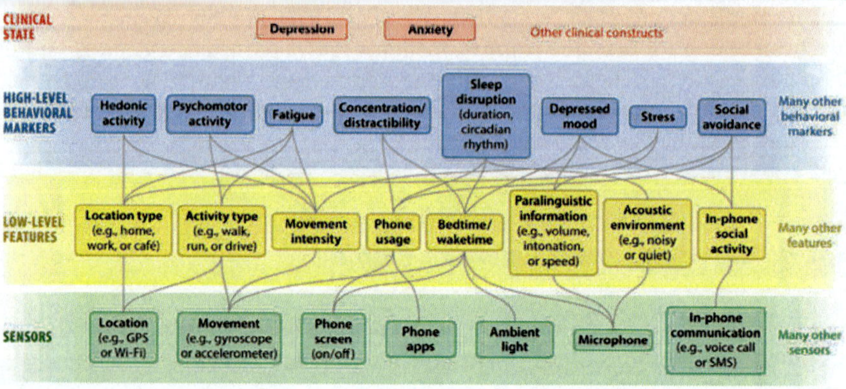

Fig. 11.1 Example of a layered, hierarchical sensemaking framework used in [11]. Boxes in blue are high-level behavioral markers. Boxes in yellow are features. Boxes in green are inputs to the sensing platform

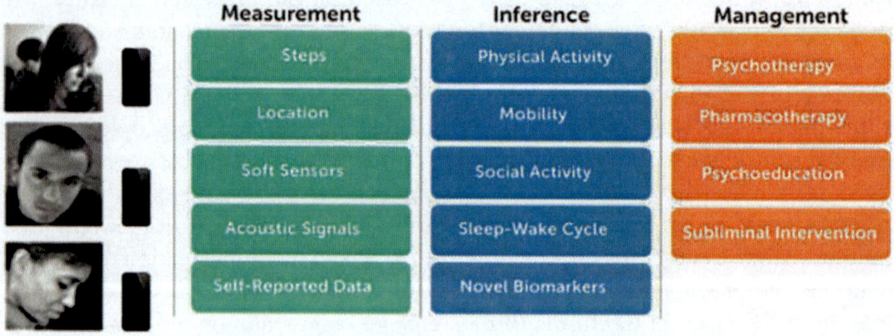

Fig. 11.2 Framework for using behavioral sensing for detection of psychiatric illness health used in [73]

Aung et al. [73] propose a more comprehensive and inclusive three-stage framework for integrating behavior sensing into the domain of mental health. This model can take into account user data from various physical sensors as well as self-reported data. Figure 11.2 shows the entire process. The first stage takes into account data from sensors as well as self-reported procedures over a time to become more inclusive. Then, this raw data is processed using machine learning or other methods to create new features and gain useful insights into the data. The final phase works on integrating the inferences from the middle step toward the management of the condition if detected. This could include using the inferences alongside traditional mental health therapies to create personalized digital interventions and chrono-therapeutic interventions.

11.5 Discussion

The existing technologies for sensing mental health condition suffer from a number of limitations. First, studies do not demonstrate a significant level of effectiveness for and correlation with improving patient detection and care for mental health patients. The dearth of clinical evidence can be linked back to the insufficient amount of research, lack of significant sample size or population, an insignificant time over which studies were live (both in short term and medium term), as well as a lack of funding opportunities, which can again lead to a lack of awareness regarding the severity and spread of these problems in different societies. These issues can be addressed by improving the study design and procedures and seeking more funding [6]. Increasing awareness about mental health problems is another wing of solving these issues.

Second, not many studies strive to combine the effects of various types of sensing. If data is being collected about a single patient or the same group of patients and the result inferred from these sources are consistent, then the system could be more confident about its inference. The challenge of combining data from different streams is chiefly computational, where machine learning systems could provide to be a helping hand. However, machine learning methods also suffer from the lack of reproducibility [74]. These techniques used for mental health sensing suffer from a lack of expiration date as well as the curse of variability [11]. Additionally, how the errors associated with the predictions of a machine learning system will be explained, addressed, and incorporated in the future iterations of the same model is something that needs more significant research, which is presently absent. Such user-facing errors need to be addressed properly and with a convincing methodology, lest we should face affecting the quality of the experience of people using technology for sensing.

Third, the nature of sensing technologies dictate that they will need to obtain a gigantic amount of data that is related to personal use and has a potential to sensitive in nature (especially when the data is related to personal behavior or health problems). Furthermore, wearable sensing technologies are not advanced enough to differentiate between target participant and non-participants and hence, due to the availability and ease of use in any setting, can risk obtaining unexpected, irrelevant, and unnecessary data [75] that can lead to false diagnosis, false triggers, and lack of care for patients. Researchers should strive to identify potentially sensitive data items to deploy a plan of action of protecting this data from malicious parties. In addition, researchers should also think about how they can identify unexpected, irrelevant, and unnecessary data and separate valuable data from all the clutter.

Fourth, related to the previous concern is another that is the issue of privacy and security for passively collected data. Unfortunately, the existing research community members are in a disagreement regarding what to do about this risk [76]. A crucial aspect that may often get overlooked is the difficulty in stripping identifying information from data collected by sensors in mobile phone and wearables. Even seeming innocuous data such as location information [77], when obtained in sufficient quality, can expose the identification of a victim, exposing to a risk of facing social stigma [78]. While there are numerous existing techniques to help de-identify data (especially location data), they are not full-proof in preserving privacy as well as usefulness of data at the same time [79].

While an exponentially increasing amount of data is being captured from mobile and wearable sensors around the world, there are other, less structured challenges that can pose significant barriers toward capturing and treating mental illness using mobile devices. In Global South, mental health is a vastly neglected domain rife with misconceptions, maltreatment, and lack of treatment options [80]. Sometimes, people consult the local witches instead of medical doctors to treat illnesses that seem unusual to the community (like mental illness) [81]. Rural areas especially suffer from the lack of medical infrastructure and mental health facilities [82] and if we plan to offset this restriction by employing mobile devices, we face another different set of challenges [75, 83]. Furthermore, the low rate of literacy is often a hurdle for people to use smartphones [84]. These challenges should also be considered along with the more "high-tech" obstacles described above if we want to capture a holistic picture of the domain where we want to treat and manage psychiatric illnesses with sensors.

References

1. Brundtland, G.H.: Mental health: new understanding, new hope. JAMA **286**(19), 2391–2391 (2001)
2. Organization WH, et al.: Investing in mental health (2003)
3. Walker, E.R., McGee, R.E., Druss, B.G.: Mortality in mental disorders and global disease burden implications: a systematic review and meta-analysis. JAMA Psychiat. **72**(4), 334–341 (2015)
4. Insel, T.: Mental health awareness month: by the numbers. National Institute of Mental Health Blog (2015)
5. Morriss, R., Vinjamuri, I., Faizal, M.A., Bolton, C.A., McCarthy, J.P.: Training to recognize the early signs of recurrence in schizophrenia. Schizophrenia Bull. **39**(2), 255 (2013)
6. Abdullah, S., Choudhury, T.: Sensing technologies for monitoring serious mental illnesses. IEEE MultiMedia **25**(1), 61–75 (2018)
7. Adibi, S.: Mobile Health: A Technology Road Map, vol. 5. Springer (2015)
8. Cerwall, P., Jonsson, P., Möller, R., Bävertoft, S., Carson, S., Godor, I.: Ericsson Mobility Report. On the Pulse of the Networked Society Hg v Ericsson (2015)
9. Ben-Zeev, D., Davis, K.E., Kaiser, S., Krzsos, I., Drake, R.E.: Mobile technologies among people with serious mental illness: opportunities for future services. Admin. Policy Mental Health Mental Health Serv. Res. **40**(4), 340–343 (2013)
10. Gaggioli, A., Riva, G.: From mobile mental health to mobile wellbeing: opportunities and challenges. In: MMVR, pp. 141–147 (2013)
11. Mohr, D.C., Zhang, M., Schueller, S.M.: Personal sensing: understanding mental health using ubiquitous sensors and machine learning. Annu. Rev. Clin. Psychol. **13**, 23–47 (2017)
12. Or, F., Torous, J., Onnela, J.P.: High potential but limited evidence: using voice data from smartphones to monitor and diagnose mood disorders. Psychiat. Rehabil. J. **40**(3), 320 (2017)
13. WHO: Mental disorders by World Health Organization. https://www.who.int/news-room/fact-sheets/detail/mental-disorders. Accessed 24 Dec 2019 (2019)
14. Lester, J., Choudhury, T., Borriello, G.: A practical approach to recognizing physical activities. In: International Conference on Pervasive Computing, pp. 1–16. Springer (2006)

15. Rabbi, M., Ali, S., Choudhury, T., Berke, E.: Passive and in-situ assessment of mental and physical well-being using mobile sensors. In: Proceedings of the 13th international conference on Ubiquitous Computing, pp. 385–394. ACM (2011)
16. De Choudhury, M., Gamon, M., Counts, S., Horvitz, E.: Predicting depression via social media. In: Seventh international AAAI Conference on Weblogs and Social Media (2013)
17. Gur, R.E., Kohler, C.G., Ragland, J.D., Siegel, S.J., Lesko, K., Bilker, W.B., Gur, R.C.: Flat affect in schizophrenia: relation to emotion processing and neurocognitive measures. Schizophrenia Bull. **32**(2), 279–287 (2006)
18. Tron, T., Peled, A., Grinsphoon, A., Weinshall, D.: Automated facial expressions analysis in schizophrenia: a continuous dynamic approach. In: International Symposium on Pervasive Computing Paradigms for Mental Health, pp. 72–81. Springer (2015)
19. Laksana, E., Baltrušaitis, T., Morency, L.P., Pestian. J.P.: Investigating facial behavior indicators of suicidal ideation. In: 2017 12th IEEE International Conference on Automatic Face & Gesture Recognition (FG 2017), pp. 770–777. IEEE (2017)
20. Valstar, M., Schuller, B., Smith, K., Almaev, T., Eyben, F., Krajewski, J., Cowie, R., Pantic, M.: Avec 2014: 3d dimensional affect and depression recognition challenge. In: Proceedings of the 4th International Workshop on Audio/Visual Emotion Challenge, pp. 3–10. ACM (2014)
21. Wang, R., Campbell, A.T., Zhou, X.: Using opportunistic face logging from smartphone to infer mental health: challenges and future directions. In: Adjunct Proceedings of the 2015 ACM International Joint Conference on Pervasive and Ubiquitous Computing and Proceedings of the 2015 ACM International Symposium on Wearable Computers, pp. 683–692. ACM (2015)
22. Hennekens, C.H., Hennekens, A.R., Hollar, D., Casey, D.E.: Schizophrenia and increased risks of cardiovascular disease. Am. Heart J. **150**(6), 1115–1121 (2005)
23. Weiner, M., Warren, L., Fiedorowicz, J.G.: Cardiovascular morbidity and mortality in bipolar disorder. Annals Clin. Psychiat.: Off. J. Am. Acad. Clin. Psychiat. **23**(1), 40 (2011)
24. Pratt, L.A., Ford, D.E., Crum, R.M., Armenian, H.K., Gallo, J.J., Eaton, W.W.: Depression, psychotropic medication, and risk of myocardial infarction: prospective data from the baltimore eca follow-up. Circulation **94**(12), 3123–3129 (1996)
25. Kemp, A.H., Quintana, D.S., Gray, M.A., Felmingham, K.L., Brown, K., Gatt, J.M.: Impact of depression and antidepressant treatment on heart rate variability: a review and meta-analysis. Biol. Psychiat. **67**(11), 1067–1074 (2010)
26. Tan, G., Dao, T.K., Farmer, L., Sutherland, R.J., Gevirtz, R.: Heart rate variability (hrv) and posttraumatic stress disorder (PTSD): a pilot study. Appl. Psychophysiol. Biofeedback **36**(1), 27–35 (2011)
27. Chalmers, J.A., Quintana, D.S., Abbott, M.J., Kemp, A.H., et al.: Anxiety disorders are associated with reduced heart rate variability: a meta-analysis. Front. Psychiat. **5**, 80 (2014)
28. Quintana, D.S., Westlye, L.T., Kaufmann, T., Rustan, Ø., Brandt, C.L., Haatveit, B., Steen, N.E., Andreassen, O.A.: Reduced heart rate variability in schizophrenia and bipolar disorder compared to healthy controls. Acta Psychiatrica Scandinavica **133**(1), 44–52 (2016)
29. Bai, Y., Hibbing, P., Mantis, C., Welk, G.J.: Comparative evaluation of heart rate-based monitors: apple watch versus fitbit charge HR. J. Sports Sci. **36**(15), 1734–1741 (2018)
30. Levy, D.L., Sereno, A.B., Gooding, D.C., O'Driscoll, G.A.: Eye tracking dysfunction in schizophrenia: characterization and pathophysiology. In: Behavioral Neurobiology of Schizophrenia and Its Treatment, pp. 311–347. Springer, (2010)
31. Winograd-Gurvich, C., Georgiou-Karistianis, N., Fitzgerald, P.B., Millist, L., White, O.B.: Ocular motor differences between melancholic and non-melancholic depression. J. Effect. Disord. **93**(1–3), 193–203 (2006)
32. Alghowinem, S., Goecke, R., Wagner, M., Parker, G., Breakspear, M.: Eye movement analysis for depression detection. In: 2013 IEEE International Conference on Image Processing, pp. 4220–4224. IEEE (2013)
33. Dhuliawala, M., Lee, J., Shimizu, J., Bulling, A., Kunze, K., Starner, T., Woo, W.: Smooth eye movement interaction using EOG glasses. In: Proceedings of the 18th ACM International Conference on Multimodal Interaction, pp. 307–311. ACM (2016)

34. Cano, L.A.M., Beltrán, J., Navarro, R., García-Vázquez, M.S., Castro, L.A.: Towards early dementia detection by oculomotor performance analysis on leisure web content. In: Proceedings of the 2017 ACM International Joint Conference on Pervasive and Ubiquitous Computing and Proceedings of the 2017 ACM International Symposium on Wearable Computers, pp. 800–804. ACM (2017)
35. Critchley, H.D.: Electrodermal responses: what happens in the brain. Neuroscientist **8**(2), 132–142 (2002)
36. Schell, A.M., Dawson, M.E., Rissling, A., Ventura, J., Subotnik, K.L., Gitlin, M.J., Nuechterlein, K.H.: Electrodermal predictors of functional outcome and negative symptoms in schizophrenia. Psychophysiology **42**(4), 483–492 (2005)
37. Lanata, A., Greco, A., Valenza, G., Scilingo, E.P.: A pattern recognition approach based on electrodermal response for pathological mood identification in bipolar disorders. In: 2014 IEEE International Conference on Acoustics, Speech and Signal Processing (ICASSP), pp. 3601–3605. IEEE (2014)
38. Greco, A., Valenza, G., Lanata, A., Rota, G., Scilingo, E.P.: Electrodermal activity in bipolar patients during affective elicitation. IEEE J. Biomed. Health Inf. **18**(6), 1865–1873 (2014)
39. Jandl, M., Steyer, J., Kaschka, W.P.: Suicide risk markers in major depressive disorder: a study of electrodermal activity and event-related potentials. J. Affect. Disord. **123**(1–3), 138–149 (2010)
40. Thorell, L.H., Wolfersdorf, M., Straub, R., Steyer, J., Hodgkinson, S., Kaschka, W., Jandl, M.: Electrodermal hyporeactivity as a trait marker for suicidal propensity in uni-and bipolar depression. J. Psychiat. Res. **47**(12), 1925–1931 (2013)
41. Roshanaei-Moghaddam, B., Katon, W.J., Russo, J.: The longitudinal effects of depression on physical activity. Gener. Hospital Psychiat. **31**(4), 306–315 (2009)
42. Canzian, L., Musolesi, M.: Trajectories of depression: unobtrusive monitoring of depressive states by means of smartphone mobility traces analysis. In: Proceedings of the 2015 ACM International Joint Conference on Pervasive and Ubiquitous Computing, pp. 1293–1304. ACM (2015)
43. Saeb, S., Zhang, M., Karr, C.J., Schueller, S.M., Corden, M.E., Kording, K.P., Mohr, D.C.: Mobile phone sensor correlates of depressive symptom severity in daily-life behavior: an exploratory study. J. Med. Internet Res. **17**(7), e175 (2015)
44. Wang, R., Aung, M.S., Abdullah, S., Brian, R., Campbell, A.T., Choudhury, T., Hauser, M., Kane, J., Merrill, M., Scherer, E.A., et al.: Crosscheck: toward passive sensing and detection of mental health changes in people with schizophrenia. In: Proceedings of the 2016 ACM International Joint Conference on Pervasive and Ubiquitous Computing, pp. 886–897. ACM (2016)
45. Nilsonne, Å.: Acoustic analysis of speech variables during depression and after improvement. Acta Psychiatrica Scandinavica **76**(3), 235–245 (1987)
46. Moore, E., Clements, M., Peifer, J., Weisser, L.: Comparing objective feature statistics of speech for classifying clinical depression. In: The 26th Annual International Conference of the IEEE Engineering in Medicine and Biology Society, vol. 1, pp. 17–20. IEEE (2004)
47. Ozdas, A., Shiavi, R.G., Silverman, S.E., Silverman, M.K., Wilkes, D.M.: Investigation of vocal jitter and glottal flow spectrum as possible cues for depression and near-term suicidal risk. IEEE Transa. Biomed. Eng. **51**(9), 1530–1540 (2004)
48. Faurholt-Jepsen, M., Munkholm, K., Frost, M., Bardram, J.E., Kessing, L.V.: Electronic self-monitoring of mood using it platforms in adult patients with bipolar disorder: a systematic review of the validity and evidence. BMC Psychiat. **16**(1), 7 (2016)
49. Lu, H., Frauendorfer, D., Rabbi, M., Mast, M.S., Chittaranjan, G.T., Campbell, A.T., Gatica-Perez, D., Choudhury, T.: Stresssense: Detecting stress in unconstrained acoustic environments using smartphones. In: Proceedings of the 2012 ACM Conference on Ubiquitous Computing, pp. 351–360. ACM (2012)
50. Muaremi, A., Gravenhorst, F., Grünerbl, A., Arnrich, B., Tröster, G.: Assessing bipolar episodes using speech cues derived from phone calls. In: International Symposium on Pervasive Computing Paradigms for Mental Health, pp. 103–114. Springer (2014)

51. Abdullah, S., Matthews, M., Murnane, E.L., Gay, G., Choudhury, T.: Towards circadian computing: early to bed and early to rise makes some of us unhealthy and sleep deprived. In: Proceedings of the 2014 ACM International Joint Conference on Pervasive and Ubiquitous Computing, pp. 673–684. ACM (2014)
52. Frost M, Doryab A, Faurholt-Jepsen M, Kessing LV, Bardram JE (2013) Supporting disease insight through data analysis: refinements of the monarca self-assessment system. In: Proceedings of the 2013 ACM international joint conference on Pervasive and ubiquitous computing, ACM, pp 133–142
53. Matthews, M., Murnane, E., Snyder, J., Guha, S., Chang, P., Doherty, G., Gay, G.: The double-edged sword: a mixed methods study of the interplay between bipolar disorder and technology use. Comput. Hum. Behav. **75**, 288–300 (2017)
54. Alvarez-Lozano, J., Osmani, V., Mayora, O., Frost, M., Bardram, J., Faurholt-Jepsen, M., Kessing, L.V.: Tell me your apps and i will tell you your mood: correlation of apps usage with bipolar disorder state. In: Proceedings of the 7th International Conference on Pervasive Technologies Related to Assistive Environments, p. 19. ACM (2014)
55. Wolff, E.A., Putnam, F.W., Post, R.M.: Motor activity and affective illness: the relationship of amplitude and temporal distribution to changes in affective state. Archiv. Gener. Psychiat. **42**(3), 288–294 (1985)
56. Walther, S., Stegmayer, K., Horn, H., Razavi, N., Müller, T.J., Strik, W.: Physical activity in schizophrenia is higher in the first episode than in subsequent ones. Front. Psychiat. **5**, 191 (2015)
57. John, D., Freedson, P.: Actigraph and actical physical activity monitors: a peek under the hood. Med. Sci. Sports Exer. **44**(1 Suppl 1), S86 (2012)
58. Wu, W., Dasgupta, S., Ramirez, E.E., Peterson, C., Norman, G.J.: Classification accuracies of physical activities using smartphone motion sensors. J. Med. Internet Res. **14**(5), e130 (2012)
59. Osmani, V., Maxhuni, A., Grünerbl, A., Lukowicz, P., Haring, C., Mayora, O.: Monitoring activity of patients with bipolar disorder using smart phones. In: Proceedings of International Conference on Advances in Mobile Computing & Multimedia, , p. 85. ACM (2013)
60. Beiwinkel, T., Kindermann, S., Maier, A., Kerl, C., Moock, J., Barbian, G., Rössler, W.: Using smartphones to monitor bipolar disorder symptoms: a pilot study. JMIR Mental Health **3**(1), e2 (2016)
61. Aharony, N., Pan, W., Ip, C., Khayal, I., Pentland, A.: Social FMRI: investigating and shaping social mechanisms in the real world. Perva. Mobile Comput. **7**(6), 643–659 (2011)
62. Ben-Zeev, D., Wang, R., Abdullah, S., Brian, R., Scherer, E.A., Mistler, L.A., Hauser, M., Kane, J.M., Campbell, A., Choudhury, T.: Mobile behavioral sensing for outpatients and inpatients with schizophrenia. Psychiatr. Serv. **67**(5), 558–561 (2015)
63. Faurholt-Jepsen, M., Vinberg, M., Frost, M., Debel, S., Margrethe Christensen, E., Bardram, J.E., Kessing, L.V.: Behavioral activities collected through smartphones and the association with illness activity in bipolar disorder. Int. J. Methods Psychiat. Res. **25**(4), 309–323 (2016)
64. Reece, A.G., Reagan, A.J., Lix, K.L., Dodds, P.S., Danforth, C.M., Langer, E.J.: Forecasting the onset and course of mental illness with twitter data. Sci. Rep. **7**(1), 13006 (2017)
65. Abdullah, S., Murnane, E.L., Costa, J.M., Choudhury, T.: Collective smile: Measuring societal happiness from geolocated images. In: Proceedings of the 18th ACM Conference on Computer Supported Cooperative Work & Social Computing, , pp. 361–374. ACM (2015)
66. Reece, A.G., Danforth, C.M.: Instagram photos reveal predictive markers of depression. EPJ Data Sci. **6**(1), 15 (2017)
67. Breiman, L.: Randomizing outputs to increase prediction accuracy. Mach. Learn. **40**(3), 229–242 (2000)
68. Lane, N.D., Mohammod, M., Lin, M., Yang, X., Lu, H., Ali, S., Doryab, A., Berke, E., Choudhury, T., Campbell, A.: Bewell: a smartphone application to monitor, model and promote wellbeing. In: 5th International ICST Conference on Pervasive Computing Technologies for Healthcare, pp. 23–26 (2011)
69. Abdullah, S., Matthews, M., Frank, E., Doherty, G., Gay, G., Choudhury, T.: Automatic detection of social rhythms in bipolar disorder. J. Am. Med. Inf. Assoc. **23**(3), 538–543 (2016)

70. Martínez, H.P., Yannakakis, G.N.: Deep multimodal fusion: combining discrete events and continuous signals. In: Proceedings of the 16th International Conference on Multimodal Interaction, pp. 34–41. ACM (2014)
71. Consolvo, S., McDonald, D.W., Toscos, T., Chen, M.Y., Froehlich, J., Harrison, B., Klasnja, P., LaMarca, A., LeGrand, L., Libby, R., et al.: Activity sensing in the wild: a field trial of UbiFit garden. In: Proceedings of the SIGCHI Conference on Human Factors in Computing Systems, pp 1797–1806. ACM (2008)
72. Costa, J., Adams, A.T., Jung, M.F., Guimbretière, F., Choudhury, T.: Emotioncheck: leveraging bodily signals and false feedback to regulate our emotions. In: Proceedings of the 2016 ACM International Joint Conference on Pervasive and Ubiquitous Computing, pp. 758–769. ACM (2016)
73. Aung, M.H., Matthews, M., Choudhury, T.: Sensing behavioral symptoms of mental health and delivering personalized interventions using mobile technologies. Depress. Anxiety **34**(7), 603–609 (2017)
74. Asselbergs, J., Ruwaard, J., Ejdys, M., Schrader, N., Sijbrandij, M., Riper, H.: Mobile phone-based unobtrusive ecological momentary assessment of day-to-day mood: an explorative study. J. Med. Internet Res. **18**(3), e72 (2016)
75. Ahmed, S.I., Haque, M.R., Chen, J., Dell, N.: Digital privacy challenges with shared mobile phone use in Bangladesh. In: Proceedings of the ACM on Human-Computer Interaction 1(CSCW), pp. 1–20 (2017)
76. Shilton, K., Sayles, S.: "We aren't all going to be on the same page about ethics": ethical practices and challenges in research on digital and social media. In: 2016 49th Hawaii International Conference on System Sciences (HICSS), pp. 1909–1918. IEEE (2016)
77. De Montjoye, Y.A., Hidalgo, C.A., Verleysen, M., Blondel, V.D.: Unique in the crowd: the privacy bounds of human mobility. Sci. Rep. **3**, 1376 (2013)
78. Sweeney, L.: Simple demographics often identify people uniquely. Health (San Francisco) **671**, 1–34 (2000)
79. Brush, A., Krumm, J., Scott, J.: Exploring end user preferences for location obfuscation, location-based services, and the value of location. In: Proceedings of the 12th ACM International Conference on Ubiquitous Computing, pp. 95–104. ACM (2010)
80. Tushar, A.K., Antara, I.J., Das, D., Chandra, P., Soron, T.R., Haque, M.M., Ahamed, S.I., Ahmed, S.I.: "We need more power to stand up": designing to combat stigmatization of the caregivers of children with autism in urban Bangladesh. In: Proceedings of the 11th International Conference on Information and Communication Technologies and Development (2020) (to appear)
81. Sultana, S., Ahmed, S.I.: Witchcraft and HCI: morality, modernity, and postcolonial computing in rural Bangladesh. In: Proceedings of the 2019 CHI Conference on Human Factors in Computing Systems, pp. 1–15 (2019)
82. Sultana, S., Ahmed, S.I., Fussell, S.R.: "Parar-daktar understands my problems better" disentangling the challenges to designing better access to healthcare in rural Bangladesh. In: Proceedings of the ACM on Human-Computer Interaction, vol. 3(CSCW), pp. 1–27 (2019)
83. Ahmed, S.I., Haque, M.R., Guha, S., Rifat, M.R., Dell, N.: Privacy, security, and surveillance in the global south: a study of biometric mobile SIM registration in Bangladesh. In: Proceedings of the 2017 CHI Conference on Human Factors in Computing Systems, pp. 906–918 (2017)
84. Ahmed, S.I., Jackson, S.J., Zaber, M., Morshed, M.B., Ismail, M.H.B., Afrose, S.: Ecologies of use and design: individual and social practices of mobile phone use within low-literate rickshawpuller communities in urban Bangladesh. In: Proceedings of the 4th Annual Symposium on Computing for Development, pp. 1–10 (2013)

Chapter 12
Artificial Intelligence, Machine Learning and Reasoning in Health Informatics—Case Studies

Mobyen Uddin Ahmed, Shaibal Barua, and Shahina Begum

Abstract To apply Artificial Intelligence (AI), Machine Learning (ML) and Machine Reasoning (MR) in health informatics are often challenging as they comprise with multivariate information coming from heterogeneous sources e.g. sensor signals, text, etc. This book chapter presents the research development of AI, ML and MR as applications in health informatics. Five case studies on health informatics have been discussed and presented as (1) advanced Parkinson's disease, (2) stress management, (3) postoperative pain treatment, (4) driver monitoring, and (5) remote health monitoring. Here, the challenges, solutions, models, results, limitations are discussed with future wishes.

Keywords Artificial Intelligence (AI) · Machine Learning (ML) and Machine Reasoning (MR) · Health informatics · Case studies · Advanced Parkinson's disease · Stress management · Postoperative pain treatment · Driver monitoring · Remote health monitoring

12.1 Introduction

In recent years, applications of AI and ML in health informatics domain has emerged and become a popular research topic within the researcher community. Intelligent monitoring, diagnosis and treatment support are important issues that come in literature in different ways as presented in the previous chapter. This book chapter includes five different application areas in health informatics namely, (1) Parkinson's disease, (2) stress management, (3) postoperative pain, (4) driver monitoring, and (5) remote health monitoring. In *Parkinson's*, a web-enabled decision support system (DSS) is

M. U. Ahmed (✉) · S. Barua · S. Begum
School of Innovation, Design and Engineering, Mälardalen University, Västerås, Sweden
e-mail: mobyen.ahmed@mdh.se

S. Barua
e-mail: shaibal.barua@mdh.se

S. Begum
e-mail: shahina.begum@mdh.se

M. A. R. Ahad and M. U. Ahmed (eds.), *Signal Processing Techniques for Computational Health Informatics*, Intelligent Systems Reference Library 192,
https://doi.org/10.1007/978-3-030-54932-9_12

developed by applying fuzzy rule-based reasoning (RBR) as a machine reasoning approach to provide assistance in dose alteration of Duodopa infusion based on the data from motor state (i.e. −3 to +3) assessments and dosage information. In *stress*, a multi-modal and multipurpose-oriented clinical decision support system is developed to detected stress and also to provide biofeedback treatment. Here, case-based reasoning (CBR), a machine reasoning approach together with textual information retrieval, fuzzy logic, and rules have been applied to heterogeneous data sources, i.e. figure temperature sensor signals and textual questionnaires. DSS in *postoperative pain treatment*, consist of numerical, textual and Numerical Visual Analogue Scale (NVAS) information. Here, CBR is applied as a core technique to enable experience reuse and decision explanation by retrieving the previous "similar" cases. Again, besides CBR, several clustering techniques are applied to identify rare cases. In *driver monitoring* application, multivariate data analysis is conducted by applying and combining several machine learning approaches to detect drivers' levels of sleepiness, cognitive load, and stress. Here, several physiological signals, namely, electrocardiography (ECG), galvanic skin response (GSR), finger temperature, electroencephalography (EEG), electrooculography (EOG), and respiration were used together with other contextual and demographic information. Again, in remote health monitoring, we represented an Internet of Things (IoT) based generic system-level framework for a self-serving health monitoring system. This health monitoring system acts as a DSS for providing a personalized report on persons' health condition considering vital signs' observation, where vital signs are obtained daily basis. Here, the proposed framework combines general rules with case-based reasoning (CBR) approach.

12.2 Related Work in Health Informatics

Clinical decision support system relating AI started in the early 1970s and the MYCIN [1] is one famous example. The HELP [2] system is one of the longest-running and most successful clinical information systems. According to a literature study presented in [3], different AI techniques have been applied in the clinical DSSs such as (1) rule-based reasoning [1, 4, 5], (2) Bayesian theory [6], (3) Bayesian belief networks [7], (4) heuristic, (5) semantic network, (6) neural networks [8], (7) genetic algorithms [9] (7) fuzzy logic [4, 6] and (8) case-based reasoning. Recent medical DSSs using CBR approach to name a few are: (1) ExpressionCBR [10] is a decision support system for *cancer diagnosis* and *classification;* (2) GerAmi [11] 'Geriatric Ambient Intelligence', is an intelligent system that purposes to *support healthcare facilities for the elderly, Alzheimer's patients and people with other disabilities*; (3) geneCBR [12, 13], is focusing on the *classification of cancer*, based on a gene expression profile of microarray data; (4) ISOR [14], the system *identifies the causes of ineffective therapies and advises better recommendations* to avoid inefficacy to support *long-term therapies in the endocrine domain*; (5) the KASIMIR project [15], is an effort to provide decision support for *breast cancer treatment based on a protocol in Oncology*; (6) Song et al. [16], proposes a DSS in *radiotherapy for dose planning in prostate cancer;* (7) Marling et al. in [17], described a case based DSS to assist in the daily management of *patients with Type 1 diabetes on insulin pump therapy.*

12.2.1 Advanced Parkinsons Disease

In recent years, research shows that Parkinson's Disease (PD) symptom can be monitored by using wearable sensors [18, 19]. There are also some commercial products available, e.g. Kinesia™ [20] and Parkinson's Kineti-Graph™ (PKG) [21], these systems generate scores to detect bradykinesia, tremor, dyskinesia and motor fluctuations. Data mining and artificial intelligence have been applied to recognize the presence and severity of motor fluctuations in patients with Parkinson's disease (PD) [22]. To classify or predict PD, statistical, machine learning e.g. both for supervised and unsupervised learning algorithms have been applied. Based on Artificial Neural Networks (ANNs) and Support Vector Machines (SVMs) have been used to aid in the diagnosis of PD [23, 24], and Social-Spider Optimization algorithm is applied to improve the training phase of ANN with Multilayer perceptron [25]. A model of a fuzzy expert system is applied to Parkinson's disease diagnosis [26]. Recently, deep learning e.g. a convolutional neural network is applied to classify PD; here, the results show the CNN method outperformed compare to other state-of-the-art machine learning algorithms [27]. To predict an Unified Parkinson's Disease Rating Scores (UPDRS), scores from digital voice recordings a regression analysis has been used [28], again, to monitor motor fluctuations in PD a Support vector machines (SVM) is used in accelerometer data, [29], and also artificial neural network is used to detect gait disturbances [30]. ML is well-known to use for identification of motor states based on waist sensors [31].

12.2.2 Stress Management

According to Hans Selye, stress can be defined as "the rate of wear and tear within the body" [32]. He first introduced the term 'stress' in the 1950s when he noticed that patients suffer physically without having only a disease or a medical condition. He defined stress as "the non-specific response of the body to any demand" [32]. We have an inborn reaction to stressful situations called the "fight or flight" response. That means we can react to certain events or facts that may produce stress and our body's nervous system activates and then stress hormones are released to protect ourselves. The wear and tear are a physiological reaction such as rise in blood pressure, rise in heart rate, increased respiration rate and muscles get ready for action [33–35]. The diagnosis and biofeedback treatment of stress are often multi-factorial, complex and uncertain due to large variations and personalization. According to [36], there are three methods that can be used for the diagnosis of stress: questionnaires, biochemical measures and physiological measures. Since the autonomic nervous system is activated by a stress response various physiological parameter of the SNS can be used in the diagnosis of stress. The physiological parameters are commonly measured using skin conductance, skin temperature, respiration e.g. end-tidal carbon dioxide ($ETCO_2$), electromyography (EMG), electrocardiography (ECG), heart rate e.g. calculating respiratory sinus arrhythmia (RSA) and heart rate variability (HRV), electroencephalography (EEG), brain imaging techniques, oculomotor and pupillometric measures etc. In this research, both stress diagnosis and biofeedback treatment have been conducted using the skin temperature i.e. finger temperature (FT) since the intention of the research was to design and develop a CDSS for stress management which should be simple, inexpensive and easy to use. Stress diagnosis using questionnaires can be found in [37, 38], which is mainly to calculate and identify the level of stress (i.e. work and physical related stress). A procedure for diagnosing stress-related disorders using physiological parameters has been put forward by Nilsson et al. [39], where stress-related disorders are diagnosed by classifying the Respiratory Sinus Arrhythmia (RSA) i.e. the interaction of the heartbeat with breathing cycle. DSS for only diagnosing stress based on the finger temperature (FT) measurement is addressed in Begum et al. 2009 [40], the authors have also included Heart Rate Variability (HRV) in order to measure individual stress levels and is addressed in [41].

12.2.3 *Post-operative Pain Treatment*

According to Hawthorn and Redmond [42], the pain might often be a useful thing, a "protective mechanism", a biological signal, which is essential when we, for example, learn not to touch a stove in order to protect us from being injured. The measurement of pain is very subjective and multidimensional experience and unique to every individual [43, 44]. In practice, a number of factors such as clinical, local and patient-related questions are asked to a patient by a healthcare provider before the operation to decide a proper treatment plan in pain relief. There are different pharmacological options that are used in pain treatment, such as non-opioid analgesics, weak opioids, strong opioids, and adjuvants. These opioids are given in different modes such as intravenous with continuous or incessant infusion, infusion, orally and by injection. The detailed information about different drugs, drug combination, quantity and application methods are used in pain treatment can be found in [45, 46].

Recent advancements of clinical DSSs in pain treatment have been investigated through a literature study. The authors in [47] have presented a review on DSS for chronic pain management in primary care, where 8 systems are studied. According to the paper, all 8 DSSs are designed to assist physicians in pain management. Most of them have applied artificial intelligence techniques such as CBR, RBR, and fuzzy logic. A DSS in pain management for cancer patients is described in [48]. In their proposed system, daily pain assessment has been conducted through an NVAS and the system assists physicians in recommending correct deviations from pain therapy guidelines. A recent DSS in the domain of palliative care addressed by Houeland and Aamodt [49] is an advice-giving system that supports physicians to improve pain treatment in lung cancer patients. The proposed system incorporates rule-based and model-based methods into the CBR approach. Elvidge in [50] also describes a system to help healthcare providers in improved pain and symptom management for advanced cancer patients. His web-based DSS incorporated CBR with evidence-based standards for end-of-life cancer care.

12.2.4 Driver Monitoring

Inter- and intra-individual variability [51, 52] that is the acquired physiological signals fluctuate both between people and (over time) within an individual. Because of the inter- and intra-individual variability which leads to drowsiness, cognitive load or stress profiles that evolve even for individual drivers, generalizing a driver-state detection model becomes a major challenge [51]. The difficulties of classifying driver sleepiness at very high accuracy were addressed in [51–54]. According to Yoshida et al. [55], for cognitive load classification, essential features are time series values; and tendency and stability of the time series data. The authors considered vehicular data and eye-tracking data to classify cognitive load using an RF classifier. Under different settings, the classifier achieved an average accuracy of 78% in classifying cognitive load levels. The performance of cognitive load classification became poor when there were uncertainties—such as participants failing to perform some task or, in a real-time system, where improvements could choose, for example, a suitable window size, which influences the delay that occurs between the onset of a cognitive load task and when changes are detected in the driver's performance due to higher cognitive load [56, 57]. In many sleepiness, cognitive load and stress studies suggested using multimodal data when using machine learning models to classify these driver states [51, 57, 58].

Over the years many ML methods have been used to detect driver state including the support vector machines [56, 59–66], linear discriminant analysis [67], artificial neural network [57, 68–71], logistic regression [72], and k-mean clustering [73], fuzzy c-means clustering [74], random forest [55, 75], and case-based reasoning [76–78].

12.2.5 Remote Health Monitoring

Remote health monitoring or E-health systems can reduce the physical travel of caregiver staff, replacing travel with virtual visits in the homes through computerized support systems [79, 80], and the development of such system are increased day by day with the help of Internet of Things (IoT) [79, 81, 82]. Thus, the health monitoring system for the elderly is not limited to take place in primary care facilities simply due to deployment of ICT as addressed in the reviews [79, 83, 84]. Such systems are useful in several areas, from Ambient Assisted Living (AAL) environments for elderly [80, 85, 86] to healthy people for monitoring their health regularly i.e. athletes or sportsmen [87]. Many current projects are considering the issue; such as the H@H system [88] gathers the wearable sensors data, which continuously monitor patients' physio-pathological cardiovascular and respiratory parameters. Similarly, authors in [89], presented an intelligent home-based platform, i.e. the iHome Health-IoT, where a framework is implemented through IoT. Research also shows that several projects like eCAALYX and HELP are on-going which provide home healthcare for the elderly [90]. Again, care@home[1] and ESS-H[2] current projects are focussing on the remote health monitoring [91–94]. Similarly, due to the need of ICT and globalization, several web sites or online-based healthcare service providers are available in the market, which provides possibilities to monitor health parameters such as blood pressure, blood glucose [95, 96], and activity [97]. However, most of them provide feedback, recommendation, alarm messages based on a set of general rules for an individual health-related parameter [80, 86].

12.3 Case Studies

Five case studies on health informatics have been discussed and presented as case studies (1) on advanced Parkinson's disease, (2) on stress management, (3) on postoperative pain treatment, (4) on driver monitoring, and (5) on remote health monitoring. Here, several AI and NL algorithms have been investigated together with some machine reasoning approach on multivariate data coming from heterogeneous sources. The following sub-sections contain a detailed description of each case studies.

12.3.1 Advanced Parkinson's Disease

Parkinson is a slowly progressive neurological disease. It affects a miniature area of cells in the midbrain. Gradual degeneration of these cells reduces a vital chemical called "dopamine". This can fabricate one or more of the classic signs of PD such as stiffness, tremor and pain. Parkinson disease affects about 1% of all persons over the age of 60 and 15% of the patients were diagnosed before age 50 [98]. There is an estimation, about seven to 10 million people worldwide have Parkinson's disease

[1] http://ecareathome.se/.

[2] http://www.es.mdh.se/projects/324-ESS_H___Embedded_Sensor_Systems_for_Health_Research_Profile.

according to the estimates of the https://parkinsonsnewstoday.com/. Ordinary treatment at the initial stage of this disease is 'artificial dopamine' (levodopa) in tablet form. Treatment of PD with levodopa was begun in 1960. [99] Levodopa is the main medicine used to treat Parkinson's disease. Medication must be individually tuned since too high dose leads to problems with uncontrolled movements. So, adjusting their dopamine levels to function smoothly in their daily life is a problem. For the PD patient, it is very important to tune levodopa doses quickly to adjust their dopamine levels. Fluctuating plasma concentrations of levodopa become increasingly linked to variability in motor response with advanced PD. Motor fluctuations and dyskinesias are at least partially related to variations in blood levodopa concentrations, so fluctuation can be reduced by keeping levodopa plasma concentrations constant [100, 101]. Significantly lower variability in plasma levodopa levels can be achieved with infusion of the stabilized carbidopa/levodopa (Duodopa) suspension compared with oral sustained-release tablets [102].

The main purpose of this research work is to develop a web-enabled decision support system (DSS) based on a fuzzy logic inference system (FIS) as an artificial intelligent (AI) approach to assist in dose alteration of Duodopa infusion in patients with advanced Parkinson's disease, given data from motor state assessments and dosage. It is very important to design systems to support individual decision making for this dose optimization tasks. A decision support system (DSS) can be any system that helps decision makers to make the decisions. Further, a web application with an interactive graphical user interface that presented alerts indicating no optimal dosage, dose summary information, advice for new dosage and options to calculate initial dose and evaluation of the DSS is implemented States were defined from + 3 to −3 in various times of the day. This scale (TRS) is further described in [103]. A patient (sample in Fig. 12.1) is to start their treatment by taking a morning dose (2 ml at 7:15 a.m. and the flow rate was 1.6 ml/h 7:45 a.m.) At that time, the state was −3 but after a few hours, at 8:30 a.m., it was 0 (normal). At 9:30 a.m. state was −2.5 so the patient had taken one extra dose as 1 ml and also increased his/her flow rate by 0.1 ml/h. At 10:00 a.m. it was still in negative condition, so the patient had again taken one extra dose as 1 ml and also increased flow rate by 0.2 ml/h. Now at 11:30 a.m. to 13:45 a.m. state was in zero that means in the normal position.

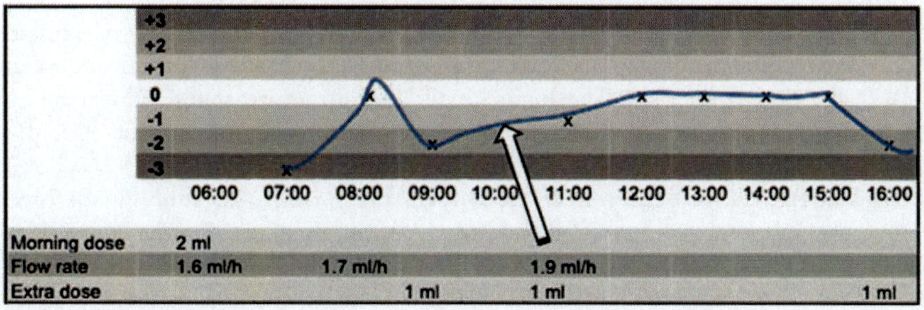

Fig. 12.1 Raw data format for checking state in time of observation study [104]

Table 12.1 Rules of the FIS [4]

Category	Rules to generate new dose
Morning dose	1. If after dose state is negative (−), then the new Morning dose is increased 20% 2. If after dose state is positive (+), then the new Morning dose is decreased 20%
Extra dose	1. If after dose state is negative (−), then the new Extra dose is increased 20% 2. If after dose state is positive (+), then the new Extra dose is decreased 20%
Flow rate	1. If after dose state is falling (−), then the new Flow rate is increased 20% 2. If after dose state is rising (+), then the new Flow rate is decreased 20%

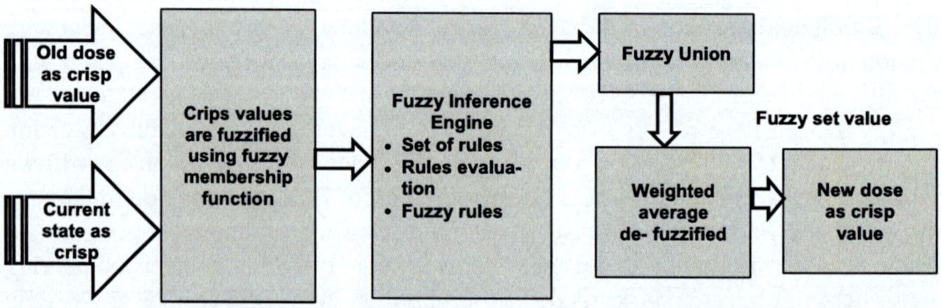

Fig. 12.2 Fuzzy inference system for DSS [105]

The fuzzy rule-based system consisted of three conceptual components: a rule base that consists of a collection of fuzzy IF–THEN rules (Table 12.1); a database that defines the membership functions (MF) used in the fuzzy rules; and a reasoning mechanism that combines these rules into a mapping routine from the inputs to the outputs of the system, to derive an output conclusion as presented in Fig. 12.2. A single-input single-output fuzzy model was extracted from the expert's knowledge. 'Negative', 'positive', 'falling' and 'rising' were linguistic values determined by the fuzzy sets "RightLinearFuzzySet" and "LeftLinearFuzzySet" associated with the fuzzy variable TRS state (or slope of TRS vs. time regression line for flow rate). Increased and decreased were linguistic values determined by the fuzzy sets "SingletonFuzzySet" associated with the fuzzy variable new dose.

Manual tuning of membership function parameters was performed to minimize the mean absolute difference between the advised dose and the next relevant taken dose in the design data set. The logic for finding after-dose states, typical doses and advice and for generating alerts based on expert knowledge was included in the business level as presented in Table 12.2.

Evaluation data were taken from the DireQt study [103]. This study was a three + three weeks crossover study of Duodopa vs. conventional anti-Parkinson medications with blinded assessment of Parkinson symptoms and side effects from video recordings of patients and using the TRS. Only the days when the patients were on Duodopa were used as evaluation data. In this case, doses had already been stabilized at the time of data collection. Dosage of Duodopa was tailored to each patient's

Table 12.2 A list of logic rules for dose, advice and alerts

After-dose state logic	Morning dose	• If patients had not taken any extra doses within one hour after morning dose, then states were considered • The state was considered for decision making from 45 min to 90 min after the dose. If found, priority order was 60, 75, 45 and 90 min
	Extra dose	• If patients had not taken any other extra doses within two hours after taking an extra dose, then states were considered • The state was considered from 45 min to 90 min after the dose with the same priority as morning dose described above
	Flow rate	• If patients had not taken any extra doses or a morning dose within four hours after last changing flow rate, then state and dose time were scanned • If the number of states were more than one within 4 h interval, then states and times were considered for calculation of a regression slope used for decision making
Typical dose and advice	• Median of old dose values or the nearest upper of median dose value for a period was considered the typical dose • Median of new dose values related to the typical dose value was considered the typical advice for the typical dose of a period	
Alerts	Dose alerts	• If extra doses were taken more than three times in a day • If the flow rate was changed more than three times during a day • If total daily dose differed more than (20%) from the previous day
	State alerts	• If states were more than 2 or less than −2 • If regression slopes were more than 0.5 or less than -0.5 TRS units per hour

need based on the practice we tried to capture in our DSS. The Goodness of fit (R^2), between advised and taken doses were calculated for all categories of doses: morning dose, extra dose, flow rate and this was done for both design and evaluation data sets. Advice of 'no change' were excluded from calculations. Overall goodness-of-fit for the design data set (Duodopa untreated) was 0.64 and for the evaluation data set (Duodopa stabilized), 0.97. For the design data set the R^2 was 0.85 for flow rate but for morning dose and extra doses it was only 0.28 and 0.30 respectively. For the evaluation data set R^2 for the flow rate and extra dose was 0.87 and 0.91 respectively which showed that the system behaved much better in case of the evaluation data compared to the design data. There was no result for morning dose in the evaluation data since that data came from non-consecutive days. The worse performance in the new patients can be explained by the fact that the rules were designed for ongoing patients, usually needing only minor adjustments. The initial acclimatization period for new patients often requires bigger changes and a more individual approach by the treating doctor [4, 105].

12.3.2 Stress Management

This research work presents a multi-modal and multipurpose-oriented clinical decision support system for the stress management i.e. stress diagnosis and biofeedback treatment. The stress management system is based on the finger temperature (FT) sensor data and also it considers contextual information i.e. human perception and feelings in textual format. The system applies CBR as a core technique to facilitate experience reuse and decision explanation by retrieving the previous "similar" profiles. Reliability of the performance for the diagnosis and decision-making tasks into the system is further improved through textual information retrieval (IR) with ontology [106]. Again, a three-phase computer-assisted sensor-based DSS for treatment i.e. biofeedback training in stress management is proposed herein [107]. The system incorporates fuzzy techniques with CBR to handle vagueness, uncertainty inherently existing in clinicians reasoning [108]. Diagnosis and treatment of stress is an example of a complex application domain. It is well known that an increased stress level can lead to serious health problems. Medical investigations have shown that the finger temperature (FT) has a correlation with stress for most people [109]. During stress, the sympathetic nervous system of our body is activated, causing a decrease in the peripheral circulation which in turn decreases the skin temperature [109, 110]. During relaxation, the reverse effect occurs (i.e. parasympathetic nervous systems activates) and increases the finger temperature. Thus, finger skin temperature responds to stress. In clinical practice, the balances between the sympathetic and parasympathetic nervous systems are monitored as a part of diagnosis and treatment of psychophysiological dysfunctions. Hence, the rise (increase) and fall (decrease) of the finger temperature (FT) can help to diagnose stress-related dysfunctions [111]. However, the behaviour of the FT is individual for each individual due to health factors, metabolic activity etc. Interpreting/analyzing the FT and understanding large variations of measurements from diverse patients require knowledge and experience. Without having adequate support, the erroneous judgment could be made by less experienced staff. Since there are large individual variations when looking at FT, it is a worthy challenge to find a computational solution to apply it in a computer-based system. The demand for a computer-aided system in the stress domain is increasing day-by-day in our present world [112]. The schematic diagram of the proposed CBR stress management system presented in Fig. 12.3.

Step 1: The signal employed in this research is finger temperature (FT) and clinical studies show that the FT is decreased with stress in general. This is one of the psychophysiological parameters clinically used to determine stress-related disorders [61].

Step 2 and 3: The measurement is collected from 31 subjects using a temperature sensor in six steps (i.e. Baseline, Deep-breath, Verbal-stress, Relax with positive thinking, Math-stress and Relax) in the calibration phase [76]. Eight women and twenty-three men within the age range of 24–51 are participating in this study. The number of individual parameters identified, and features extracted from the complex data format are briefly presented in [113].

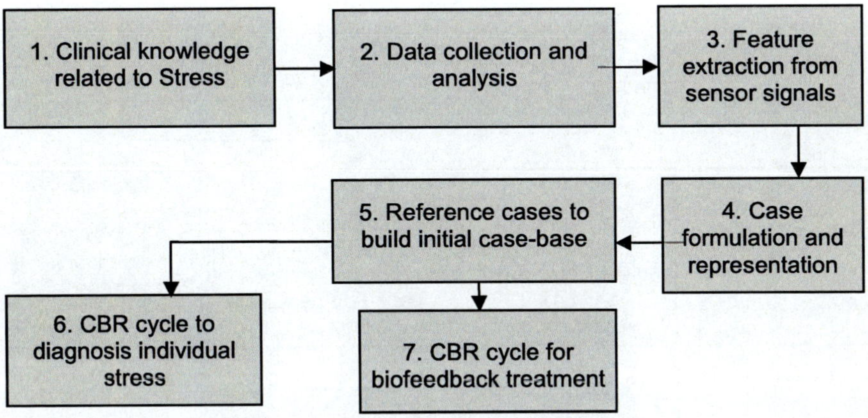

Fig. 12.3 Schematic diagram of the stress management system

Step 4 and 5: A new problem case is formulated by the 19 features (17 extracted features from the signal and 2 other features) in total. The levels of stress are denoted as *Very Relaxed*, *Relaxed*, *Normal/Stable*, *Stressed* and *Very Stressed* and the initial case base, with 53 reference cases from 31 subjects, is classified by a domain expert.

Step 6: To diagnose individual stress level [76], a new FT measurement (formulated as a problem case) is inputted into the CBR cycle as presented in Fig. 12.4. The new problem case is then matched using three different matching algorithms: (1) modified distance function, (2) similarity matrix and (3) fuzzy similarity. The nearest neighbour (NN) algorithm is applied for the retrieval of similar cases. Finally, the topmost case or the case selected by a clinician will provide a classification of the FT measurement as output. A detailed description about the diagnosis of stress is presented in [113].

Step 7: The last step is focuses on the CBR system in biofeedback treatment. A three phase CBR framework [107] is deployed to classify a patient, estimate initial parameters and to make recommendations for biofeedback training as presented in Fig. 12.5.

The average outcome across the seven subsets in terms of the goodness-of-fit (R^2), evaluating the three algorithms comparing the expert's in two aspects: cases ranked by the system as well by the expert and similarity values given by the expert and the system [113]. Here, 80% of the cases are classified correctly by the system.

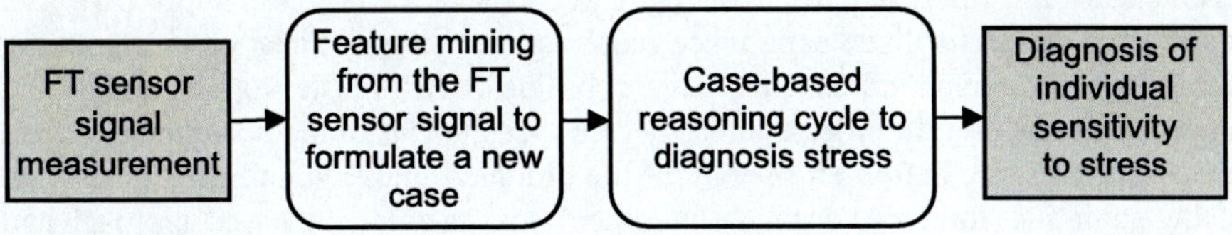

Fig. 12.4 Schematic diagram of the steps in stress diagnosis

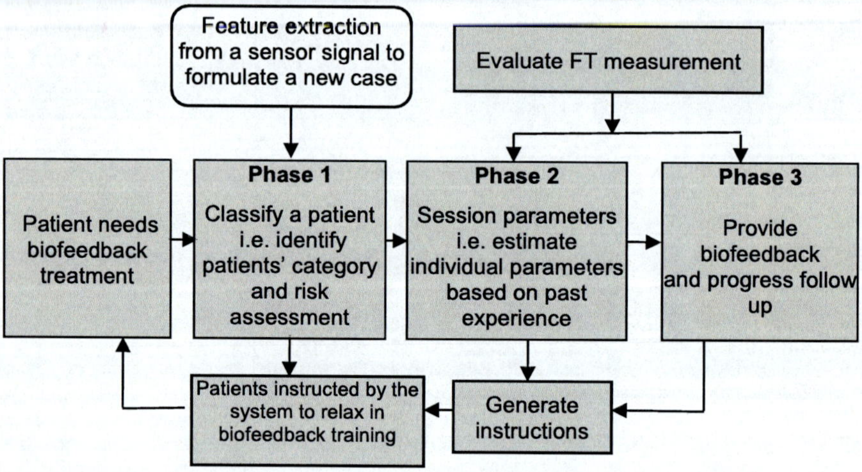

Fig. 12.5 A schematic diagram of the steps in the biofeedback treatment cycle

Among the 20% misclassified cases there are 5% low false positive i.e. cases are one step over classified; 10% are low false negative i.e. cases that are one step over misclassified and 5% are serious false negative i.e. cases that are two steps more misclassified. Compare to the trainee clinicians, the test group setA, the system classifies correctly 81% and the trainee clinicians classify correctly 64% and 55% respectively. The number of the correctly classified cases for setB in percentage is 79 by the system whereas the trainee clinicians have succeeded to classify correctly as 57 in percentage. For both the test groups (setA and setB), when comparing the system against a senior clinician, the obtained Goodness-of-fit (R^2) values are 92% (setA) and 83% (setB). Thus, the case study shows that the system provides results close to a human expert and the system could be useful both for trainee and senior clinicians [113].

12.3.3 Post-operative Pain Treatment

In developing DSS in postoperative pain treatment, (1) information is collected through questionnaires both in numerical and textual formats and (2) pain measurements using a Numerical Visual Analogue Scale (NVAS). The DSS apply CBR as a core technique to facilitate experience reuse and decision explanation by retrieving the previous "similar" cases [114]. Again, besides CBR, clustering techniques and approaches are used in order to identify rare cases [115]. In the postoperative pain treatment domain, before an operation, the clinician makes a pain treatment plan using guideline (following a standard protocol) and an evidence-based approach and makes observations to the patient's response afterwards. However, approximately

30% of the population does not fit the recommended pain treatment procedures due to some hidden individual factors or unusual clinical situations. Cases that do not follow the standard protocol can be classified as a "rare case". These "rare cases" often need personalized adaptation to standard procedures. A CDSS that uses these rare cases and generates a warning by providing references to similar bad or good cases is often beneficial. This will help a clinician to formulate an individual treatment plan [116].

Experience can be represented as a contextualized piece of knowledge in a case. A case can be constructed in traditional ways with symptoms and a solution (treatment) and added outcome (recovery success) in an innovative way. In this article cases that do not follow any standard protocol are regarded as outliers and classified in the "rare case" group. The "rare case" group contains exceptionally good cases and/or unusually bad cases.

Figure 12.6 illustrates a scenario of the experience reuse in the context of post-operative pain treatment (both regular and rare cases). Here, the physician finds 90% of the regular cases with treatment and outcome (a new structure is used in postoperative pain treatment) similar to the new problem. However, 10% of the similar cases are presented as rare, some cases among them have severe outcomes (i.e. 4%) and defined as unusual, on the other hand, some have a (6%) better outcome than expected (may use a new medication) and are presented as exceptional cases.

One common and easy way is to cluster all the cases in a case library and then identify the rare cases. In this system, the rare case identification is done offline in two steps: (1) all cases in the case library are clustered using a Fuzzy C-Means Clustering (FCM) algorithm and (2) the cases from each cluster are again grouped by applying the Hierarchical algorithm. Figure 12.7 illustrates the steps that are taken into consideration while searching rare cases. A data pre-processing step including a feature abstraction step is performed on the records of post-operative pain patients [114]. The *1st order clustering* has been done using FCM as a multi-variant clustering.

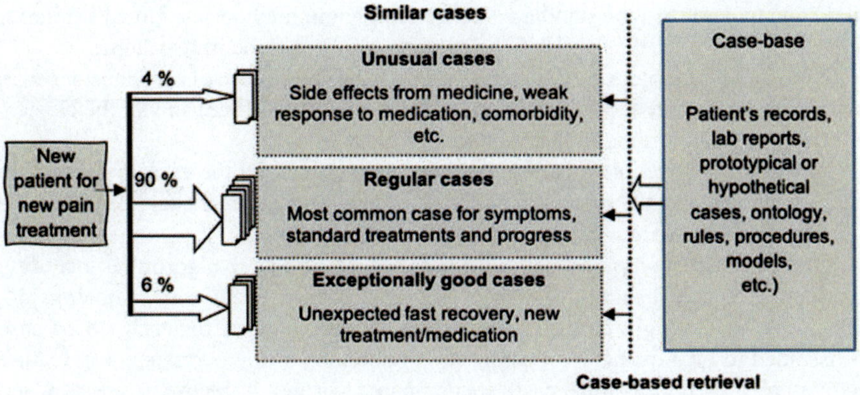

Fig. 12.6 An example of an experience reusing system in post-operative pain treatment

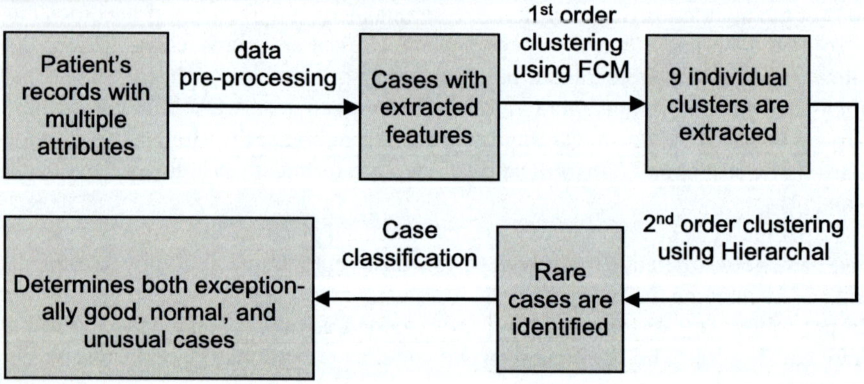

Fig. 12.7 Steps of the approach in order to identify rare cases

Here, the percentage of average variance is used as a function to determine the number of clusters. The lowest percentage of average variance is achieved when the number of clusters is 9. [115]. In the *2nd order clustering*, the Hierarchical clustering algorithm is applied with the distance between pairs of objects is calculated using Euclidean distance as a default parameter of the MATLAB function 'pdist'. The linkage function applies 'single' (i.e. shortage distance) as a default parameter which determines the objects in the data set that should be grouped into clusters. Finally, a cluster function is applied to group the sample data set into clusters by specifying the cluster's number. Then, the clusters with small sizes (i.e. less than 10%) are selected as the rare case cluster and thus the approach has achieved $\approx$18% as rare cases. The last step in Fig. 12.7, determines the $\approx$18% cases whether they are exceptionally good (0–3.9) or unusual bad (6–10) according to the pain outcome (the threshold for good/bad may be changed) [115].

In this CBR system, similarity measurements are used to assess the degrees of matching by applying the standard Nearest Neighbour method as a global similarity algorithm. However, the similarity calculation has been done in two steps:

Step 1: a new problem case is compared with the centre case of each cluster (note, all the clustering and outlier detection has been made on offline) and all the clusters are then sorted according to their similarity value.

Step 2: the new problem case is compared again with all the cases belonging to each cluster. Hence, the system only considers the top nearest clusters define by the user threshold to the new problem case.

Two cases are compared using different local similarity algorithms including modified distance function; similarity matrix and fuzzy similarity matching [40, 106]. The local weight defined by the case author or owner for each stored case is assumed to be a quantity reflecting the importance of the corresponding feature individually. The most similar cases are compared to a new problem case are retrieved and presented in 9 different clusters. A case outcome has a value between 0 and 10, where “0” defines no pain at all and “10” defines severe pain. Note that, in the domain of postoperative pain treatment, similar solutions have different outcomes.

The proposed approach combines a CBR approach with a 2nd order clustering approach in order to retrieve and present rare cases together with regular ones. Here, the retrieval step is conducted in two steps; 1st similarity values have been calculated between a new problem case with the center case of each cluster identified by applying Fuzzy C-Means and 2nd similarity values have been calculated between all the cases in the top clusters and the new problem case. Finally, the most similar cases in the clusters are structured in regular, exceptionally good and unusually bad cases are presented together.

12.3.4 Driver Monitoring

Road transportation is a complex system and poses challenges in safe transportation due to dynamic environment changes and adaptation of driving according to the dynamic traffic environment is challenging. Driving a vehicle is a task that requires continuous adjustment of cognitive activities synchronises with a complex manifold of physiological events [51]. One’s ability to adapt, predict and react to upcoming traffic events can be affected due to impaired driving, for example, for example, sleepiness, inattention, cognitive load or stress. In fact, in more than 90% of traffic crashes, it has been reported that human error is a major contributing factor. [117]. The human related error includes recognition (41%), performance (11%) and non-performance errors (7%); destruction, cognitive load is a consequence of recognition error, overcompensation and poor directional control contributed to performance error, and health-related factors such as sleepiness, stress cause non-performance errors. Physiological parameters acquired by sensors widely used and become reliable and useful objective measures for driver state monitoring. Signal patterns (i.e., changes in physiological signals corresponding to different impaired states) have been widely studied [118].

In this work, multivariate data analysis has been done using machine learning to detect drivers’ levels of sleepiness, cognitive load, and stress. Several physiological signals, namely, electrocardiography (ECG), galvanic skin response (GSR), finger temperature, electroencephalography (EEG), electrooculography (EOG), and respiration were used. In addition, driving behavioural data obtained from the vehicle and contextual information obtained from the driving scenarios are also incorporated. An overview of the driver monitoring framework is shown in Fig. 12.8. Various data preprocessing, data analysis methods are applied to handled noise and artifacts [118, 119]. Different statistical and information-theoretic methods are used for feature extraction and selection that provide understanding of the patterns in the data [118]. Finally, machine learning methods are used to detect and classify the driver state i.e., sleepiness, cognitive load and stress. The goal of this work is to offer a research mechanism that can add value to the following driver monitoring scenarios:

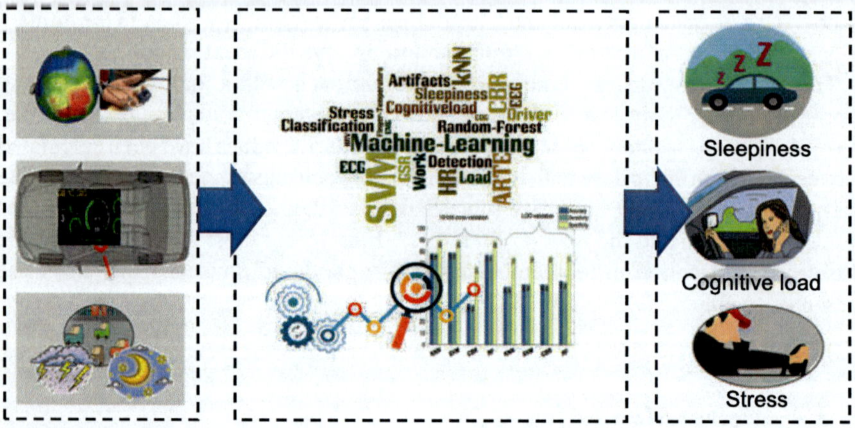

Fig. 12.8 Driver monitoring framework

- Research is interested in investigating various contextual factors such as driving environment, light conditions, emotions, etc.
- The research focused on the non-obtrusive or non-contact-based driver-state detection systems, for example, computer vision-based driver monitoring.
- Evaluating different countermeasures for sleepiness, fatigue, cognitive load, and stress, such as rumble strips, rest breaks, caffeine and napping.

Three different datasets were acquired to address sleepiness, cognitive load, and stress classification problem. Sleepiness and cognitive load data were acquired from the Vehicle Driver Monitoring (VDM) project [120]. The study was approved by the regional ethics committee at Linköping University, Sweden (Dnr 2014/309-31). Both physiological and vehicular data are acquired while participants were driving in a high-fidelity moving base driving simulator at the Swedish National Road and Transport Research Institute (VTI). Sleepiness study consists of three driving scenarios: (1) a rural road with a speed limit of 80 km/h in daylight, (2) a suburban road in daylight and (3) the same rural road in darkness. Cognitive load study also consists of three driving scenarios: (1) a hidden exit on the right side of the road with a warning sign (HE), (2) four-way crossing with an oncoming bus and a car approaching the crossing from the right (CR), and (3) a strong side wind in open terrain (SW). Contextual information from these scenarios is extracted as a feature and used in the building of machine learning models. The Karolinska Sleepiness Scale (KSS) [121] is used at the target variable in the sleepiness study and whereas n-back task [122], which indicates cognitive load task is used on the cognitive load study. The stress study was conducted under the research project "IMod-Intelligent Concentration Monitoring and Warning System for Professional Drivers," [123]. During the data collection session, each participant performed two tests: (1) Psychophysiological Stress Profile (PSP) tests [76] and (2) operating a wheel loader. The duration of PSP was approximately 15 min, afterwards, participants operated the wheel loader. Each participant received ten minutes of self-training called "adapt" to familiarize themselves with the machine setup and wheel loader operation, followed by 5 min of live test driving termed "sharp", where they had to perform a bucket filling task considering some preconditions.

The overall data analysis process for supervised machine learning setup is divided into four phases as depicted in Fig. 12.9 [124]. The first phase deals with problem

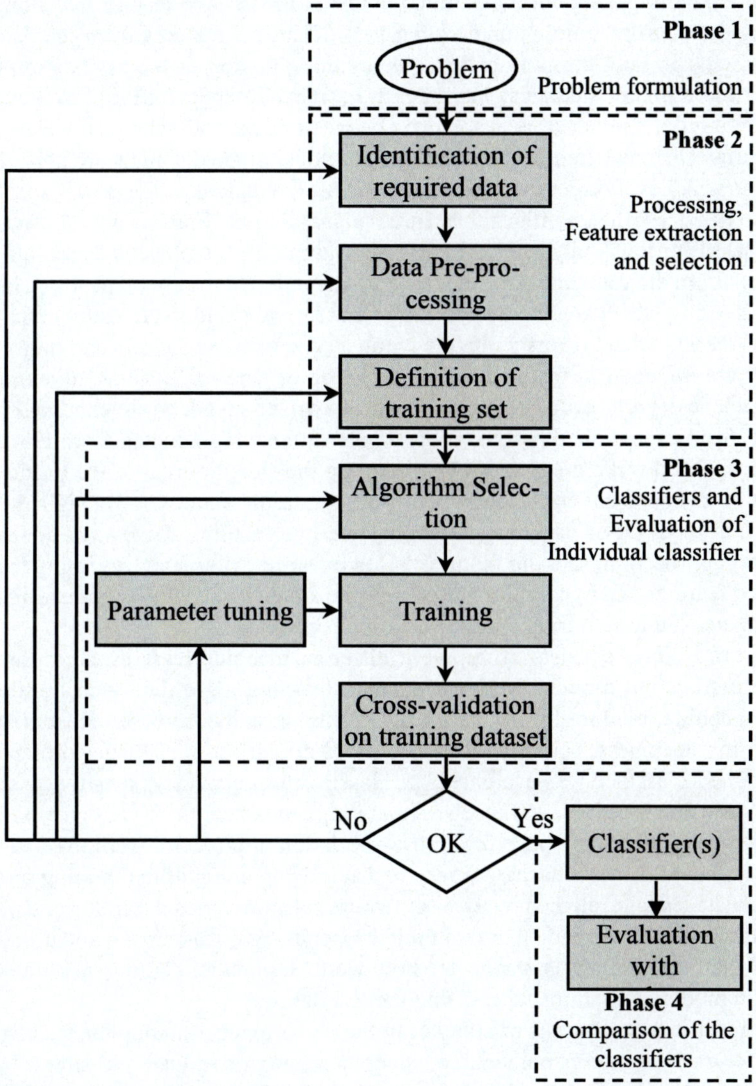

Fig. 12.9 Supervised machine learning approach. Adapted from [124], modified with phases to fit the research process

formulation to define each of the phenomena in the context of driving, the hypotheses behind physiological and other measures, and literature review to understand and outline the state-of-the-art.

In the second phase, the data processing, feature extraction and feature selection are conducted. Since the outcome of data analytics depends on the quality of the input data (e.g., incorrect values, missing data, noisy signal), there are several steps involved in the data processing prior to feature vector construction, e.g., data cleaning and noise handling, data normalization, feature extraction and feature selection, and creating datasets for training and testing [118]. Various features from the datasets are extracted in both the time and frequency domains for each classification task. In the time domain, statistical measures (i.e., mean, standard deviation, kurtosis, peak amplitude, number of peaks, slopes between peaks and valleys, are estimated as features. Different frequency spectra of the physiological signals are considered as features. A Fast Fourier transform (FFT) is used to calculate the power spectrum density (PSD). Further, nonlinear measures such as Sample Entropy and Multivariate Multiscale Entropy Analysis [125] are used to quantify the physiological signal as features. From the vehicular data, the standard deviation of the lateral position, lateral speed, steering wheel angle, yaw, yaw rate, and lateral position are estimated.

The steering wheel reversal rate the number of zero crossings and steering wheel entropy are obtained as features. Lanex (fraction of lane exit) values are extracted from the lane departure signal, which indicates a driver's tendency to exit the driving lane [126]. As mentioned before, contextual features are extracted from the study scenarios. Sleep/wake predictor [127] based on the sleep journal of the participant (only used in sleepiness classification), driving conditions such as day or night driving (driving in daylight or darkness) are considered as features. Two ways of feature selection approach: a) ranking features based on some criteria and selecting the top n-ranked features and b) combining features into smaller subsets and evaluating their performance are used during feature selection process [118].

The third phase consists of applying different machine learning algorithms to build classification models. Various machine learning algorithm such as support vector machine, random forest, k-nearest neighbour, and case-based reasoning are applied for sleepiness, cognitive load and stress classification. The performance of each trained classifier was evaluated for classification accuracy, sensitivity, specificity, confusion matrices, and receiver operating characteristic (ROC) curves. Both leave-one-out validation and k-fold cross-validation approaches were used to validate the models. A test dataset was reserved at the beginning of the training process to avoid data leakage; all the processes of feature selection, model training and model evaluation were performed on the training dataset using k-fold cross-validation. The goal of the final evaluation was to see how well each model could generalize (i.e., based on model predictions when using the test dataset).

The fourth phase consists of comparing the performances among the tested classifiers for each of the phenomena i.e., sleepiness, cognitive load and stress. In the sleepiness, classification results show that by 10-fold cross-validation, the SVM performed best than other classifiers [128]. The SVM achieved 79% and 93% accuracies for multiclass and binary classification respectively. We also investigated the individual differences and with the leave one subject out approach, it is found that a 10% increase in accuracy when data from the individual was included in the training dataset. Interestingly, by adding contextual information to the physiological features, the classification accuracies improved by 4% in multiclass classification and by 5% in binary classification [128]. On the other hand, results of cognitive load classification show that for each individual scenario as well as using data combined from the different scenarios, CBR achieved classification accuracy over 70% [129]. Last but not least, results of stress classification showed that for the PSP data the classifier could classify 'stressed' and 'healthy' subjects 83.33% correctly compared to an expert's classification. On the data for the wheel loader operators, the classifier achieved an accuracy of 83.30% when classifying two different conditions, 'adapt' (training) and 'sharp' (real-life driving) [77].

The driver monitoring framework described here is of interest for multivariate data analysis using machine learning. One of the significances of this work is the use of data- and feature- fusion for feature engineering that is found to be beneficial for improving the classification accuracy of the machine learning models. This the framework presented in this work could yield substantial benefits in developing a knowledge-based or decision support system and could provide a reasonable means for physiological sensor signal-based applications, such as those in other health care domains.

12.3.5 Remote Health Monitoring

Remote health monitoring aims to develop a remote healthcare system that monitors and track the health status of the elderly in a home environment. This research work presents a Health-IoT system where an intelligent healthcare service is developed to monitor vital signs in daily life. Here, a generic Health-IoT framework with a Clinical Decision Support System (CDSS) is presented. The generic system-level framework for a self-serve health monitoring system is mainly focused on the supporting sensors, communication media, secure and safe data communication, storage, and remote accesses of the data. The CDSS is used for a personalized report on persons' health condition based on daily basis observation on vital signs. Here, the proposed framework combines general rules with a case-based reasoning (CBR) approach [130, 131] to a personalized self-served health-monitoring system for elderly in the home environment. A set of general rules has used to classify individual health parameters such as 'blood pressure is high' is an instance/value for the health parameter blood pressure. However, the message is not personal as well as not provides the overall status of the user's health condition.

A case-based reasoning (CBR) [107, 132] approach can work in a way close to human reasoning e.g. solves a new problem applying previous experiences, which is more common for doctors, clinicians or engineers. The system also provides real-time feedback, and enable historical information, reminder and recommendations. A rule-based classification method is applied to classify the measurements and generate real-time feedback; a blood pressure measurement 142/92 mmHg could be classified as "High blood pressure" is one example. The goal of the historical information is to provide to the user a possibility to see and compare the summary in a graph for a specific range of dates. For example, considering medication compliance "total number of medications is taken", and "total number of medications are skipped" are presented. Reminders are generated which helps to monitor several health parameters regularly such as 'Devices_Not_Used' (if there is no measurement received over a week), 'Medications_skipped' (if a certain number of medications is skipped). Similarly, recommendations are generated such as 'Out_Of_Normal_Range' (if 70% of the measurements classes are outside the normal range considering a week), 'Fluctuation' (if the measurements over a week show fluctuation in more than 70%), 'Weight_Loss' (if the current weight is less than 3 kg then weight received 3 months ago), 'Activity_Increased/Activity_Decreased' (considering one week measurements and a calculated slope value), etc. Moreover, a monthly summary is generated where maximum, minimum, average and standard deviation is considered.

As can be seen from Fig. 12.10, an elderly user uses several sensor devices to measure blood pressure, blood glucose, heart rate, pulse, weight etc. to monitor vital signs. The remote intelligent health server where a Decision Support System (DSS) and an Expert System (ES) is running which analysis the sensor readings and provides recommendations and reminders to the user. The system also generates emergency alarms if it is necessary and sends them to clinicians/doctors. A generic system-level framework is proposed which enables different kinds of sensor devices, communications, storages, users, services, gateways, switches, etc. [91]. The system has implemented three different kinds of healthcare services: (1) real-time feedback

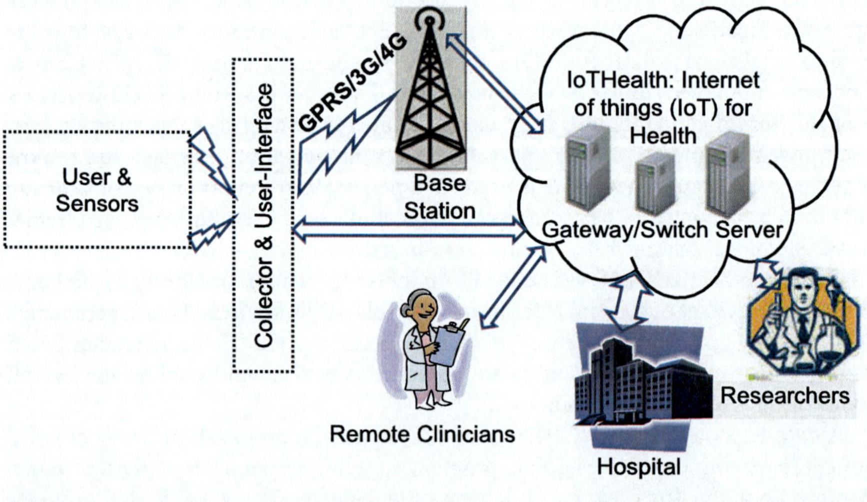

Fig. 12.10 An overview of the self-served health monitoring system through Internet of Things (IoT)

generation service, (2) historical summary calculation service and (3) recommendation generation service [80, 86]. Data were collected from six participants from Spain (n = 3) and Slovenia (n = 3) have used the system for 8 weeks. After 8 weeks, 339 cases are collected, among them, only 323 cases are selected to evaluate the proposed approach and the rest of them are ignored due to missing values in the cases. The reason for missing values is due to the bad connection of Bluetooth or Wi-Fi. An expert in the domain classifies the cases into three classes (e.g. 'Healthy', 'More or Less Healthy' and 'Need Further Diagnosis') and the evaluation results are presented in the result section.

To promote a personalized self-served health-monitoring the proposed approach combines general rules and case-based reasoning (CBR) approach. The steps in process diagram of the proposed system for personalized health monitoring service are presented in Fig. 12.11.

Step 1 is used to collect sensor readings, there are different sensor devices are used to collect measurements for different vital signs of a user i.e., (1) Blood Pressure (BP), (2) Blood Glucose (BG), (3) Weight (WGT), (4) Activity (AC), (5) Heart Rate (HR) (6) Oxygen Saturation (SpO_2), etc.

In *Step 2*, user contextual information such as height, age, gender, etc.; medical and health-related information such as diseases, comorbidity is collected.

Similarly, *Step 3* collects user preferences on the sensitivity of the vital signs and self-assessment about their health condition. To conclude the user's current health

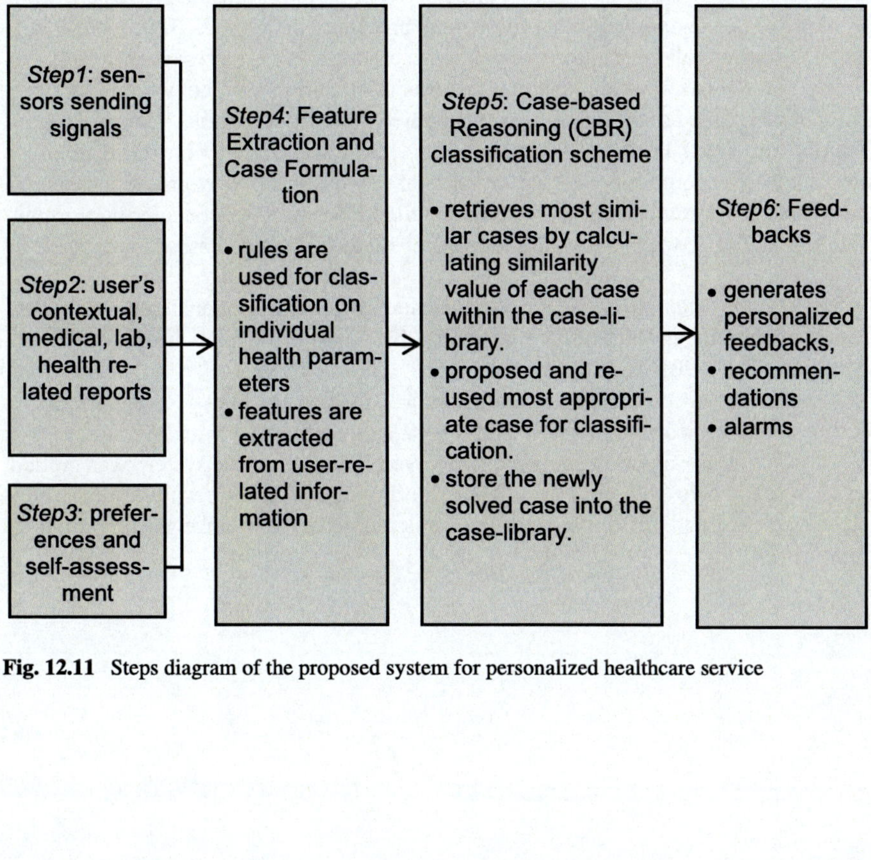

Fig. 12.11 Steps diagram of the proposed system for personalized healthcare service

Table 12.3 Rules are used to classify the blood pressure (e.g. systolic/diastolic as mmHg) and activity

Health parameters	Rules to generate real time feedback
Blood pressure (BP)	1. If Systolic < 90 (mm Hg) or Diastolic < 60 (mm Hg) then BP_class = "Low" 2. If Systolic is 90–119 (mm Hg) and Diastolic is 60–79 (mm Hg) then BP_class = "Normal" 3. If Systolic is 120–139 (mm Hg) or Diastolic is 80–89 (mm Hg) then BP_class = "Pre-High" 4. If Systolic > 140 (mm Hg) or Diastolic > 90 (mm Hg) then BP_class = "High"
Weight (WGT)	1. If BMI < 18.5 then WGT_class = "Underweight" 2. If BMI > 18.5 and BMI < 24.9 then WGT_class = "Normal" 3. If BMI > 25.0 then WGT_class = "Overweight"

condition, the users were asked the following question:" How do you assess your overall health?" The user was to choose one out of five options: 1. perfect, 2. good, 3. fair, 4. poor, 5. could not respond.

Step 4 is used for feature extraction where a rule-based classification method is applied to classify the sensor signal measurements. For example, a blood pressure measurement 142/92 mmHg could be classified as "High" and/or BMI 26.1 by measuring user's weight could be classified "Overweight". A set of rules used in the classification method is mainly collected from the literature study, one example for blood pressure and weight monitoring is presented in Table 12.3 [95, 133–136], which is further validated through healthcare practitioners are presented in [91].

Step 5 is the case-based reasoning (CBR) classification scheme, which identifies the overall health condition of a user whether they are 'Healthy', 'More or Less Healthy' or 'Need Further Diagnosis'. Here, the retrieval function retrieves most similar cases by computing similarity value of two cases (i.e. new problem case and one solved case from case-library). The detailed case retrieval considering normalized Manhattan distance between the feature values of the two cases is presented in [91].

Step 6 is the outcome of the proposed system, where the personalized feedbacks, recommendations and alarms are generated based on the overall health condition identified by the CBR classification scheme.

A sensitivity, specificity and overall accuracy are also calculated, considering $k = 2$ criteria. The values obtained is Sensitivity 90%, Specificity 97% and Accuracy 96% [137]. Also, user evaluation shows that the overall quality of the system was graded between 6 and 8 in both countries. Thus, the initial evaluation result demonstrates the competence and performance of the implemented system through the proposed framework [91].

12.4 Summary and Discussion

This book chapter presents the research development of AI, ML and MR in 5 different application domains in health informatics to develop DSS as case studies. The case studies are: (1) advanced Parkinson's disease, (2) stress management, (3) postoperative pain treatment, (4) driver monitoring, and (5) remote health monitoring. Several AI and ML algorithms such as fuzzy logic, supervised ML, clustering approaches have been applied and/or investigated together with several machine reasoning techniques, for example, fuzzy rule-based reasoning and case-based reasoning in a hybrid manner. A multi-modal approach is exploited to develop the more robust system based on multivariate data analysis, here, both numerical data, sensors signals, textual information are combined together. Information fusion both in data level, feature level and decision level have been conducted. Artifact, noise is also handled using AI and ML approaches. Feature extraction and selection are conducted together with remote data management framework.

As we have shown multivariate data are used in these five application domains, there are different challenges that need to be addressed for applying AI, ML and MR algorithms. We can categorize these challenges as follows:

- Dealing with *noise and artifacts* in the collected data. Physiological data can be affected by the noise or artifacts when acquired in a dynamic situation compared to the laboratory setting. One example is the EEG signals that are most prone to artifacts [138] in driver monitoring. Therefore, robust methods for handling artifacts is crucial in non-stationary environments.
- *Features* extracted from physiological signals are a direct and objective measure of functional state and reliable source for detecting various phenomena in healthcare application. However, often data from a single source do not efficiently reflect the condition that is in scrutiny. Data from multiple sources can improve the classification accuracy as we have shown in different applications. However, multivariate data could include duplicated information or irrelevant information in the feature space, which is a problem in many machine learning applications. Feature engineering using data- and feature-fusion, feature selection and dimensionality reduction considered to make accurate classifications
- Two major problems in machine learning are *Overfitting* and *class noise*, which occur due to subjective self-ratings are often used for labelling the training data. To overcome these problems, one possible approach is to use multimodal data and develop a multimodule solution consisting of several models with different algorithms.

In this book chapter, data analytics, and classification approached on multivariate data for several healthcare applications are presented. Recent trend shows that there is a need for a robust system. Thanks to the proliferation of the Internet of Things (IoT), connected services, it is now possible to acquire data from heterogeneous sources. Thus, IoT and cloud-based distributed system that connects these heterogeneous data can benefit the society and the healthcare providers, and most importantly can bring the healthcare services at the door of each individual.

Acknowledgements The authors would like to acknowledge the projects named ESS-H: Embedded Sensor Systems for Health Research Profile is funded by Knowledge Foundation and SAAPHO: Secure Active Aging: Participation and Health for the Old (aal-2010-3-035) is funded by the Call AAL (Ambient Assisted Living) within the Call 3. Authors would also like to acknowledge the Swedish Governmental Agency for Innovation Systems (VINNOVA), Volvo Car Corporation, and VTI for financing the Vehicle Driver Monitoring (VDM) project. Authors also acknowledge the funding agency KKS and project partners for the IMod and the SafeDriver project.

References

1. Buchanan, B., Shortliffe, E.: Rule-based expert system. The MYCIN Experiments of the Stanford Heuristic Programming Project (1984)
2. Gardner, R.M., Pryor, T.A., Warner, H.R.: The HELP hospital information system: update 1998. Int. J. Med. Informatics **54**(3), 169–182 (1999). https://doi.org/10.1016/S1386-5056(99)00013-1
3. Kong, G., Xu, D.-L., Yang, J.-B.: Clinical decision support systems: a review on knowledge representation and inference under uncertainties. In. J. Comput. Intell. Syst. **1**(2), 159–167 (2008). https://doi.org/10.1080/18756891.2008.9727613
4. Ahmed, M., Westin, J., Nyholm, D., Dougherty, M., Groth, T.: A fuzzy rule-based decision support system for Duodopa treatment in Parkinson. In: 23rd Annual Workshop of the Swedish Artificial Intelligence Society, Umeå, May, 2006 (2006)
5. Alayón, S., Robertson, R., Warfield, S.K., Ruiz-Alzola, J.: A fuzzy system for helping medical diagnosis of malformations of cortical development. J. Biomed. Inform. **40**(3), 221–235 (2007). https://doi.org/10.1016/j.jbi.2006.11.002
6. Casas, F., Orozco, A., Smith, W.A., De Abreu-García, J.A., Durkin, J.: A fuzzy system cardio pulmonary bypass rotary blood pump controller. Expert Syst. Appl. **26**(3), 357–361 (2004). https://doi.org/10.1016/j.eswa.2003.09.006
7. Lindgaard, G.: Intelligent decision support in medicine: back to bayes? In: Proceedings of the 14th European conference on Cognitive Ergonomics: Invent! Explore!, pp. 7–8. ACM (2007)
8. Kahn, C.E., Roberts, L.M., Shaffer, K.A., Haddawy, P.: Construction of a Bayesian network for mammographic diagnosis of breast cancer. Comput. Biol. Med. **27**(1), 19–29 (1997). https://doi.org/10.1016/S0010-4825(96)00039-X
9. Podgorelec, V., Kokol, P., Zavrsnik, J.: Medical diagnosis prediction using genetic programming. In: Proceedings 12th IEEE Symposium on Computer-Based Medical Systems (Cat. No. 99CB36365), 18–20 June 1999, pp. 202–207 (1999). https://doi.org/10.1109/cbms.1999.781271
10. Paz, J.F.D., Rodríguez, S., Bajo, J., Corchado, J.M.: Case-based reasoning as a decision support system for cancer diagnosis: A case study. Int. J. Hybrid. Intell. Syst. **6**(2), 97–110 (2009)
11. Corchado, J.M., Bajo, J., Abraham, A.: GerAmi: improving healthcare delivery in geriatric residences. IEEE Intell. Syst. **23**(2), 19–25 (2008). https://doi.org/10.1109/MIS.2008.27
12. Díaz, F., Fdez-Riverola, F., Corchado, J.M.: gene-CBR: a case-based reasonig tool for cancer diagnosis using microarray data sets. Comput. Intell. **22**(3–4), 254–268 (2006). https://doi.org/10.1111/j.1467-8640.2006.00287.x
13. Glez-Peña, D., Díaz, F., Hernández, J.M., Corchado, J.M., Fdez-Riverola, F.: geneCBR: a translational tool for multiple-microarray analysis and integrative information retrieval for

aiding diagnosis in cancer research. BMC Bioinf. **10**(1), 187 (2009). https://doi.org/10.1186/1471-2105-10-187
14. Schmidt, R., Vorobieva, O.: Case-based reasoning investigation of therapy inefficacy. In: Applications and Innovations in Intelligent Systems XIII, pp. 13–25. Springer London (2006)
15. D'Aquin, M., Lieber, J., Napoli, A.: Adaptation knowledge acquisition: a case study for case-based decision support in oncology. Comput. Intell. **22**(3–4), 161–176 (2006). https://doi.org/10.1111/j.1467-8640.2006.00281.x
16. Song, X., Petrovic, S., Sundar, S.: A Case-based reasoning approach to dose planning in Radiotherapy (2007)
17. Marling, C., Shubrook, J., Schwartz, F.: Case-based decision support for patients with type 1 diabetes on insulin pump therapy. In: Advances in Case-Based Reasoning, pp 325–339. Springer Berlin Heidelberg (2008)
18. Maetzler, W., Klucken, J., Horne, M.: A clinical view on the development of technology-based tools in managing Parkinson's disease. Mov. Disord. **31**(9), 1263–1271 (2016). https://doi.org/10.1002/mds.26673
19. Espay, A.J., Bonato, P., Nahab, F.B., Maetzler, W., Dean, J.M., Klucken, J., Eskofier, B.M., Merola, A., Horak, F., Lang, A.E., Reilmann, R., Giuffrida, J., Nieuwboer, A., Horne, M., Little, M.A., Litvan, I., Simuni, T., Dorsey, E.R., Burack, M.A., Kubota, K., Kamondi, A., Godinho, C., Daneault, J.-F., Mitsi, G., Krinke, L., Hausdorff, J.M., Bloem, B.R., Papapetropoulos, S., Technology obotMDSTFo: Technology in Parkinson's disease: challenges and opportunities. Mov. Disord. **31**(9), 272–1282 (2016). https://doi.org/10.1002/mds.26642
20. Giuffrida, J.P., Riley, D.E., Maddux, B.N., Heldman, D.A.: Clinically deployable Kinesia™ technology for automated tremor assessment. Mov. Disord. **24**(5), 723–730 (2009). https://doi.org/10.1002/mds.22445
21. Griffiths, R.I., Kotschet, K., Arfon, S., Xu, Z.M., Johnson, W., Drago, J., Evans, A., Kempster, P., Raghav, S., Horne, M.K.: Automated assessment of bradykinesia and dyskinesia in Parkinson's disease. J. Parkinson's Dis. **2**(1), 47–55 (2012)
22. Bonato, P., Sherrill, D.M., Standaert, D.G., Salles, S.S., Akay, M.: Data mining techniques to detect motor fluctuations in Parkinson's disease. In: The 26th Annual International Conference of the IEEE Engineering in Medicine and Biology Society, 1–5 Sept 2004, pp. 4766–4769 (2004). https://doi.org/10.1109/iembs.2004.1404319
23. Gil, D., Johnson, M.: Diagnosing Parkinson by using artificial neural networks and support vector machines. **9** (2009)
24. Soleimanian Gharehchopogh, F., Mohammadi, P.: A case study of Parkinson's disease diagnosis using artificial neural networks. Int. J. Comput. Appl. **73**, 1–6 (2013). https://doi.org/10.5120/12990-9206
25. Pereira, L.A.M., Rodrigues, D., Ribeiro, P.B., Papa, J.P., Weber SAT social-spider optimization-based artificial neural networks training and its applications for Parkinson's disease identification. In: 2014 IEEE 27th International Symposium on Computer-Based Medical Systems, 27–29 May 2014, pp. 14–17 (2014). https://doi.org/10.1109/cbms.2014.25
26. Geman, O.: A fuzzy expert systems design for diagnosis of Parkinson's disease. In: 2011 E-Health and Bioengineering Conference (EHB), 24–26 Nov. 2011, pp. 1–4 (2011)
27. Eskofier, B.M., Lee, S.I., Daneault, J., Golabchi, F.N., Ferreira-Carvalho, G., Vergara-Diaz, G., Sapienza, S., Costante, G., Klucken, J., Kautz, T., Bonato, P.: Recent machine learning advancements in sensor-based mobility analysis: Deep learning for Parkinson's disease assessment. In: 2016 38th Annual International Conference of the IEEE Engineering in Medicine and Biology Society (EMBC), 16–20 Aug 2016, pp. 655–658 (2016). https://doi.org/10.1109/embc.2016.7590787
28. Tsanas, A., Little, M.A., McSharry, P.E., Ramig, L.O.: Accurate telemonitoring of Parkinson's disease progression by noninvasive speech tests. IEEE Trans. Biomed. Eng. **57**(4), 884–893 (2010). https://doi.org/10.1109/TBME.2009.2036000
29. Patel, S., Lorincz, K., Hughes, R., Huggins, N., Growdon, J., Standaert, D., Akay, M., Dy, J., Welsh, M., Bonato, P.: Monitoring motor fluctuations in patients with Parkinson's disease using wearable sensors. IEEE Trans. Inf. Technol. Biomed. **13**(6), 864–873 (2009). https://doi.org/10.1109/TITB.2009.2033471

30. Nancy Jane, Y., Khanna Nehemiah, H., Arputharaj, K.: A Q-backpropagated time delay neural network for diagnosing severity of gait disturbances in Parkinson's disease. J. Biomed. Inform. **60**, 169–176 (2016). https://doi.org/10.1016/j.jbi.2016.01.014
31. Lopane, G., Mellone, S., Chiari, L., Cortelli, P., Calandra-Buonaura, G., Contin, M.: Dyskinesia detection and monitoring by a single sensor in patients with Parkinson's disease. Mov. Disord. **30**(9), 1267–1271 (2015). https://doi.org/10.1002/mds.26313
32. Selye, H.: The Stress of Life. McGraw-Hill, New York, NY, US (1956)
33. Won, E., Kim, Y.-K.: Stress, the autonomic nervous system, and the immune-kynurenine pathway in the etiology of depression. Curr. Neuropharmacol. **14**(7), 665–673 (2016). https://doi.org/10.2174/1570159x14666151208113006
34. Guan, L., Collet, J.-P., Mazowita, G., Claydon, V.E.: Autonomic nervous system and stress to predict secondary ischemic events after transient ischemic attack or minor stroke: possible implications of heart rate variability. Front. Neurol. **9**(90) (2018). https://doi.org/10.3389/fneur.2018.00090
35. Landis, C., Cannon, W.B.: Bodily Changes in Pain, Hunger, Fear and Rage, 2nd ed., revised and enlarged., pp. xvi + 404. Appleton, New York, 1929 (1930). Pedagogical Sem. J. Genet. Psychol. **38**(1–4), 527–531. https://doi.org/10.1080/08856559.1930.10532290
36. Noble, R.E.: Diagnosis of stress. Metabol. Clin. Exp. **51**(6), 37–39 (2002). https://doi.org/10.1053/meta.2002.33190
37. Begum, S., Ahmed, M.U., Schéele, B., Olsson, E., Funk, P.: Development of a stress questionnaire: a tool for diagnosing mental stress. Technical Report, MRTC (2010)
38. Cohen, S., Kessler, R.C., Gordon, L.U.: Measuring stress: A Guide for Health and Social Scientists. Oxford University Press on Demand (1997)
39. Perner, P.: An architecture for a CBR image segmentation system. Eng. Appl. Artif. Intell. **12**(6), 749–759 (1999). https://doi.org/10.1016/S0952-1976(99)00038-X
40. Begum, S., Ahmed, M.U., Funk, P., Xiong, N., Von Schéele, B.: A case-based decision support system for individual stress diagnosis using fuzzy Y similarity matching. Computational Intelligence **25**(3), 180–195 (2009). https://doi.org/10.1111/j.1467-8640.2009.00337.x
41. Begum, S., Ahmed, M.U., Funk, P.: ECG sensor signal analysis to represent cases in a case-based stress diagnosis system. In: Proceedings of the 10th IEEE International Conference on Information Technology and Applications in Biomedicine, 3–5 Nov 2010, pp. 1–5 (2010). https://doi.org/10.1109/itab.2010.5687657
42. Hawthorn, J., Redmond, K.: Pain: causes and management. J. Psychiatr. Ment. Health Nurs. **6**(5), 409–410 (1999). https://doi.org/10.1046/j.1365-2850.1999.00227-8.x
43. Crawford Clark, W., Yang, J.C., Tsui, S.-L., Ng, K.-F., Bennett Clark, S.: Unidimensional pain rating scales: a multidimensional affect and pain survey (MAPS) analysis of what they really measure. Pain **98**(3), 241–247 (2002). https://doi.org/10.1016/S0304-3959(01)00474-2
44. Kumar, S., Tandon, O., Mathur, R.: Pain measurement: a formidable task. Ind. J. Physiol. Pharmacol. **46**(4), 396–406 (2002)
45. Rothaug, J., Zaslansky, R., Schwenkglenks, M., Komann, M., Allvin, R., Backström, R., Brill, S., Buchholz, I., Engel, C., Fletcher, D., Fodor, L., Funk, P., Gerbershagen, H.J., Gordon, D.B., Konrad, C., Kopf, A., Leykin, Y., Pogatzki-Zahn, E., Puig, M., Rawal, N., Taylor, R.S., Ullrich, K., Volk, T., Yahiaoui-Doktor, M., Meissner, W.: Patients' perception of postoperative pain management: validation of the international pain outcomes (IPO) questionnaire. J. Pain **14**(11), 1361–1370 (2013). https://doi.org/10.1016/j.jpain.2013.05.016
46. Jose, D., Fischer, H., Ivani, G., Mogensen, T., Narchi, P., Singelyn, F., Stienstr, R., Wulf, H.: Postoperative pain management—good clinical practice. European Society of Regional Anaesthesia and Pain therapy (2011)
47. Smith, M.Y., DePue, J.D., Rini, C.: Computerized decision-support systems for chronic pain management in primary care. Pain Med. **8**(suppl_3), S155–S166 (2007). https://doi.org/10.1111/j.1526-4637.2007.00278.x
48. Bertsche, T., Askoxylakis, V., Habl, G., Laidig, F., Kaltschmidt, J., Schmitt, S.P.W., Ghaderi, H., Bois, A.Z.-d., Milker-Zabel, S., Debus, J., Bardenheuer, H.J., Haefeli, W.E.: Multidisciplinary pain management based on a computerized clinical decision support system in cancer pain patients. PAIN® **147**(1), 20–28 (2009). https://doi.org/10.1016/j.pain.2009.07.009

49. Houeland, T.G., Aamodt, A.: Towards an introspective architecture for meta-level reasoning in clinical decision support systems. In: Proceedings of the Workshop on CBR in the Health Sciences, 8th International Conference on Case-Based Reasoning, pp. 235–244 (2009)
50. Elvidge, K.: Improving pain & symptom management for advanced cancer patients with a clinical decision support system. Stud. Health Technol. Inf. **136**, 169–174 (2008). https://doi.org/10.3233/978-1-58603-864-9-169
51. Jacobé de Naurois, C., Bourdin, C., Stratulat, A., Diaz, E., Vercher, J.-L.: Detection and prediction of driver drowsiness using artificial neural network models. Accid. Anal. Prev. (2017). https://doi.org/10.1016/j.aap.2017.11.038
52. Wang, X., Xu, C.: Driver drowsiness detection based on non-intrusive metrics considering individual specifics. Acc. Anal. Prevent. **95**(Part B), 350–357 (2016). doi:https://doi.org/10.1016/j.aap.2015.09.002
53. Balandong, R.P., Ahmad, R.F., Saad, M.N.M., Malik, A.S.: A review on EEG-based automatic sleepiness detection systems for driver. IEEE Access **6**, 22908–22919 (2018). https://doi.org/10.1109/ACCESS.2018.2811723
54. Fu, R., Wang, H., Zhao, W.: Dynamic driver fatigue detection using hidden Markov model in real driving condition. Expert Syst. Appl. **63**, 397–411 (2016). https://doi.org/10.1016/j.eswa.2016.06.042
55. Yoshida, Y., Ohwada, H., Mizoguchi, F.: Extracting tendency and stability from time series and random forest for classifying a car driver's cognitive load. In: 2014 IEEE 13th International Conference on Cognitive Informatics and Cognitive Computing, 18–20 Aug 2014, pp. 258–265 (2014). https://doi.org/10.1109/icci-cc.2014.6921469
56. Liang, Y., Reyes, M.L., Lee, J.D.: Real-time detection of driver cognitive distraction using support vector machines. IEEE Trans. Intell. Transp. Syst. **8**(2), 340–350 (2007). https://doi.org/10.1109/TITS.2007.895298
57. Solovey, E.T., Zec, M., Perez, E.A.G., Reimer, B., Mehler, B.: Classifying driver workload using physiological and driving performance data: two field studies. In: Paper presented at the Proceedings of the 32nd annual ACM conference on Human factors in computing systems, Toronto, Ontario, Canada (2014)
58. Kartsch, V.J., Benatti, S., Schiavone, P.D., Rossi, D., Benini, L.: A sensor fusion approach for drowsiness detection in wearable ultra-low-power systems. Inf. Fusion (2017). https://doi.org/10.1016/j.inffus.2017.11.005
59. Yeo, M.V.M., Li, X., Shen, K., Wilder-Smith, E.P.V.: Can SVM be used for automatic EEG detection of drowsiness during car driving? Saf. Sci. **47**(1), 115–124 (2009). https://doi.org/10.1016/j.ssci.2008.01.007
60. Chen, L.-L., Zhao, Y., Ye, P.-F., Zhang, J., Zou, J.-Z.: Detecting driving stress in physiological signals based on multimodal feature analysis and kernel classifiers. Expert Syst. Appl. **85**(Supplement C), 279–291 (2017). https://doi.org/10.1016/j.eswa.2017.01.040
61. Hu, S., Zheng, G.: Driver drowsiness detection with eyelid related parameters by Support Vector Machine. Expert Syst. Appl. **36**(4), 7651–7658 (2009). https://doi.org/10.1016/j.eswa.2008.09.030
62. Chui, K.T., Tsang, K.F, Chi, H.R., Wu, C.K., Ling, B.W.K.: Electrocardiogram based classifier for driver drowsiness detection. In: 2015 IEEE 13th International Conference on Industrial Informatics (INDIN), 22–24 July 2015, pp. 600–603 (2015). https://doi.org/10.1109/indin.2015.7281802
63. Yoshizawa, A., Nishiyama, H., Iwasaki, H., Mizoguchi, F.: Machine-learning approach to analysis of driving simulation data. In: 2016 IEEE 15th International Conference on Cognitive Informatics & Cognitive Computing (ICCI*CC), 22–23 Aug 2016, pp. 398–402 (2016). https://doi.org/10.1109/icci-cc.2016.7862067
64. Liao, Y., Li, S.E., Li, G., Wang, W., Cheng, B., Chen, F.: Detection of driver cognitive distraction: an SVM based real-time algorithm and its comparison study in typical driving scenarios. In: 2016 IEEE Intelligent Vehicles Symposium (IV), 19–22 June 2016, pp. 394–399 (2016). https://doi.org/10.1109/ivs.2016.7535416

65. Soman, K., Sathiya, A., Suganthi, N.: Classification of stress of automobile drivers using Radial Basis Function Kernel Support Vector Machine. In: International Conference on Information Communication and Embedded Systems (ICICES2014), 27–28 Feb 2014, pp. 1–5 (2014). https://doi.org/10.1109/icices.2014.7034000
66. Munla, N., Khalil, M., Shahin, A., Mourad, A.: Driver stress level detection using HRV analysis. In: 2015 International Conference on Advances in Biomedical Engineering (ICABME), 16–18 Sept 2015, pp. 61–64 (2015). https://doi.org/10.1109/icabme.2015.7323251
67. Vicente, J., Laguna, P., Bartra, A., Bailón, R.: Drowsiness detection using heart rate variability. Med. Biol. Eng. Comput. **54**(6), 927–937 (2016). https://doi.org/10.1007/s11517-015-1448-7
68. Garcés Correa, A., Orosco, L., Laciar, E.: Automatic detection of drowsiness in EEG records based on multimodal analysis. Med. Eng. Phys. (0) (2013). http://dx.doi.org/10.1016/j.medengphy.2013.07.011
69. Ma J, Murphey YL, Zhao H Real Time Drowsiness Detection Based on Lateral Distance Using Wavelet Transform and Neural Network. In: 2015 IEEE Symposium Series on Computational Intelligence, 7–10 Dec 2015, pp. 411–418 (2015). https://doi.org/10.1109/ssci.2015.68
70. Dwivedi, K., Biswaranjan, K., Sethi, A.: Drowsy driver detection using representation learning. In: 2014 IEEE International Advance Computing Conference (IACC), 21–22 Feb 2014, pp. 995–999 (2014). https://doi.org/10.1109/iadcc.2014.6779459
71. Manawadu, U.E.: Kawano, T., Murata, S., Kamezaki, M., Muramatsu, J., Sugano, S.: Multiclass classification of driver perceived workload using long short-term memory based recurrent neural network. In: 2018 IEEE Intelligent Vehicles Symposium (IV), 26–30 June 2018, pp. 1–6 (2018). https://doi.org/10.1109/ivs.2018.8500410
72. Babaeian, M., Bhardwaj, N., Esquivel, B., Mozumdar, M.: Real time driver drowsiness detection using a logistic-regression-based machine learning algorithm. In: 2016 IEEE Green Energy and Systems Conference (IGSEC), 6–7 Nov 2016, pp. 1–6 (2016) https://doi.org/10.1109/igesc.2016.7790075
73. Gurudath, N., Riley, H.B.: Drowsy driving detection by EEG analysis using wavelet transform and K-means clustering. Procedia Comput. Sci. **34**, 400–409 (2014). https://doi.org/10.1016/j.procs.2014.07.045
74. Ming, J., Zhelong, W.: A method for stress detection based on FCM algorithm. In: 2nd International Congress on Image and Signal Processing, 2009. CISP'09, 17–19 Oct 2009, pp. 1–5 (2009). https://doi.org/10.1109/cisp.2009.5304150
75. El Haouij, N., Poggi, J.-M., Ghozi, R., Sevestre-Ghalila, S., Jaïdane, M.: Random forest-based approach for physiological functional variable selection for driver's stress level classification. Stat. Methods Appl. (2018). https://doi.org/10.1007/s10260-018-0423-5
76. Begum, S., Ahmed, M., Funk, P., Xiong, N., Schéele, B.V.: Using calibration and fuzzification of cases for improved diagnosis and treatment of stress (2006)
77. Begum, S., Barua, S., Filla, R., Ahmed, M.U.: Classification of physiological signals for wheel loader operators using Multi-scale Entropy analysis and case-based reasoning. Expert Syst. Appl. **41**(2), 295–305 (2014). https://doi.org/10.1016/j.eswa.2013.05.068
78. Begum, S., Ahmed, M.U., Funk, P., Filla, R.: Mental state monitoring system for the professional drivers based on Heart Rate Variability analysis and Case-Based Reasoning. In: Paper presented at the Computer Science and Information Systems (FedCSIS), 2012 Federated Conference on 9–12 Sept 2012 (2012)
79. Kulkarni, A., Sathe, S.: Healthcare applications of the Internet of Things: a review. Int. J. Comput. Sci. Inf. Technol. **5**(5), 6229–6232 (2014)
80. Ahmed, M., Espinosa, J., Reissner, A., Domingo, A., Banaee, H., Loutfi, A., Rafael-Palou, X,: Self-serve ICT-based health monitoring to support active ageing (2015). https://doi.org/10.13140/2.1.4956.1921
81. Simonov, M., Zich, R., Mazzitelli, F.: Personalized healthcare communication In Internet of Things (2008)
82. Sidén, J., Skerved, V., Gao, J., Forsstr, S., #246, Nilsson, H.-E., Kanter, T., Gulliksson, M.: Home care with NFC sensors and a smart phone. In: Paper presented at the Proceedings of the 4th International Symposium on Applied Sciences in Biomedical and Communication Technologies, Barcelona, Spain (2011)

83. Salih, A., Abraham, A.: A review of ambient intelligence assisted healthcare monitoring. Int. J. Comput. Inf. Syst. Ind. Manage. (IJCISIM) **5**, 741–750 (2013)
84. Patel, S., Park, H., Bonato, P., Chan, L., Rodgers, M.: A review of wearable sensors and systems with application in rehabilitation. J. Neuro Eng. Rehabil. **9**(1), 21 (2012). https://doi.org/10.1186/1743-0003-9-21
85. Parra, J., Hossain, M.A., Uribarren, A., Jacob, E.: Restful discovery and eventing for service provisioning in assisted living environments. Sensors (Basel, Switzerland) **14**(5), 9227–9246 (2014). https://doi.org/10.3390/s140509227
86. Ahmed, M.U., Banaee, H., Rafael-Palou, X., Loutfi, A.: Intelligent healthcare services to support health monitoring of elderly. In: Internet of Things. User-Centric IoT, pp. 178–186. Springer, Cham (2015)
87. Armstrong, S.: Wireless connectivity for health and sports monitoring: a review. Br. J. Sports Med. **41**(5), 285–289 (2007). https://doi.org/10.1136/bjsm.2006.030015
88. System, H.H.: Health@Home. http://www.aal-europe.eu/projects/healthhome/ (2016). Accessed 27 June 2016
89. Yang, G., Xie, L., Mäntysalo, M., Zhou, X., Pang, Z., Xu, L.D., Kao-Walter, S., Chen, Q., Zheng, L.: A health-IoT platform based on the integration of intelligent packaging, unobtrusive bio-sensor, and intelligent medicine box. IEEE Trans. Ind. Inf. **10**(4), 2180–2191 (2014). https://doi.org/10.1109/TII.2014.2307795
90. Projects Co.: Ambient Assisted Living Joint Programme (AAL JP) (2011)
91. Ahmed, M.: An intelligent healthcare service to monitor vital signs in daily life—A case study on health-IoT. Int. J. Eng. Res. Appl. **7**, 43 (2017). https://doi.org/10.9790/9622-0703024345
92. Ahmed, M.U., Banaee, H., Loutfi, A.: Health Monitoring for elderly: an application using case-based reasoning and cluster analysis. ISRN Artif. Intell. **2013**, 11 (2013). https://doi.org/10.1155/2013/380239
93. Tsiftes, N., Duquennoy, S., Voigt, T., Ahmed, M.U., Köckemann, U., Loutfi, A.: The E-Care@Home infrastructure for IoT-enabled healthcare. In: Internet of Things Technologies for HealthCare, pp. 138–140. Springer, Cham (2016)
94. Ahmed, M., Björkman, M., Lindén, M.: A Generic System-Level Framework for Self-Serve Health Monitoring System through Internet of Things (IoT), vol. 211 (2015). https://doi.org/10.3233/978-1-61499-516-6-305
95. Strowig, S., Raskin, P.: Improved glycemic control in intensively treated type 1 diabetic patients using blood glucose meters with storage capability and computer-assisted analyses. Diabetes Care **21**, 1694–1698 (1998). https://doi.org/10.2337/diacare.21.10.1694
96. Association AH: Understanding blood pressure readings. http://www.heart.org/HEARTORG/Conditions/HighBloodPressure/AboutHighBloodPressure/Understanding-Blood-Pressure-Readings_UCM_301764_Article.jsp. Accessed 02 Dec 2019
97. Ahmed, M.U., Loutfi, A.: Physical activity identification using supervised machine learning and based on pulse rate. Int. J. Adv. Comput. Sci. Appl. (IJACSA) **4**(7) (2013). http://dx.doi.org/10.14569/IJACSA.2013.040730
98. Mariann, D.: Parkinson's Disease Clinic and Research Center at the University of California SF The National Parkinson Foundation, Inc. http://www.parkinson.org/pdedu.htm. Accessed 05 July 2005
99. Shefrin, S.L.: Therapeutic advances in idiopathic Parkinsonism. Expert Opin. Investig. Drugs **8**(10), 1565–1588 (1999). https://doi.org/10.1517/13543784.8.10.1565
100. Bredberg, E., Tedroff, J., Aquilonius, S.-M., Paalzow, L.: Pharmacokinetics and effects of levodopa in advanced Parkinson's disease. Eur. J. Clin. Pharmacol. **39**(4), 385–389 (1990). https://doi.org/10.1007/bf00315415
101. Harder, S., Baas, H., Rietbrock, S.: Concentration-effect relationship of Levodopa in patients with Parkinson's disease. Clin. Pharmacokinet. **29**(4), 243–256 (1995). https://doi.org/10.2165/00003088-199529040-00004
102. Nyholm, D., Askmark, H., Gomes-Trolin, C., Knutson, T., Lennernäs, H., Nyström, C., Aquilonius, S.-M.: Optimizing levodopa pharmacokinetics: intestinal infusion versus oral sustained-release tablets. Clin. Neuropharmacol. **26**(3), 156–163 (2003)

103. Nyholm, D., Nilsson Remahl, A.I.M., Dizdar, N., Constantinescu, R., Holmberg, B., Jansson, R., Aquilonius, S.-M., Askmark, H.: Duodenal levodopa infusion monotherapy versus oral polypharmacy in advanced Parkinson disease. Neurology **64**(2), 216–223 (2005). https://doi.org/10.1212/01.Wnl.0000149637.70961.4c
104. Sättler, M.: On off Schedule. Uppsala, Sweden
105. Ahmed, M.U.: A web enabled fuzzy rule-based decision support system for dose adjustments of Duodopa infusion to patients with advanced Parkinsons disease. Computer Engineering, Dalarna University, Dalarna, Sweden (2005)
106. Ahmend, M.U., Begum, S., Funk, P., Xiong, N., Von Schéele, B.: Case-based reasoning for diagnosis of stress using enhanced cosine and fuzzy similarity. Trans. Case-Based Reason. Multimedia Data **1**(1), 3–19 (2008)
107. Ahmed, M.U., Begum, S., Funk, P., Xiong, N., von Scheele, B.: A multi-module case-based biofeedback system for stress treatment. Artif. Intell. Med. **51**(2), 107–115 (2011). https://doi.org/10.1016/j.artmed.2010.09.003
108. Ahmed, M.U., Begum, S., Funk, P., Xiong, N.: Fuzzy rule-based classification to build initial case library for case-based stress diagnosis. In: The Proceedings of 9th International Conference on Artificial Intelligence and Applications (AIA), pp 225–230 (2009)
109. AAPB: The Association for Applied Psychophysiology and Biofeedback. http://www.aapb.org/i4a/pages/index.cfm?pageid=336. Accessed 30 Nov 2019
110. Stress TPo A Guide to Psychology and its Practice. http://www.guidetopsychology.com/stress.htm. Accessed 30 Nov 2019
111. Healey, J.A., Picard, R.W.: Detecting stress during real-world driving tasks using physiological sensors. IEEE Trans. Intell. Transport. Syst. **6**(2), 156–166 (2005). https://doi.org/10.1109/TITS.2005.848368
112. Begum, S., Ahmed, M.U., Funk, P., Xiong, N.: Intelligent signal analysis using case-based reasoning for decision support in stress management. In: Bichindaritz, I., Vaidya, S., Jain, A., Jain, L.C. (eds.) Computational Intelligence in Healthcare 4: Advanced Methodologies. Springer, Berlin, Heidelberg, Berlin, Heidelberg, pp 159–189. (2010). https://doi.org/10.1007/978-3-642-14464-6_8
113. Ahmed, M.U.: A case-based multi-modal clinical system for stress management. Mälardalen University (2010)
114. Ahmed, M., Funk, P.: A case-based retrieval system for post-operative pain treatment (2011)
115. Ahmed, M., Funk, P.: Mining rare cases in post-operative pain by means of outlier detection (2011). https://doi.org/10.1109/ISSPIT.2011.6151532
116. Ahmed, M.U.: Multimodal Approach for Clinical Diagnosis and Treatment. Mälardalen University (2011)
117. Singh, S.: Critical reasons for crashes investigated in the National Motor Vehicle Crash Causation Survey. Traffic Safety Facts Crash. Report No. DOT HS 812 115. National Highway Traffic Safety Administration, Washington, DC (2015)
118. Barua, S.: Multivariate Data Analytics to Identify Driver's Sleepiness, Cognitive Load, and Stress. Mälardalen University (2019)
119. Barua, S., Ahmed, M.U., Ahlstrom, C., Begum, S., Funk, P.: Automated EEG artifact handling with application in driver monitoring. IEEE J. Biomed. Health Inf. (99), 1–1 (2017). https://doi.org/10.1109/jbhi.2017.2773999
120. Nilsson, E., Ahlström, C., Barua, S., Fors, C., Lindén, P., Svanberg, B., Begum, S., Ahmed, M.U., Anund, A.: Vehicle Driver Monitoring: Sleepiness and Cognitive Load (Driver Monitoring: sömnighet och kognitiv belastning (swe)). VTI rapport. Statens väg- och transportforskningsinstitut, Linköping (2017)
121. Åkerstedt, T., Anund, A., Axelsson, J., Kecklund, G.: Subjective sleepiness is a sensitive indicator of insufficient sleep and impaired waking function. J. Sleep Res. **23**(3), 242–254 (2014). https://doi.org/10.1111/jsr.12158
122. Mehler, B., Reimer, B, Wang, Y.: A comparison of heart rate and heart rate variability indices in distinguishing single-task driving and driving under secondary cognitive workload. In: Paper presented at the 6th International Driving Symposium on Human Factors in Driver

Assessment, Training, and Vehicle Design, Olympic Valley - Lake Tahoe, California, USA, June 27–30 (2011)
123. Filla, R., Olsson, E., von Schéele, B., Ohlsson, K.: A case study on quantifying the workload of working machine operators by means of psychophysiological measurements. In: The 13th Scandinavian International Conference on Fluid Power, SICFP2013, 3–5 June 2013, Linköping, Sweden (2013)
124. Kotsiantis, S.B.: Supervised machine learning: a review of classification techniques. In: Paper presented at the Proceedings of the 2007 conference on Emerging Artificial Intelligence Applications in Computer Engineering: Real Word AI Systems with Applications in eHealth, HCI, Information Retrieval and Pervasive Technologies (2007)
125. Ahmed, M.U., Mandic, D.P.: Multivariate multiscale entropy: a tool for complexity analysis of multichannel data. Phys. Rev. E **84**(6), 061918 (2011)
126. Sandberg, D., Åkerstedt, T., Anund, A., Kecklund, G., Wahde, M.: Detecting driver sleepiness using optimized nonlinear combinations of sleepiness indicators. IEEE Transactions on Intelligent Transportation Systems **12**(1) (2011)
127. Åkerstedt, T., Connor, J., Gray, A., Kecklund, G.: Predicting road crashes from a mathematical model of alertness regulation—The sleep/wake predictor. Accid. Anal. Prev. **40**(4), 1480–1485 (2008). https://doi.org/10.1016/j.aap.2008.03.016
128. Barua, S., Ahmed, M.U., Ahlström, C., Begum, S.: Automatic driver sleepiness detection using EEG, EOG and contextual information. Expert Syst. Appl. **115**, 121–135 (2019). https://doi.org/10.1016/j.eswa.2018.07.054
129. Barua, S., Ahmed, M.U., Begum, S.: Classifying drivers' cognitive load using EEG signals. Stud. Health Technol. Inf. **237**, 99–106 (2017)
130. Aamodt, A., Plaza, E.: Case-based reasoning: foundational issues, methodological variations, and system approaches. AI Commun **7**(1), 39–59 (1994)
131. Watson, I.: Applying case-based reasoning: techniques for enterprise systems. Morgan Kaufmann Publishers Inc. (1998)
132. Montani, S., Portinale, L., Leonardi, G., Bellazzi, R., Bellazzi, R.: Case-based retrieval to support the treatment of end stage renal failure patients. Artif. Intell. Med. **37**(1), 31–42 (2006). https://doi.org/10.1016/j.artmed.2005.06.003
133. Association AH: Understanding Blood Pressure Readings. Updated November 7 (2014)
134. Culhane, K.M., O'Connor, M., Lyons, D., Lyons, G.M.: Accelerometers in rehabilitation medicine for older adults. Age Ageing **34**(6), 556–560 (2005). https://doi.org/10.1093/ageing/afi192
135. World Health O: Definition, diagnosis and classification of diabetes mellitus and its complications: report of a WHO consultation. Part 1, Diagnosis and Classification of Diabetes Mellitus. World Health Organization, Geneva (1999)
136. Deurenberg, P., Weststrate, J.A., Seidell, J.C.: Body mass index as a measure of body fatness: age- and sex-specific prediction formulas. Br. J. Nutr. **65**(2), 105–114 (1991). https://doi.org/10.1079/BJN19910073
137. Ahmed, M.U.: A personalized health-monitoring system for elderly by combining rules and case-based reasoning. In: pHealth, pp. 249–254 (2015)
138. Minguillon, J., Lopez-Gordo, M.A., Pelayo, F.: Trends in EEG-BCI for daily-life: requirements for artifact removal. Biomed. Signal Process. Control **31**, 407–418 (2017). https://doi.org/10.1016/j.bspc.2016.09.005

Chapter 13
Risk Prediction with Machine Learning in Cesarean Section: Optimizing Healthcare Operational Decisions

Shelia Rahman, Md. Imran Khan, Md. Shahriare Satu, and Mohammad Zoynul Abedin

Abstract In recent years, data mining is becoming very popular in healthcare and medical research. With its enormous library and a large number of machine learning (ML) algorithms, it is being used for the complex, multidimensional and large data in healthcare systems. Cesarean section or C-section is the widely used method when any abnormality affects the normal birth of a child. The aim of this research is to identify the cesarean section of child birth by considering some important situations of pregnant women using different ML algorithms. In this situation, several data imbalanced techniques were implemented in the cesarean data. Then, various classifiers were applied to the derived balanced and base cesarean sample. After applying ML classifiers, we have received a success rate over 95%.

Keywords C-Section · ML · Oversampling · Classifiers

13.1 Introduction

Nowadays, healthcare industries have analyzed all sorts of medical data to predict the patient's health. The medical domain produces a large amount of data with heterogeneity and multi-dimensionality. Digital data are being produced from a number of

S. Rahman
Institute of Information Technology, Jahangirnagar University, Dhaka, Bangladesh

Md. I. Khan
Department of Computer Science and Engineering, Gono Bishawbidyalay, Dhaka, Bangladesh

Md. S. Satu
Department of Management Information Systems, Noakhali Science and Technology University, Noakhali, Bangladesh

M. Z. Abedin (✉)
Collaborative Innovation Center for Transport Studies, Dalian Maritime University, Dalian, People's Republic of China
e-mail: abedinmz@yahoo.com

Department of Finance and Banking, Hajee Mohammad Danesh Science and Technology University, Dinajpur, Bangladesh

M. A. R. Ahad and M. U. Ahmed (eds.), *Signal Processing Techniques for Computational Health Informatics*, Intelligent Systems Reference Library 192,
https://doi.org/10.1007/978-3-030-54932-9_13

sources such as electronic and personal health records, which include medical history, laboratory results, and prescriptions. The dataset, which is produced in healthcare, falls victim to bias, noise, and abnormalities. It can also suffer from improper decision-making processes and faulty treatments to patients. Machine Learning (ML) methods have been considered to be relatively inexpensive and available to collect, store, and manipulate such kinds of data. It can be used to discover regularities and patterns over the patient dataset, explore medical imaging, predict harmful diseases, and create many more using expert and intelligent models.

This discussion generally belongs to the department of obstetrics. Obstetrics is the branch of medicine and surgery which specializes in childbirth and midwifery. Whether a woman in labor, it is a very important issue to decide which methods (cesarean or a vaginal) can be used to the birth of her baby. Vaginal birth is generally called the natural birth process with shorter hospital stay and faster recovery compared with cesarean delivery. However, a cesarean (C)-section is suggested if any risk is involved with the normal delivery. If a patient will require a cesarean birth, it depends on a number of situations. Doctors and patients generally try to avoid C-sections as it is major surgery and involves opening up a pregnant woman's abdomen and removing the baby from her uterus. ML methods can be useful to assess the situation of pregnant women and take a decision about C-section. In [1], these algorithms were used to detect the risk of developing gestational diabetes, preterm delivery and the presence of existing preeclampsia by analyzing menstrual cycle, health history, current health status, nutrition habits, exercise activity, symptoms, or moods of the pregnant woman. Again, researchers [2] have used ML-based analysis into MRI images to evaluate the presence of the placenta accrete spectrum (PAS), where the patient is affected with placenta preview and several algorithms were used about decision making for pregnant women to decide if a C-section is required. In this article, we discuss the prediction made by a number of ML algorithms in comparison with doctor's decisions in case of C-section.

Moreover, the methodology of this study is also applicable in the signal processing domain in which machine learning consists of a number of non-linear processing stages as well as the lower stage's output is fed into higher stages and finally generate some form of information from the learning instances. However, the rest of the chapter is organized as follows. Section 13.2 includes the background that comprises an overview of the machine learning operations regarding the current research. Section 13.3 describes the methodology and Sect. 13.4 discusses the experiment results. Finally, Sects.13.5 and 13.6 represent the discussion and conclusion, respectively.

13.2 Background

13.2.1 Theoretical Literature

13.2.1.1 Healthcare Operational Decision

To provide efficient health services, proficient healthcare operational management is very important for diagnosis, treatment, and prevention of illness, diseases or any abnormality of patients. It can be differentiated healthy patients from unhealthy ones, prescribes medical care requirements and also describes the characteristics of diseases of different patients. A doctor decides to perform C-section and make safe delivery of a child or if there are any complications involved. It is a massive surgery and also includes a number of complications itself to the patient. According to the CDC (Center for Disease Control), one woman to three womans are delivering their baby using C-section. There are happened a large number of cases where C-section has been performed, but it could have been avoided where C-section has not been needed. Faulty operational decisions can sometimes be life-threatening. ML methods are found very helpful for taking decision about operations in this case. This model can be trained with previous cases of medical operational decisions that can predict decisions more accurately. In this experiment, we used different ML algorithms for healthcare operational decisions about C-section. A brief description of this regard is given in the following.

13.2.1.2 Machine Learning

Machine learning refers to the optimization of performance metrics based on some training data or past experience. A ML model is generated some particular parameters and algorithms where the instances of the dataset are trained to estimate unknown records. It is used different statistical theories, which are both predictive and descriptive. ML differs from a general program on the properties of learning and improving. A problem calls ML when the problem is very complex and requires adaptive with the environment [3]. In the next decades, ML systems will be widely demanded in a number of large and complex data-intensive fields for example- astronomy, biology, climatology, medicine, finance, and economy. Let, we consider a training dataset $x = (x_1, x_2, \ldots, x_n)$ and the target vector as t. The result of the ML algorithms are expressed as $y(x)$ which takes an input x and generates an output vector y. The precise form of y is manipulated at the training phase that is also called the learning phase. For efficiency, the large dataset goes through a pre-processing step which is also known as feature extraction in speeding up the computation. In general, there are considered two types of ML algorithms that are supervised and unsupervised.

Supervised Versus Unsupervised Machine Learning

All the instances of the dataset can be manipulated by ML algorithms that contain different types of features such as categorical, continuous, or binary. When the instances are provided the corresponding outputs or labels, then supervised ML algorithms can be used. In contrast, when the instances are not labeled, then we have to consider the unsupervised ML algorithm. In supervised algorithms, there are included classifications when input is mapped to a specific output label and regression when input is mapped to a continuous output. A specific relation among the data can be found in both classification and regression to produce correct output effectively. In unsupervised ML algorithms, there are included clustering, density estimation, and representation learning, etc. These algorithms are also useful for exploratory analysis. Different ML algorithms have been represented useful contributions to determine healthy patients from affected along with any future possibility of affecting with any disease. They produce specific results about data analysis where perfect prediction is required.

13.2.1.3 Machine Learning for Signal Processing

For a long time, ML has been considered as an important technical area for signal and information processing. Signal processing requires to extract complex structures and build internal representation from inputs. It can process a wide variety of information, including voice, image, records, numbers, and many others [4–7]. As a result, it is gained a lot of attention from signal processing researchers. ML in signal processing consists of a number of non-linear processing stages where the lower stage's output is fed into higher stages and finally generates some form of information from the input dataset. Medical data practitioners generate the maximum advantages from ML by applying it in optimizing clinical instances, including different medical images (X-ray, CT scan, PET scan, ultrasounds, MRI, etc.) and medical records.

13.3 Empirical Literature

In recent years researchers working with medical data have shown great interest in using ML to generate models that helped them in the diagnosis and treatment of patients.

Almost every section of the medical system uses ML, and it has also been used with data regarding childbirth, pregnancy, postpartum care, natal care. However, we have found only a limited number of research works regarding caesarian operation using ML techniques. Gharehchopogh et al. [8] considered several risk factors regarding childbirth to predict if a pregnant woman requires a C-section or not. They have applied the decision tree (DT) algorithm for its negotiation strategies and diagnosed delivery method in women. Caruana et al. [9] have shown the physician's decision about C-section that varies to a great extent from the actual C-section requirement. The dataset of pregnant women was divided into a number of groups where each group is shown with a certain level of risk (requirement of C-section). On each group, DT with Bayesian smoothing and artificial neural networks (ANN) were applied to calculate the C-section rate. The behavior of five ML algorithms including random forest (RF), naïve Bayes (NB), logistic regression (LR), k-nearest neighbor (KNN), support vector machine (SVM) on caesarian data was observed in [3]. Among them, KNN and RF have successfully predicted C-section over 90% cases. Besides, ANN with fuzzy cognitive maps was used by Stylios et al. [10] to predict the procedure of the labor by regularly monitoring fetus heart signal, uterine contractions and psychological condition of the patient. Vovsha et al. [11] have proposed a model to identify women at risk of preterm birth during the course of their pregnancy at early child delivery. They have considered the preterm birth problem as a binary classification problem and applied SVM with radial basis kernel function and logistic and lasso regression. In order to allow the algorithm and handle the skewness in the dataset, they have scaled the hinge of loss penalty from the cost function proportionally to the size of each class. Maroufizadeh et al. [12] have analyzed Iranian 2120 primiparous by using LR, RF andANN and ANN shows the highest accuracy (70%). Manzanares et al. [13] developed a prediction model called Trial of labor after cesarean (TOLAC) for predicting vaginal delivery success after cesarean delivery using classification and regression tree modeling. Iftitah et al. [14] have made an android based mobile application which which predicts delivery method of a pregnant woman using NB classification with 90% accuracy. Lee et al. [15] investigated practical variance to perform epidural anesthesia for C section using ML and data-driven informatics. Besides, Lee et al. [16] analyzed 596 obstetric patients in preterm birth where six classification methods such as ANN, LR, DT, NB, RF and SVM were implemented and their outcomes were compared with ANN to explore its significant determinants based on variable importance. Saleem et al. [17] derived robust features by using multivariate extensions of EMD based on nonlinear and nonstationary neural interactions of FHR and UC signals. In this case, the fetal state prediction can be manipulated by using DT, SVM, and AdaBoost.

The dataset used in this paper contained a range of discrete values. It suffers from an imbalanced data problem, missing values, outliers, noisy data and so on. In data mining classification problems, most classifiers such as LR, DT, and ANN are worked well when their response variable of this dataset is balanced [12, 13]. According to [14] oversampling methods, it inflates the minority class using synthetic data that is used amongst the most popular techniques for resolving class imbalance problem.

Based on the above survey, this chapter asserts that no study highlights a comprehensive task of the experimented issues applying more ML classifiers to estimate C-section. Therefore, more extensive research on supervised learning is represented in this section. Along with widely used classifiers, several recent ML algorithms are included, which were not observed for C-sections in previous works.

13.4 Methodology

This proposed work aims to illustrate the performance of different ML algorithms to process C-section data. For this, we have used a caesarian dataset with attributes that represent different medical conditions of pregnant women. However, this dataset does not contain a large number of instances and not appropriately balanced. So, this data is pre-processed by implementing several data oversampling techniques to increase instances and balance it. Then, different ML classifiers are applied to baseline and various balanced datasets. Finally, a non-parametric significant test is performed to evaluate the results.

13.4.1 Dataset Description

Caesarian section dataset was collected from the University of California, Irvine (UCI) machine learning archive (http://archive.ics.uci.edu/ml/datasets/Caesarian+Section+Classification+Dataset) which includes 80 data samples about pregnant women from the healthcare of Tabriz. There are considered several attributes such as the age of the patient, no of delivery, blood pressure, heart condition, and if the delivery was C-section. These attributes are very significant determinants according to the conditional requirement of C-section. The type of each attribute are considered in Table 13.1.

We have converted some of these categorical attributes to numerical value for implementing the ML algorithms as a requirement. Our input dataset includes 80 cases of pregnant women between 18 to 40 ages. Among them, 41 women are having first time delivery, 27 women are having second time delivery and 10 women are having on their third delivery and 2 are having 4th delivery. In the case of delivery time, there are 46 timely, 17 premature, 17 latecomers. In case of blood pressure, we have 20 high, 40 normal, 20 low and 30 inept, 50 apt cases in heart condition. Finally, the dataset includes 34 no, 46 yes cases of cesarean surgery. Among the 46 patients who had C-section has 14 cases of high blood pressure, 23 cases of inept heart, but in most cases had timely delivery.

Table 13.1 Feature description

Attributes	Type
Age	Numerical
Pregnancy time	Numerical
Delivery time	Premature, Timely, Latecomer
Blood pressure	Low, Normal, High
Heart condition	Apt (normal), Inept (abnormal)
Caesarian	Yes, No

However, the dataset is divided into k equal subsets or folds where each fold is distinctly tested and the other folds are used as a training set. The common choice of k is usually 5 or 10 where, k generally is an unfixed parameter. In this work, we have set the value of $k = 10$.

13.4.2 Data Balancing Techniques

The behavior of an ML algorithm can be affected by the problem of the imbalanced dataset [18]. It depends on the extent of difference in the number of samples from distinct classes. To handle such issue, we have used different oversampling techniques such as random oversampling, SMOTE and ROSE, respectively. Then, different classification algorithms are applied to all four datasets.

13.4.2.1 Random Oversampling

Random oversampling replaces old samples with new samples that are generated by random sampling and replicated values at a random point using its nearest neighbors. It changes the priors in the training set by increasing points from minority class. It also increases the likelihood of occurring overfitting. In principle, oversampling does not add any new class into the training set. Replication of positive examples prevents the learning algorithm from pruning parts of the model that contains very few training examples of certain types.

13.4.2.2 Synthetic Minority Oversampling Technique

Synthetic Minority Over-sampling Technique (SMOTE) [19] is useful when one class dominates the other. It inserts new synthesized values of existing minority instances. It contrasts random oversampling in the sense that synthetic minority class data points are added to the training set by creating new points rather than replicating the previous ones. It comparatively works better than oversampling in some instances. If a data point x_i has k-nearest neighbors and from it, a point x_{zi} is selected then a sample is generated as follows:

$$x_{new} = x_i + \lambda \times (x_{zi} - x_i)$$

where λ is a random number in the range between [0, 1] used as a weight.

13.4.2.3 Random Over-Sampling Examples

Random Over-Sampling Examples (ROSE) [20] handle the binary classification problem where imbalanced dataset is generated artificial samples of the minority class in the neighborhood feature space. It helps the better estimation of learner accuracy and overcomes the limits of both resubstitution and holdout method. Let, we consider (x_i, y_i) which belongs to a training set T_n, size n and the class labels y_i which belongs to the set $\{Y_0, Y_1\}$. Besides, $(x_i, y_i) \in T_n$ are selected such that $y_i = y^*$ ϵ [0, 1], with probability $\frac{1}{n_j}$. Then, a^*x from $K_{Hj}(x_i)$ is sampled with K_{Hj} probability distribution that centered at x_i and covariance matrix H_j. The newly generated data point can be denoted as $(x * y)$.

13.4.3 *Machine Learning Algorithms*

Large quantities of data are produced by healthcare systems which vary in quality and complexity. The selection of appropriate algorithms is a critical issue for processing these data and decision making which ensures the correctness of the information and minimizes the cost of data processing. A number of factors affect the behavior of the algorithms, such as the size of dataset, type of accuracy, linearity, number of attributes, data type, and many others. In this research, we have chosen a medical dataset of pregnant women where the data is labeled and classify the instances into two classes named caesarian and non-caesarian. Based on the literature survey, we have used a number of classification algorithms [21, 22] which are briefly described in the following.

13.4.3.1 *K*-Nearest Neighbor

K-Nearest Neighbor (KNN) [23] is a simple and straightforward algorithm and its ability to map continuous attributes that enable it handling healthcare data. It is a non-parametric classification algorithm where a given instance is compared with k training instances and assessed similarity to it and n number of attributes is represented in n-dimensional space. KNN explores the pattern space when any unknown instance is introduced for k similar instances that are closest to the unknown one. It generally assigns a class to an unlabeled data point which is the nearest point of a previously seen labeled data [7]. The relativity between two instances or data point is called "Closeness" that can be defined by Euclidean distance between two points $x_1 = \{x_{11}, x_{12} \ldots x_{1m}\}$ and $x_2 = \{x_{21}, x_{22} \ldots x_{2m}\}$ as

$$d(x_1, x_2) = \sqrt{\sum_{m=1}^{n} (x_{1m} - x_{2m})^2}$$

Now for each such x if we define the distance in order, $d_1(x) \leq d_2(x)) \leq d_3(x)$... then $d_1(x)$ is the distance to the nearest point and $d_2(x)$ is the distance to the second nearest point and so on. The KNN density function can be defined as

$$h(x) = \frac{k}{2N d_k(x)}$$

We change the value of k that changes the number of observations. KNN works well in multimodal classes and applications where instances can have multiple labels. However, this classifier gives poor accuracy when noise or irrelevant data is present ed. Attribute weighting and pruning of noisy instances or condensing of the dataset is used to avoid this problem [8].

13.4.3.2 Decision Tree

Decision Tree (DT) [24] is a hierarchical data structure, a highly interpretable supervised learning method that uses the divide and conquers approach. It is a nonparametric method that can be used both in classification and regression problems. These methods divide the input space into local regions and a training model is created for each region separately. There are no prior parametric forms for the class densities and no fixed prior structure [10]. In a DT, each internal node, branch and leaf node represents an attribute, outcome on the test and a class label, respectively. At the top-most nodes is represented as the root node where the procedure starts from and the process is repeated until a leaf node is met. Generating a DT starts with a single node and a splitting criterion is selected to determine which attribute should be tested at that node to separate. The goodness of splitting of these trees is measured by impurity measurement. It can be done by manipulating entropy or the minimum number of bits and encoding the class code of an instance [6]. The entropy measurement function is computed a set N can be defined as follows-

$$I_m = -\sum_{l=1}^{n} p_l \log_2(p_l)$$

Here p_l is the probability of an instance belonging to a class C_l that can be determined by $\frac{|C_l,N|}{N}$. Now, if we want to split N based on an attribute T, then the amount of information required can be defined as,

$$I_m T = \sum_{i=1}^{k} \frac{|N_i|}{|N|} \times I_m(N_i)$$

The value of $\frac{|N_i|}{|N|}$ is represented as a weight function of ith partition. An information gain $g = I_m - I_m T$ that can be received by the branching of attribute T. The attribute with the highest information gain will be used as the splitting attribute.

The structure of a decision tree makes it understandable where each node of the model is precisely building. It might require pruning as it is prone to overfitting. The most well-known decision tree algorithm is considered as C4.5, which is a good tradeoff between the speed and the error rate. The decision tree can handle data with a high degree of error and missing values for both numeric and nominal input attributes.

13.4.3.3 Support Vector Machine

Support Vector Machines (SVMs) [25] are the newest proposed algorithms by Vapnik [14] in 1995 which can work on both linear and non-linear data. In brief, it uses support vectors to draw a differentiating line or hyperplane that works as a decision boundary for separating one class from another. It uses non-linear mapping to transform original data in higher-dimensional space. The support vector maximizes the separation between the data points.

A hyperplane in a linearly separable space S is described by $\{s \in S|w, s + b = 0\}$, where $w \in S$ and $b \in \mathbb{R}]$ divides the space into two subspace as $\{s \in S|w, s + b \geq 0\}$ and $\{s \in S|w, s + b < 0\}$. For a given training dataset, $\{(x_1, y_1), (x_2, y_2) \ldots (x_m, y_m)\}$ with $x_i \in S$ and $y_i \pm 1$. We aim to find a linear parameterized boundary such that:

$$w, x_i + b \geq 0, \ when\ y_i = +1$$

$$w, x_i + b \leq 0, \ when\ y_i = -1$$

From any point x_i to the hyperplane the distance can be measured by $|w, x_i + b|/\|w\|$. An optimum solution for the separating hyperplane can be found by either maximizing the norm or minimizing the squared norm of the hyperplane. That is,

$$\left.\begin{array}{r} \max_{w,b}\dfrac{1}{\|w\|} \\ \max_{w,b}\dfrac{1}{2}\|w\|^2 \end{array}\right\} where\ y_i(w, x_i + b) \geq 1\ for all\ i$$

Using these equations, an optimum hyperplane can be found and the data points that lie on the margins of the hyperplane are called the support vectors. For SVM classifier, an upper bound for the expected error rate can be determined by the number of support vectors. Even with a small number of support vectors, SVM can offer good generalization although the dimensionality of the data is high. Sometimes a kernel function is used with SVM to map new points in feature space rather than high dimensional space involving dot products. Generally, SVMs tends to perform better when dealing with the multidimensional and continuous feature. It can work in both linear and non-linear problems.

13.4.3.4 Random Forest

Random forest (RF) [26] is a type of ensemble learning which is used for classification, regression, and others. Ensemble learning uses multiple models that combined to solve a particular intelligence problem. In the same way, a random forest constitutes of a number of DTs that operates as an ensemble. In a general DT, a split is done by selecting the best criteria. In contrast to the RF, a node is split which is selected randomly among n best splits. In addition, these trees are constructed from different subsets of a node. New data is predicted by aggregating the prediction of each tree. The error rate of random forest depends on the correlation between any two trees and the strength of each tree in the forest.

A random vector Υ_k is produced for kth tree which independent of its previous random vectors and $\Phi(x, \Upsilon_k)$ classifier is generated where x is an input vector from the training data set. Given a number of such classifier trees such as $\Phi_1(x, \Upsilon_1)$, $\Phi_2(x, \Upsilon_2)$, ... and randomly drawing training set from random vector Y, X the margin function can be defined as

$$mar(X, Y) = P_\Upsilon(\Phi(X, \Upsilon) = Y) - \max_{j \neq Y} = P_\Upsilon(\Phi_k(X, \Upsilon) = j).$$

The strength of the set of classifier $\{\Phi_k(x, \Upsilon)\}$ is

$$\partial = E_{X,Y} mar(X, Y)$$

The random forest faces generalization error or prediction error when a loss function is involved. It can be denoted by,

$$P * E = P_{X,Y}(mg(X, Y) < 0)$$

The margin calculates how much the average number of votes at X, Y for the right class exceeds the average vote for all other classes where the prediction error is limited by the convergence function. As a result, the random forest doesn't overfit when the number of trees increases.

To consider a random uniform forest, the binary classification is considered where $Y \in \{0, 1\}$. Then, the decision rule for such a random uniform classifier can be denoted as,

$$g_c^B(x) = \begin{cases} 1, \ if \sum_{b=1}^{B} \mathrm{I}_{\{g_c^b(x)=1\}} > \sum_{b=1}^{B} \mathrm{I}_{\{g_c^b(x)=0\}} \\ 0, \ otherwise \end{cases}$$

And for regression

$$g_r^B(x) = \frac{1}{B} \sum_{b=1}^{B} g_r^b(x)$$

Here, B is the number of bagging times and $g_c^b(x)$ and $g_r^b(x)$ are respectively the decision tree rule for uniform classifier and uniform regression. It can handle large databases and is an effective method for estimating missing data.

13.4.3.5 Gradient Boosting and Extreme Gradient Boosting

A boosting algorithm [27, 28] trains weak learners based on past errors and generates a modified model that can avoid previous errors. The original boosting algorithm combines various weak learners to generate a strong learner. Besides, a strong learner has represented less error probability than a weak learner. The knowledge of Adaboost [18] or Adaptive Boost helps to understand the gradient boosting. This algorithm assigns equal weight to each observation and the weights are gradually changed and new tree is generated. Subsequent trees have classified the observations which are misclassified by the previous trees. This prediction made by the previous trees that are used to the prediction of the final ensemble model. Gradient Boosting algorithm works in a similar manner. However, it differs from AdaBoost in the sense of finding the prediction error of the prior DTs. It also detects the error using gradients in the loss function.

Let, we have a random input dataset $X = \{x_1, x_2 \ldots x_{\mathrm{m}}\}$ and they are labeled to a random number of output variables $Y = \{y_1, y_2 \ldots y_{\mathrm{n}}\}$. According to Jerome H. Friedman [19], a training set is used for the joint distribution of all values from (*x*, *y*) and the goal is to find a function $\mathrm{P}^*(x)$ such that the expected value of some loss functions $\Gamma(y, \mathrm{P}^*(x))$ is minimized

$$\mathrm{P}^*(x) = \arg\min_{\mathrm{P}^*(x)} E_{y,x}\Gamma\big(y, \mathrm{P}^*(x)\big)$$

If the model has a simple base learner function as $\omega(x; a_k)$ where $\mathrm{a_k}$ is the parameters of x and the Gradient boosting approximates $\mathrm{P}^*(x)$ using an additive expansion of the form

$$\mathrm{P}(x) = \sum_{k=0}^{K} \beta_k \omega(x; a_k)$$

Gradient boosting is quite successful algorithm used for both classification and regression. However it requires large dataset for training. Besides, it does not provide any fast and efficient model and there is no smooth continuous base-learner that captures non-trivial interactions. However, its high flexibility offers a large number of algorithms making it efficient in using in healthcare field.

Extreme Gradient Boosting or XGboost [28] is a special implementation of the Gradient Boosting which generates a more regularized model to control overfitting. It calculates the second-order gradients or partial derivatives of the loss function, which offers more detailed view on the direction of the gradient and minimization of the loss function as a result minimizing error of the overall model. Training with XGboost is faster and can be both parallelized and distributed across clusters.

13.4.3.6 Extreme Learning Machine

Extreme Learning Machine (ELM) [29] is a type of single feed-forward network with faster learning speed and lower training error with excellent generalization performance. A single layer feed-forward network (SLFN) consists of a single layer of output and the input nodes that are fed directly to the output nodes using a series of weights. This requires tuning of parameters at each step, which causes dependency between different layers of weights and biases. On the contrary, no tuning is performed and the weights between inputs and hidden nodes that are randomly assigned and never updated in ELM which remains constant throughout the training and predicting phases.

Let, we consider a set of *N* arbitrary distinct samples (x_i, s_i) where $x_i = [x_{i1}, x_{i2}, \ldots, x_{in}] \in R^n$ and $t_i = [s_{i1}, s_{i2}, \ldots s_{im}] \in R^m$ with *m* samples and *n* input units, ELM model output is written as follows-

$$\Omega(s) = M_i^S h(s)$$

Here, $M_i \in R^q$ is the weight connecting the hideous input to the *i*th output layer neurons and $h(s) \in R^q$ represents the vector of outputs of hidden neurons for a certain input pattern $x_i \in R^q$. Then, $h(s)$ can be defined as follows

$$h(s) = \left[\mathcal{F}\left(\omega_1^S x(s) + b_1\right), \mathcal{F}\left(\omega_2^S x(s) + b_2\right) + \cdots + \mathcal{F}\left(\omega_q^S x(s) + b_q\right)\right]$$

Here ω_k and $b_k \in R^q$ represent the weight and bias of *k*th hidden neuron and $\mathcal{F}(\cdot)$ is the activation function, respectively. According to Guang-Bin Huang who proposed ELM in 2005 if the activation functions in the hidden layer are infinitely differentiable, then the weights can randomly assigned to the hidden nodes.

13.4.4 Evaluation Metrics

We have used seven ML classifiers which have been analyzed the labeled caesarian dataset and effectively predict decision for C-section. The classes are predicted by the classifier which is categorized instances using confusion matrix in Table 13.2 and represented as follow.

Table 13.2 Confusion matrix

	Positive prediction	Negative prediction
Actual positive	True Positive (TP)	False Negative (FN)
Actual Negative	False Positive (FP)	True Negative (TN)

Table 13.3 Measurement formula

Measure	Formula
Accuracy	$\frac{TP+TN}{TP+TN+FN+FP}$
F-measure	$\frac{2TP}{2TP+FP+FN}$
Geometric mean	$\frac{TP}{\sqrt{(TP+FP)*(TP+FN)}}$
Sensitivity	$\frac{TP}{TP+FN}$
Specificity	$\frac{TN}{TN+FP}$
False Alarm Rate (FAR)	$1-\frac{TN}{TN+FP}$
Miss Rate (MR)	$1-\frac{TP}{TP+FN}$

True positive (TP) is when the classifier has predicted caesarian, False negative (FN) is when a caesarian case has been predicted non-caesarian, False positive (FP) represents a non-caesarian prediction that is actually a caesarian case and finally the true negative (TN) is when a non-caesarian case has been predicted the same. These values are used to determine the accuracy of prediction by each algorithm. For a more detailed and efficient insight into the performance of classifiers, we have calculated some other measurements [30] illustrating in Table 13.3 such as Accuracy, Area under Receiver Operating Characteristics (AUROC), F-measure, Geometric mean (G-Mean), Sensitivity, Specificity, False Alarm Rate (FAR) and Miss Rate (MR).

The value of accuracy represents the rate of correct prediction against all predictions. F-measure (or F1-score or F-score) is also indicated the harmonic mean of precision and recall. Sensitivity and specificity indicate the proportion of positive results that have been predicted as positive and the proportion of negative results that have been predicted as negative respectively. FAR also called the false positive rate (FPR) that indicates the rate of negative case predicted as positive and MR or false-negative rate (FNR) denoted the rate of a positive result is predicted as negative. Therefore, we have implemented ML algorithms using the scikit-learn ML library in python.

Moreover, ROC is created by putting the cumulative distributive function of true positive rate (TPR) against the cumulative distributive function of false-positive rate (FPR). It represents the sensitivity as a function of TPR showing a tradeoff between sensitivity and specificity. In healthcare field, the importance of ROC curve analysis is more impactful because it shows the accuracy of a testing operation along with the cost. The AUROC of different classifiers is used for comparing their performance. The perfect classifier has 1.0 sensitivity and a 0.0 false-positive rate. The efficiency of an algorithm is represented by its tendency to grow closer to the positive y-axis and closer to point 1.0.

In the next and final step of this experiment, we have evaluated the efficiency of the results produced by each algorithm using the non-parametric Friedman Test including different post hoc methods such as Iman-Devanport and Holm with a significance level $\alpha = 0.05$.

13.5 Experimental Results

In this experiment, we have used seven widely used classification algorithm, namely, KNN, DT, SVM, RF, GB, XGB, and ELM on caesarian database from the healthcare of Tabriz. Before, three distinct sampling techniques such as random oversampling, SMOTE, ROSE were applied and again resampled with 10-fold cross-validation. Then, these algorithms are applied to the four datasets separately and the results are recorded in different tables.

Table 13.4 shows the result of each classifier's effectiveness on the original dataset. Considering accuracy, we observe that KNN and ELM show the best accuracy among all classifiers. Besides, ELM shows the highest f-measure, G-mean, sensitivity and lowest FAR as well as KNN represents the highest AUROC, specificity, and the lowest MR. But, the highest result of AUROC is used to represent the best classifier. Therefore, KNN has represented the best performance by considering AUROC and overall result. On the other hand, DT also shows the worst performance that contains the lowest accuracy and highest error rate. GB and XGB results are pretty closer so far RF and SVM respectively. However, the overall accuracy for all classifiers is not very high. If we observe each attribute of the dataset, then imbalance classes are found. For example, among 80 to 46 cases of timely delivery but only 17 premature, 17 latecomers and 40 patients with normal heart rate. This might be affected by the performance of the classifiers. So we have applied random oversampling, SMOTE and ROSE respectively.

The effect on the randomly oversampled data is shown in Table 13.5. Using random oversampling, it affects the result but it's still pretty unsatisfactory. We see that KNN still has the highest accuracy and the lowest MR same as SVM. On the other hand, ELM has comparatively lower accuracy comparing with others in this scenario. Besides, the performance of SVM has improved in this case. XGB shows an modrate accuracy comparing to others but it has the highest sensitivity and specificity respectively.

When we look at the classification results of SMOTE dataset in Table 13.6, all measurement has improved considerably with KNN still having the highest accuracy, F-measure and also the lowest error rate. KNN works very well on this dataset as it

Table 13.4 Classification result of different classifier on a base dataset

Classifier	Accuracy	AUROC	F-measure	G-mean	Sensitivity	Specificity	MR	FAR
DT	0.5375	0.5288	0.5934	0.5934	0.5869	0.4706	0.413	0.5294
GB	0.55	0.5396	0.6087	0.6087	0.6086	0.4705	0.3913	0.5294
RF	0.6	0.5907	0.6521	0.6521	0.6521	0.5294	0.3478	0.4705
SVM	0.625	0.6164	0.6739	0.6739	0.6739	0.5588	0.3261	0.4412
XGB	0.575	0.5691	0.6222	0.6223	0.6087	0.5295	0.3913	0.4706
ELM	0.675	0.6675	0.7173	0.7173	0.7173	0.6176	0.2826	0.3823
KNN	0.675	0.6867	0.6829	0.6881	0.6087	0.7647	0.3913	0.2353

Table 13.5 Classification result of different classifier on dataset with random oversampling

Classifier	Accuracy	AUROC	F-measure	G-mean	Sensitivity	Specificity	MR	FAR
DT	0.6847	0.6847	0.6506	0.6545	0.5869	0.7826	0.413	0.2174
GB	0.5978	0.5978	0.5747	0.5757	0.5435	0.6522	0.4565	0.3478
RF	0.6304	0.6304	0.6046	0.6061	0.5652	0.6956	0.4348	0.3043
SVM	0.7282	0.7282	0.6987	0.7029	0.6304	0.8261	0.3695	0.1739
XGB	0.663	0.663	0.6353	0.6375	0.7391	0.5869	0.413	0.2609
ELM	0.6086	0.6086	0.5813	0.5814	0.5828	0.5434	0.6739	0.4565
KNN	0.7282	0.7282	0.6988	0.7029	0.6304	0.826	0.3696	0.1739

Table 13.6 Classification result of different classifier on SMOTE dataset

Classifier	Accuracy	AUROC	F-measure	G-mean	Sensitivity	Specificity	MR	FAR
DT	0.8953	0.8917	0.9096	0.9096	0.9158	0.8676	0.0842	0.1323
GB	0.9281	0.9245	0.9382	0.9382	0.9483	0.9007	0.0516	0.0992
RF	0.9375	0.9365	0.9455	0.9455	0.9429	0.9301	0.0571	0.0698
SVM	0.9031	0.9004	0.9159	0.9159	0.9184	0.8823	0.0815	0.1176
XGB	0.9359	0.9347	0.9442	0.9442	0.9429	0.9265	0.0571	0.0735
ELM	0.8297	0.8288	0.8492	0.8493	0.8342	0.8235	0.1658	0.1765
KNN	0.9453	0.9428	0.9527	0.9528	0.9592	0.9265	0.0407	0.0735

received nearly 95% of accuracy with 95% f-score and only 4% FAR and 7% MR. It has also shown the best performance regarding sensitivity and specificity. GB, RF, SVM, and XGB show modest performance greater than 90% except error rate. After that, DT and ELM comparatively represent their performance scores where ELM show 83% accuracy. ELM also shows the highest generalization error for both FAR and MR.

In the case of ROSE, DT, KNN, RF, and GB provide around 90% accuracy along with other metrics except FAR and MR that represents in Table 13.7. DT contains the highest accuracy similar to KNN. However, it falls behind KNN regarding other measurements such as sensitivity, specificity, FAR and MR. SVM and XGB also work pretty well but comparatively lower than the first-mentioned ones. The performance of ELM is significantly reduced where it shows only around 67% accuracy along with 32% FAR and approximately 34% MR (see Table 13.7).

Now if we consider the entire four scenarios together, KNN is represented as the best classifier for estimating decision about C-section. After KNN, RF shows good performance. The results of GB and XGB seem to be quite similar nature. SVM shows the stable performance throughout the whole experiment. DT doesn't work well on the original data, but it performs better on the ROSE and SMOTE dataset. Though ELM shows comparatively low result regarding random oversampling, SMOTE, and ROSE where it shows the highest accuracy for original dataset. This indicates that

Table 13.7 Classification result of different classifier on ROSE dataset

Classifier	Accuracy	ROC	F-measure	G-mean	Sensitivity	Specificity	FAR	MR
DT	0.9245	0.9253	0.9242	0.9247	0.8957	0.9549	0.1043	0.0451
GB	0.9025	0.9036	0.9012	0.902	0.8649	0.9423	0.1351	0.0576
RF	0.9245	0.9246	0.926	0.926	0.9194	0.9298	0.0806	0.0702
SVM	0.8063	0.8077	0.801	0.8023	0.7583	0.8571	0.2417	0.1428
XGB	0.8782	0.8799	0.8734	0.8755	0.8175	0.9423	0.1825	0.0576
ELM	0.6699	0.6695	0.68	0.68	0.6825	0.6566	0.3175	0.3433
KNN	0.9245	0.9241	0.9272	0.9272	0.936	0.9122	0.0639	0.0877

ELM performs well with imbalanced dataset compared to the other six classifiers in this experiment.

Figures 13.1, 13.2, 13.3 and 13.4 represent the ROC curves of classifiers on original, random oversampling, SMOTE, and ROSE dataset respectively. In all figures, the ROC of KNN has a higher tendency to grow closer to the positive *y*-axis. Therefore using KNN for this cesarean section prediction has a higher accuracy with the least cost involved.

Table 13.8 represents the ranking, *z*-score, an unadjusted and adjusted *p*-value of post hoc methods of various classifiers which we have used in this experiment. The unadjusted *p*-value of different post hoc methods are also investigated the conditions and detected which classifiers reject the null hypothesis. When the unadjusted *p*-value is compared with Holm's post hoc method, no classifier's hypotheses are rejected.

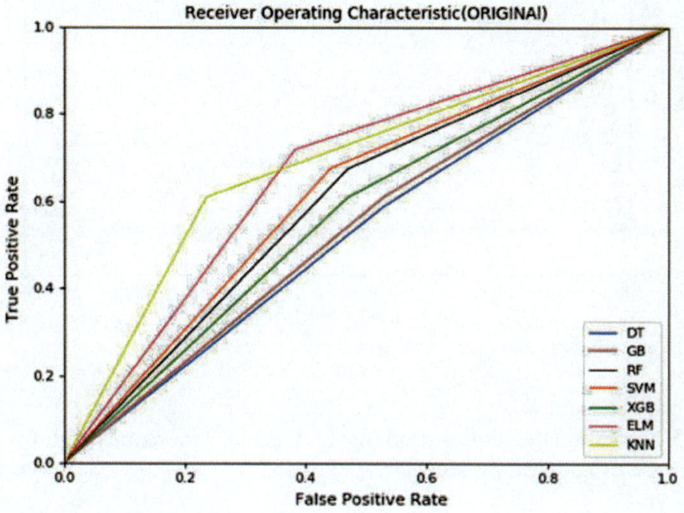

Fig. 13.1 ROC curves (original)

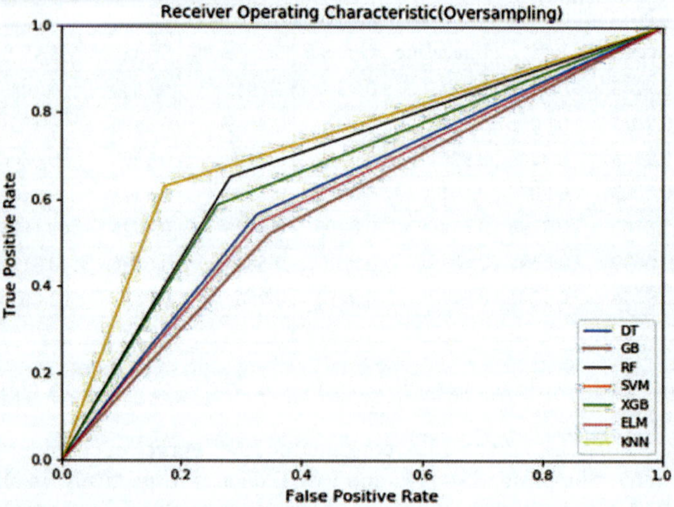

Fig. 13.2 ROC curves (random oversampling)

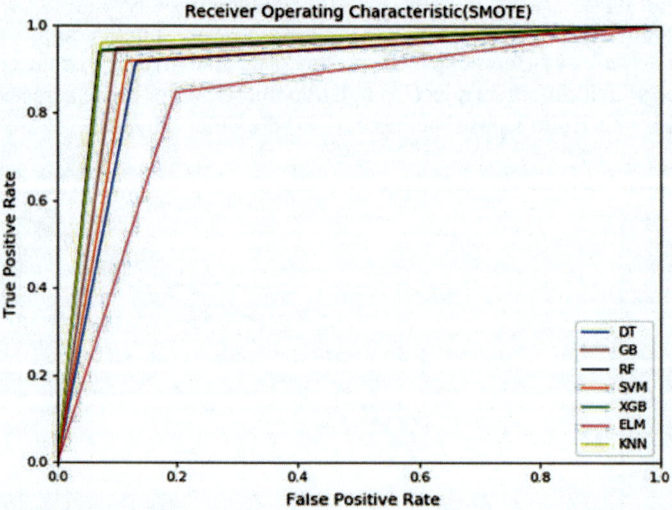

Fig. 13.3 ROC curves (SMOTE)

However, KNN shows the highest-ranking; and receives the same result for post hoc method in case of adjusted p-values.

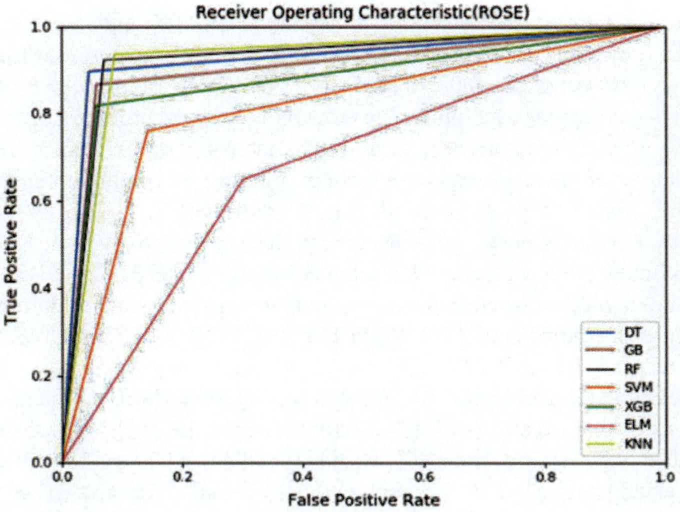

Fig. 13.4 ROC curves (ROSE)

Table 13.8 Classifiers accuracy ranking and adjusted *p*-values using post hoc methods (Friedman)

S/N	Algorithms	Ranking	$z = \frac{R_0 - R_i}{SE}$	p	p_{Holm}
0	KNN	1.5	–	–	–
1	RF	3.2	1.145644	0.251943	0.251943
2	SVM	3.87	1.554802	0.119993	0.239986
3	XGB	4.25	1.800298	0.071814	0.215441
4	DT	4.5	1.963961	0.04953	0.198138
5	GB	5.25	2.454951	0.01409	0.070452
6	ELM	5.375	2.536783	0.011188	0.067126

(1) Friedman statistic (distributed according to chi-square with 6 degrees of freedom): 9.080357 (2) *P*-value computed by Friedman test: 0.169109 (3) Iman-Davenport statistic (distributed according to F-distribution with 6 and 18 degrees of freedom): 1.825853. *P*-value computed by Iman-Daveport test: 0.150392066222 (4) $\alpha = 0{:}05$(Friedman). Holm's procedure rejects those hypotheses that have an unadjusted *p*-value $\leq 0{:}00833$

13.6 Discussion

The prediction of C-section is important to take emergency decision for the safety of both mother and child respectively. Therefore, more extensive research is required to enhance the quality of the cesarean service. In this paper, different data balancing techniques were used to balance C-section dataset and generated three datasets from base dataset. Then, classification techniques were used to evaluate the result [3–6]. There were happening several works about cesarean data using ML. Most of these work such as Gharehchopogh et al. [8], Stylios et al. [10] and Iftitah et al. [14] were used a few numbers of classifiers to identify factors related to caesarian cases. Besides, some of works like Saleem et al. [17] were used cardiotocographic signals with other physiological data but not given early solutions before treatment. In this case, we want to explore a new dimension in ML where a few attributes are used to identify the risk of the caesarean case early in different pregnant women. Different existing ML models (e.g., Amin et al. [3], Maroufizadeh et al. [12]) were implemented into various balanced and imbalanced datasets and found that KNN is the best algorithm to predict result. We implemented some latest and well-performing ML algorithms in this C-section dataset, which were performed well in other fields (Maji et al. [31], Ahmed et al. [29], Sridharan et al. [32]). In addition, we also evaluated this result based on different metrics such as accuracy, ROC area, f-measure, g-mean, sensitivity, specificity, FAR and MR which were absent in the most of the previous works (e.g., Amin et al. [3], Maroufizadeh et al. [12], Manzanares et al. [13], Iftitah et al. [14]). In Amin et al. [3], they found that KNN and RF can be generated 95% accuracy to predict C-section. We also found KNN and RF can predict C-section data which accuracy was being approximately better result (95% for KNN and 94% for RF) by analyzing the base and three balanced C-section data. Furthermore, Friedman Test is a non-parametric statistical significant test, which is also indicated that KNN is the best classifier to predict C-section in emergency cases.

13.7 Conclusion

Identification of delivery type is very critical as both the mother and the child's health which depends on it to a great extent. The delivery type of a patient shows relevance to the patient's heart rate, blood pressure, age and previous record of delivery. This relevance can be used for data mining to generate a model for cesarean prediction. In this paper, we have proposed a ML model where we have analyzed the caesarian dataset from the healthcare of Tabriz with seven ML classifiers such as KNN, DT, RF, GB, XGB,SVM and ELM. The performance of each algorithm is recorded and compared based on accuracy, roc, error rate and other vital factors.

The seven algorithms are applied to the original and random oversampled, SMOTE and ROSE dataset to avoid the effect of imbalanced data. These algorithms are already proven to be good classifiers in many fields; therefore we have used them to predict cesarean data. To manipulate significant test of individual classifiers, we used Friedman test to compare their performance.

The classifiers show a significant level of classifying capability in separating cesarean delivery from normal ones. After comparing the result, we have found KNN is the best classifier for caesarian prediction. Among the other classifiers, RF also showed excellent performance, and ELM offers the weakest performance by analyzing individual C-section datasets.

However, the dataset has been used here is not large enough, and the number of attributes considered is also not adequate to have a more detailed view on the requirement of C-section for childbirth. Here we have only considered the risk factors related to pregnant women; nevertheless, the condition of the child is also essential. In the future work, we expect to consider these limitations and improve our model. We will include some other algorithms to our model and find out their classifying ability with such cases.

References

1. Bradley, D., Landau, E., Wolfberg, A., Baron, A.: Predicting obstetric disease with machine learning applied to patient-reported data. J. Med. Internet Res. **20**(9) (2018)
2. Romeo, V., Ricciardi, C., Cuocolo, R., Stanzione, A., Verde, F., Sarno, L., Maurea, S.: Machine learning analysis of MRI-derived texture features to predict placenta accreta spectrum in patients with placenta previa. Magn. Reson. Imaging (2019)
3. Amin, M., Ali, A.: Performance Evaluation of Supervised Machine Learning Classifiers for Predicting Healthcare Operational Decisions. Wavy AI Research Foundation, Lahore, Pakistan (2018)
4. Polat, K.: A hybrid approach to parkinson disease classification using speech signal: the combination of SMOTE and random forests. In: 2019 Scientific Meeting on Electrical-Electronics & Biomedical Engineering and Computer Science (EBBT), pp. 1–3. IEEE (2019)
5. Lakhani, P., Prater, A.B., Hutson, R.K., Andriole, K.P., Dreyer, K.J., Morey, J., Prevedello, L.M., Clark, T.J., Geis, J.R., Itri, J.N., Hawkins, C.M.: Machine learning in radiology: applications beyond image interpretation. J. Am. Coll. Radiol. **15**(2), 350–359 (2018)
6. Liu, S., Liu, S., Cai, W., Pujol, S., Kikinis, R., Feng, D.: Early diagnosis of Alzheimer's disease with deep learning. In 2014 IEEE 11th International Symposium on Biomedical Imaging (ISBI), pp. 1015–1018. IEEE (2014)
7. Lama, R.K., Gwak, J., Park, J.S., Lee, S.W.: Diagnosis of Alzheimer's disease based on structural MRI images using a regularized extreme learning machine and PCA features. J. Healthcare Eng. (2017)
8. Gharehchopogh, F.S., Mohammadi, P., Hakimi, P.: Application of decision tree algorithm for data mining in healthcare operations: a case study. Int. J. Comput. Appl. **52**(6), 326–337 (2012)
9. Caruana, R., Niculescu, R.S., Rao, R.B., Simms, C.: Machine learning for sub-population assessment: evaluating the C-section rate of different physician practices. In Proceedings of the AMIA Symposium, p. 126. American Medical Informatics Association (2002)
10. Stylios, C.D., Georgoulas, G., Groumpos, P.P.: The challenge of using soft computing for decision support during labour. In: 2001 Conference Proceedings of the 23rd Annual International Conference of the IEEE Engineering in Medicine and Biology Society, vol. 4, pp. 3835–3838. IEEE (2001)
11. Vovsha, I., Rajan, A., Salleb-Aouissi, A., Raja, A., Radeva, A., Diab, H., Tomar, A., Wapner, R.: Predicting preterm birth is not elusive: machine learning paves the way to individual wellness. In 2014 AAAI Spring Symposium Series (2014)
12. Maroufizadeh, S., Amini, P., Hosseini, M., Almasi-Hashiani, A., Mohammadi, M., Navid, B., Omani-Samani, R.: Determinants of cesarean section among primiparas: a comparison of classification methods. Iran. J. Public Health **47**(12), 1913 (2018)
13. Manzanares, S., Ruiz-Duran, S., Pinto, A., Pineda, A., Puertas, A.: An integrated model with classification criteria to predict vaginal delivery success after cesarean section. J. Maternal-Fetal Neonatal Med. 1–7 (2018)
14. Iftitah, E.N., Rulaningtyas, R.: The baby delivery method estimation using Naïve Bayes classification model for mobile application. J. Phys.: Conf. Ser. **1120**(1), 012049 (2018) (IOP Publishing)

15. Lee, E. K., Tian, H., Wei, X., Lee, J., Smith, K. D., Neeld, J., Kaplan, A.R.: Factors influencing epidural anesthesia for cesarean section outcome. In: 2018 IEEE International Conference on Bioinformatics and Biomedicine (BIBM), pp. 1062–1069. IEEE (2018)
16. Lee, K.S., Ahn, K.H.: Spontaneous preterm labor and birth and its major determinants: artificial neural network analysis of general hospital data. J. Korean Med. Sci. **34**(16), 134–147 (2019)
17. Saleem, S., Naqvi, S.S., Manzoor, T., Saeed, A., Mirza, J.: A strategy for classification of vaginal versus cesarean section' delivery: bivariate empirical mode decomposition of cardiotocographic recordings. Front. Physiol. **10**, 246–257 (2019)
18. Yap, B.W., Rani, K.A., Rahman, H.A.A., Fong, S., Khairudin, Z., Abdullah, N.N.: An application of oversampling, undersampling, bagging and boosting in handling imbalanced datasets. In Proceedings of the First International Conference on Advanced Data And Information Engineering (DaEng-2013), pp. 13–22. Springer, Singapore (2014)
19. Gao, R., Peng, J., Nguyen, L., Liang, Y., Thng, S., Lin, Z. Classification of non-tumorous facial pigmentation disorders using deep learning and SMOTE. In: 2019 IEEE International Symposium on Circuits and Systems (ISCAS), pp. 1–5. IEEE (2019)
20. Zhang, J., Chen, L.: Clustering-based undersampling with random over sampling examples and support vector machine for imbalanced classification of breast cancer diagnosis. Comput. Assis. Surg. 1–11 (2019)
21. Akter, T., Satu, M.S., Khan, M.I., Ali, M.H., Uddin, S., Lió, P., Quinn, J.M., Moni, M.A.: Machine learning-based models for early stage detection of autism spectrum disorders. IEEE Access **7**, 166509–166527 (2019)
22. Eftekhar, H., Hossain, M.F., Rahaman, M.A: A Color and texture based approach for the detection and classification of plant leaf disease using KNN classifier. In: 2019 International Conference on Electrical, Computer and Communication Engineering (ECCE). IEEE (2019)
23. Satu, M.S., Ahamed, S., Hossain, F., Akter, T., Farid, D.M.: Mining traffic accident data of N5 national highway in Bangladesh employing decision trees. In: 2017 IEEE Region 10 Humanitarian Technology Conference (R10-HTC), pp. 722–725. IEEE (2017)
24. Abedin, M.Z., Guotai, C., Moula, F E.: Weighted SMOTE-ensemble algorithms: Evidence from Chinese imbalance credit approval instances. In: Proceedings of IEEE Xplore: The 2nd International Conference on Data Intelligence and Security, 28–30 June 2019, South Padre Island, Texas, USA, pp. 208–211 (2019). https://doi.org/10.1109/icdis.2019.00038
25. Moula, F.E., Guotai, C., Abedin, M.Z.: Credit default prediction modeling: application of support vector machine. Risk Manage. **19**(2), 158–187 (2017)
26. Satu, M.S., Sathi, F.F., Arifen, M.S., Ali, M.H., Moni, M.A.: Early detection of autism by extracting features: a case study in Bangladesh. In: 2019 International Conference on Robotics, Electrical and Signal Processing Techniques (ICREST), pp. 400–405. IEEE (2019)
27. Xie, Y., Jiang, B., Gong, E., Li, Y., Zhu, G., Michel, P., Zaharchuk, G.: Use of gradient boosting machine learning to predict patient outcome in acute ischemic stroke on the basis of imaging, demographic, and clinical information. Am. J. Roentgenol. **212**(1), 44–51 (2019)
28. Chen, T., Guestrin, C.: Xgboost: a scalable tree boosting system. In Proceedings of the 22nd ACM SIGKDD International Conference on Knowledge Discovery and Data Mining, pp. 785–794. ACM (2016)
29. Ahmad, I., Basheri, M., Iqbal, M.J., Rahim, A.: Performance comparison of support vector machine, random forest, and extreme learning machine for intrusion detection. IEEE Access **6**, 33789–33795 (2018)
30. Abedin, M.Z., Guotai, C., Colombage, S., Moula, F.E.: Credit default prediction by using a support vector machine and a probabilistic neural network. J. Credit Risk **14**(2), 1–27 (2018)
31. Maji, S., Arora, S.: Decision tree algorithms for prediction of heart disease. In Information and Communication Technology for Competitive Strategies, pp. 447–454. Springer, Singapore (2019)
32. Sridharan, K., Komarasamy, G.: Sentiment classification using harmony random forest and harmony gradient boosting machine. Soft Comput. 1–8 (2019)

Chapter 14
Automatic Epileptic Seizures Detection and EEG Signals Classification Based on Multi-domain Feature Extraction and Multiscale Entropy Analysis

Md. Abu Sayem, Md. Sohel Rana Sarker, Md Atiqur Rahman Ahad, and Mosabber Uddin Ahmed

Abstract Epilepsy is a frequently observed neurological abnormality. In the manual method, a physician monitors the recording of Electroencephalogram (EEG) of a patient to detect epileptic seizures. But this method is time-consuming and fallible. This chapter presents an automatic epileptic seizures detection and EEG signals classification method based on multi-domain feature extraction and multiscale entropy analysis. In this method, EEG data is collected and preprocessed for artifacts removal from the original data. Then discrete Fourier transform (DFT) and discrete wavelet transform (DWT) are applied for extracting features. Multiscale entropy (MSE) with sample entropy is also applied to extract nonlinear features. Finally, supervised learning classifiers such as support vector machine (SVM), k-nearest-neighbors (k-NN) and artificial neural network (ANN) are used for epileptic seizures detection, three-class and five-class classification of the EEG signals. The dataset has been collected from the University of Bonn. This method attained an accuracy of 99.54%, sensitivity of 98.56% and specificity of 99.76% for epileptic seizures detection. For three-class and five-class classification, accuracy was 98.22% and 87.00%, respectively.

Keywords Epilepsy · EEG · Discrete wavelet transform · Multiscale entropy · Support vector machine · Artificial neural networks

14.1 Introduction

Human brain consists of billions of neurons which are intricately interconnected and use electrical signal to communicate with each other [1]. In the case of central nervous system disorder, abnormality and hypersynchronous discharge of cortical neurons cause electrical disturbance in the brain results in two or more unprovoked,

Md. Abu Sayem (✉) · Md. Sohel Rana Sarker · M. A. R. Ahad · M. U. Ahmed
Department of Electrical and Electronic Engineering, University of Dhaka, Dhaka 1000, Bangladesh
e-mail: abusayem.du14@gmail.com

M. A. R. Ahad and M. U. Ahmed (eds.), *Signal Processing Techniques for Computational Health Informatics*, Intelligent Systems Reference Library 192,
https://doi.org/10.1007/978-3-030-54932-9_14

repetitive seizures called epilepsy [2]. Epileptic seizures result in transient loss of consciousness and involuntary movement of the body. In each year, about 24 million people are diagnosed for epileptic seizures and currently the number of epileptic seizures patients in the world is approximately 50 million [3]. The most common approach uses EEG signals to detect epileptic seizures because EEG signals of a patient with epileptic seizures are aberrant. Identifying epileptic seizures manually using EEG signals is time-consuming and error-prone [4]. Thus, an automatic reliable and robust system is required to detect epileptic seizures.

A number of methods have already been introduced. Paivinen et al. [5] suggested that features extraction from linear and nonlinear realm produce better accuracy for seizures detection. Time-frequency analysis of the EEG signals and artificial neural network (ANN) based model obtained an average accuracy of 97.72% to detect epileptic seizures [4]. Kobayashi et al. [6] utilized Gabor transform and computed power difference with the background to detect seizures. Another study exploited time-frequency analysis to detect epileptic seizures [7]. Short-time Fourier transform (STFT) was exploited to detect epileptic seizures in [8–11].

Xie et al. [12] proposed wavelet-based sparse functional model to detect epileptic seizures. EEG signal decomposition level using wavelet transform was selected by a forward search algorithm. In that study, a 1-NN classifier detected epilepsy. A significant number of studies exploited wavelet transform to obtain subbands and compute popular entropy to detect epileptic seizures using supervised classifiers [13–17]. Guo et al. [18] utilized approximate entropy (ApEn) feature using multi-wavelet transform and multilayer perceptron neural network (MLPNN) to detect epileptic seizures and acquired an accuracy of 98.27%. Djemili et al. [19] introduced empirical mode decomposition to differentiate epileptic seizures from normal subject. Four statistical measurements were used to feed MLPNN. The accuracy of this method was 100% for normal vs ictal classification. Kaleem et al. [20] used the nonlinear analysis of Empirical Mode Decomposition-Modified Peak Selection (EMD-MPS) with a 1-NN classifier and got 98.2% accuracy of epileptic seizures detection. EMD and Hilbert marginal spectrum analysis (HMS) were applied on the EEG signals by Fu et al. [21] who achieved 98.80% accuracy to detect epileptic seizures.

Lina et al. [22] recommended multi-domain and nonlinear analysis based feature extraction method to detect epileptic seizures using EEG signals. The proposed method could achieve an accuracy of 99.25%. Three-level lifting DWT and the nonlinear sparse extreme learning machine (SELM) based model was offered by Yuanfa et al. [23] for epileptic seizures detection which achieved 98.4% accuracy. In [24], multiscale entropy (MSE) with sample entropy (SampEn), permutation entropy (PermEn) and Lempel-Ziv entropy (LZEn) were utilized for complexity analysis of brain electrical activity. In that study, nearest neighbor classification (NNC) and leave-one-out classification (LOOC) methods were selected for classification. For three-class classification, the highest accuracy was 90.0% and for five-class classification, the maximum accuracy was 69.2%.

Kumar et al. [25] introduced one-dimensional local binary-based epileptic seizures detection using EEG signal. In this work, EEG signal was processed by four parallel Gabor filters followed by segmentation and features extraction from each segment. Finally, features were combined from all segments and a 1-NN classifier was utilized. The highest accuracy was 98.33%. Sharma et al. [26] proposed analytic time-frequency flexible wavelet transform to decompose EEG signal into desired subbands and calculate fractal dimension from each subband as a feature for eight binary classification problems. The method utilized least square SVM and obtained 99.20% accuracy in case of epileptic seizures detection. Tiwari et al. [27] proposed to compute local binary patterns (LBP) at key points of EEG signal which were detected using a pyramid of the difference of Gaussian filter signal. Histogram of LBP was used as a feature to classify EEG using SVM. The accuracy of seizure vs seizure-free was 99.31%.

Weighted multiscale Renyi permutation entropy from each subband obtained by performing the Fourier-Bessel series expansion [28] based method was proposed by Gupta et al. [29] to detect epileptic seizures. RF, SVM classifiers were used and the obtained accuracy was 98.6%. Bhattacharyya et al. [30] proposed multivariate empirical wavelet transform based epileptic seizures detection in which the first five best channels were selected based on statistical measures and decomposed each channel into ten adaptive frequency scales. Then amplitude and frequency information of all channels were combined for a mode to get joint amplitude and frequency information. Features were extracted and processed to detect seizures. This method achieved an average accuracy of 97.91%. Recently, deep learning is exploited to detect epileptic seizures.

Ullah et al. [31] proposed pyramidal 1-D convolutional neural network (CNN) to perform ternary classification, normal vs interictal vs ictal and obtained accuracy of 99.1% $\pm$ 0.09%. To detect epileptic seizures, Hussein et al. [32] applied long short term memory (LSTM) network. In this approach, first EEG signals were segmented into non-overlapping epoch followed by learning and finally classification. Acharya et al. [33] presented a CNN composed of 13 layers which could detect seizures 88.67% accurately. Zhou et al. [34] fed time domain or frequency domain EEG signals into a CNN to detect epileptic seizures. Emami et al. [35] proposed a CNN based seizures detection model that utilized EEG plot image. In this approach, EEG signal was divided into a short given time window which was fed into CNN to detect epileptic seizure without complex feature extraction. Deep learning was also utilized in the studies of [36–38] to detect epileptic seizures.

EEG signals are complex, inherently nonlinear and nonstationary [39]. Thus, detecting epileptic seizures by analyzing EEG signals in time or frequency domain is not enough. To obtain the time-frequency domain feature, DWT was used in the manuscript. In this case, different wavelet families were applied to compute DWT coefficients. Fast Fourier transform (FFT) algorithm was used for computing DFT coefficients. The complexity of the EEG signal was studied by multiscale entropy using sample entropy. Sample entropy (SampEn) was selected for MSE analysis as it doesn't much depend on data length [40]. Sample entropy was enumerated for scale factors 1–10 and used as a feature. Time domain, frequency domain, time-frequency domain and MSE with sample entropy analysis features formed a feature vector for classification by supervised classifiers k-NN, SVM, and ANN.

Remaining of this chapter is structured as follows. Section 2 describes the datasets used in this work, elucidates the feature extraction process and the classification models. The classification performance and discussion are scrutinized in Sect. 3. Section 4 represents the conclusion of this work.

14.2 Materials and Methods

14.2.1 Datasets

The dataset used in this study was collected from the epilepsy center in Bonn, Germany [41]. The data consists of five sets (A–E). Sets A and B comprise of data collected from five normal subjects with open and closed eyes, respectively through standardized external surface electrodes placement. Data of set C were come from the hippocampal formation of the opposite hemisphere of the brain and set D included data recorded from epileptogenic zone of the brain. Sets C and D data were recorded through intracranial electrodes prior to a seizure. Data with epilepsy was recorded with intracranial electrodes and placed in set E. Each set encompasses 100 EEG segments. Each segment has a duration of 23.6 sec and collected from a single channel with a sampling rate of 173.61 Hz.

14.2.2 Methods

An automatic system for epileptic seizures detection and EEG signals classification based on multi-domain feature extraction, multiscale entropy analysis is exemplified. The system involves two phases: training the system and testing. EEG signals contain different types of artifacts that were removed first. Then five-level DWT was applied to get six subbands. DWT was exploited to extract features including standard deviation of the wavelet coefficients and relative energy from each subband of the EEG signals. MSE with sample entropy was computed for the EEG signals. Then a feature vector was formed by these extracted features. Finally, k-NN, SVM, and ANN classifiers were used to identify the epileptic seizures from the EEG signals. Figure 14.1 shows the workflow of the system.

14.2.2.1 Preprocessing

Signals which are not originated in cerebral are artifacts and can be physiological or nonphysiological [42]. Higher frequency components of EEG signals are affected by noise [43]. Thus, a Finite Impulse Response (FIR) low pass filter of order 24 and cut off frequency 64 Hz was applied to the EEG signals.

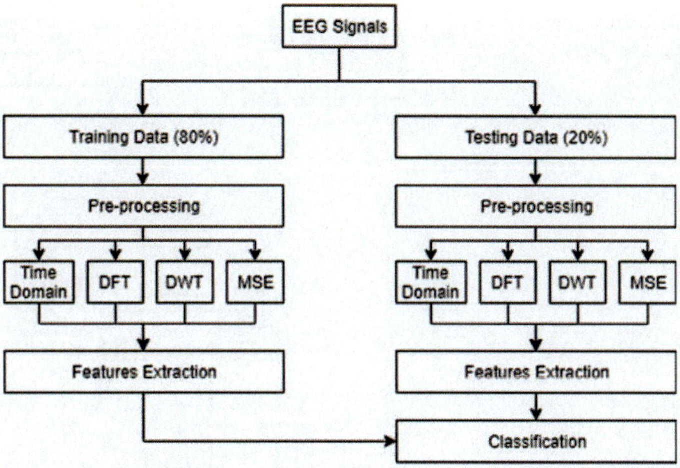

Fig. 14.1 The workflow of the system

14.2.2.2 Discrete Wavelet Transform

Wavelet transform is a time-frequency analysis which is superior over Fourier transform and short-time Fourier transform (STFT) because it changes window size-extends at low frequencies and compacts at high frequencies-depending on the frequency and conserves better time-frequency resolution at any frequency [44]. In the case of DWT, the original time series is decomposed sequentially using a high pass filter g(n) called mother wavelet and a low pass filter h(n) which is the mirror version of g(n) at a down sampling rate of 2 [45]. The output of the initial low pass filter is called approximation, A1 which is decomposed up to a specific level. A high pass filter at each level produces detailed coefficients of that level. The process of decomposition of a signal using DWT is schematically shown in Fig. 14.2.

The low pass and high pass filters define the scaling function, $\Phi_{l,k}(m)$ and wavelet function, $\Psi_{l,k}(m)$, respectively and can be expressed as follows [46]:

$$\Phi_{l,k}(m) = 2^{-l/2} h\left(2^{-l}m - k\right) \tag{14.1}$$

$$\Psi_{l,k}(m) = 2^{-l/2} g\left(2^{-l}m - k\right) \tag{14.2}$$

where $m = 0, 1, 2, 3, \ldots, M - 1$; $l = 0, 1, 2, \ldots, L - 1$; $k = 0, 1, 2, \ldots, 2^l - 1$; $L = 5$; and M is the length of the signal.

Approximation coefficients (A_i) and detailed coefficients (D_i) at the ith level are determined as below [47]:

$$A_i = \frac{1}{\sqrt{M}} \sum_m x(m)\Phi_{l,k}(m) \tag{14.3}$$

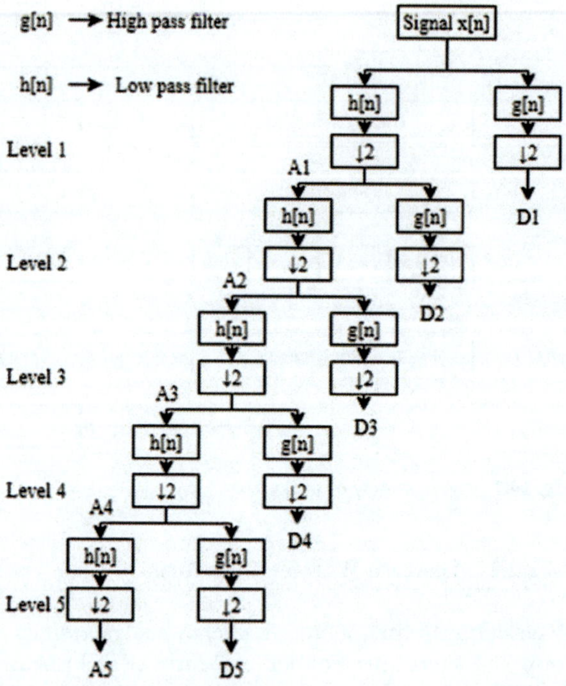

Fig. 14.2 Decomposition of a signal using five levels DWT

$$D_i = \frac{1}{\sqrt{M}} \sum_m x(m) \Psi_{l,k}(m) \tag{14.4}$$

In this work, five levels of decomposition were conducted using daubechies (db), symlets (sym), coiflets (coif), biorthogonal (bior) wavelet families. Thus, five details D1–D5 and one last approximation, A5 were obtained.

14.2.2.3 Multiscale Sample Entropy

Multiscale entropy (MSE) is applied because the time scale relevance of EEG signals is unknown. MSE with sample entropy can be applied to analyze the complexity of a physiological signal on multiple time scales [48]. MSE with sample entropy can be calculated by the coarse-grained method: allocating the given original time series, $\{x_1, x_2, x_3, \ldots, x_M\}$ into non-overlapping windows of length, τ and average the each window to form constituent $y^{(\tau)}$ at scale factor τ of coarse-grained time series as shown in Fig. 14.3.

Each element of coarse-grained time series is determined by the following equation.

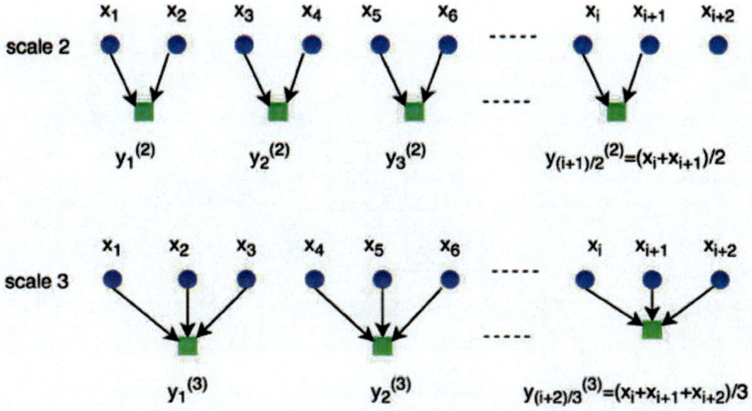

Fig. 14.3 Delineating coarse-graining method for scale 2 and 3 which was modified from reference [49]

$$y_j^{(\tau)} = \frac{1}{\tau} \sum_{i=(j-1)\tau+1}^{j\tau} x_i, \quad 1 \leq j \leq \frac{M}{\tau}$$

Then sample entropy for each coarse-grained time series, $\{y_1, \ldots, y_i, \ldots, y_N\}$ is calculated as follows [10, 12]:

N-m template vectors of dimension m are formed as $Y_m(i) = \{y(i), y(i+1), \ldots, y(i+m-1)\}$, where $1 \leq i \leq N-m$. The Chebyshev distance between two vectors $Y_m(i)$ and $Y_m(j)$ is considered and calculated as the following expression:

$$d[Y_m(i), Y_m(j)] = \max\{|y(i+k-1) - y(j+k-1)|\}, 1 \leq k \leq m.$$

If $d[Y_m(i), Y_m(j)] \leq r$ then it is considered that $Y_m(j)$ matches with $Y_m(i)$. For a particular template vector $Y_m(i)$, the number of matching vectors exclude self-matching is counted and designated as B_i. Then for $1 \leq i \leq N-m$, $B_i^m(r)$ is calculated as $\frac{1}{N-m-1}B_i$. $B^m(r)$ is defined by $\frac{1}{N-m}\sum_{i=1}^{N-m} B_i^m(r)$. The dimension of the vectors is increased to $m+1$ and A_i is calculated as the number of matches between vectors $Y_{m+1}(i)$ and $Y_{m+1}(j)$ within r, where $1 \leq j \leq N-m$ and $j \neq i$. Divide A_i by $N-m-1$ to get $A_i^m(r)$ and $A^m(r)$ is defined as $\frac{1}{N-m}\sum_{i=1}^{N-m} A_i^m(r)$. Then $B^m(r)$ is the probability that two sequences of m points are matched and $A^m(r)$ is the probability that two sequences of $m+1$ points are matched. Then sample entropy (SampEn) statistic is estimated as follows:

$$\text{SampEn(m,r,N)} = -\ln\left[\frac{A^m(r)}{B^m(r)}\right] \quad (14.5)$$

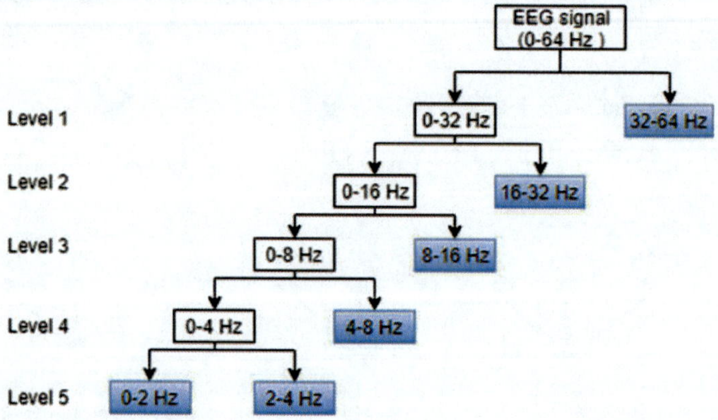

Fig. 14.4 Features were extracted from colored boxes subbands generated by five-level decomposition of an EEG signal using DWT

In this study, for calculating sample entropy, m = 2 was considered and tolerance level, r was set to 0.2 times the standard deviation of the EEG signals.

14.2.2.4 Features Extraction

Features were extracted in the time-frequency domain, frequency domain, time domain, and nonlinear domain. In this study, five levels decomposition of the EEG signals using DWT was performed by wavelets, db4, db9, coif4, bior3.9, and sym6 to get six subbands, (0–2) Hz, (2–4) Hz, (4–8) Hz, (8–16) Hz, (16–32) Hz and (32–64) Hz as shown in Fig. 14.4. In this work, the maximum amplitude of the EEG signals was selected as the time domain feature. The mean of the absolute values of DFT coefficients was picked out as a frequency-domain feature. Relative energy and statistical parameter like standard deviation of DWT coefficients of each subband were selected as a feature. MSE with sample entropy was calculated for scale factors 1–10 and used as a feature. The feature vector was composed of these 24 features. MSE complexity profiles of five datasets are depicted in Fig. 14.5.

14.2.2.5 Classification

Supervised learning method was considered for epileptic seizures detection in our manuscript. Support vector machine (SVM), k-nearest neighbor (k-NN) and artificial neural network (ANN) were applied for classification of the EEG signals to detect epileptic seizures.

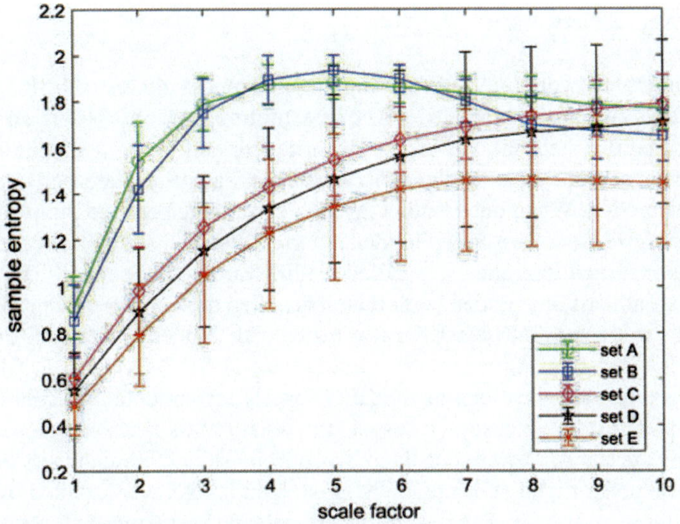

Fig. 14.5 Multiscale entropy analysis of five datasets

Support Vector Machine

Support vector machine (SVM) is a supervised learning model which is utilized for classification and regression purposes. SVM uses a kernel function to obtain a higher dimensional output feature space from low dimensional input space [50]. A hyperplane is used to separate the data into two categories. It maximizes the distance between the two categories. When a testing sample is used for classification purposes, it is characterized as the nearest category type.

k-Nearest Neighbors

k-nearest neighbors (k-NN) is a non-parametric machine learning algorithm used for classification and regression. A value of k is defined and the distances of k nearest neighbors samples from a testing sample are calculated with the help of a distance function. The testing sample is categorized as the maximum number of occurring classes within k samples. Choosing the value of k is very important and it is normally kept odd positive integer to avoid ambivalence. As $k = 1$ was selected here, it is simply called nearest neighbor algorithm.

Statistics and machine learning toolbox 11.2 in MATLAB R2017b was used for k-NN and SVM classification.

Artificial Neural Network

Artificial neural network (ANN) is a computational model motivated by the structure and functions of human brain [51]. The constituting unit of ANN is an artificial neuron. Generally, neurons are organized in layers and neurons of one layer are connected to neurons of other layers. Neurons in each layer are activated by an activation function. When one or more layers are available between input and output layers then those layers are called hidden layers. When connections between neural nodes do not form a loop then it is called feedforward neural network (FFNN) and if FFNN has at least one hidden layer then it is called multi-layer perceptron (MLP) [52]. In this study, the ANN classifier was tested with hidden layer nodes of number 5, 10, 15, 20, and 25 using neural network toolbox 11.0 in MATLAB R2017b.

In this study, classifications of the EEG signals for epileptic seizures detection were completed in three cases. In case-1, the binary classification was performed. All data in datasets A–D were considered as normal subjects and data in set E were epileptic seizures or ictal subjects. SVM, k-NN, and ANN were trained by 80 data of each dataset from A–E. The rest 20 data of each dataset from A–E were kept for testing. As a result, five-fold cross-validation was used in the case of ANN, SVM and k-NN classifiers. Epileptic seizure detection was considered as positive. In case-2, the classifiers were used for three-class classification. The data in set A and B were grouped as normal subjects, the data in set C and D were grouped as interictal subjects and the data in set E were ictal subjects. The result of classifiers could be a healthy subject or interictal subject or ictal subject. In case-3 the SVM, k-NN and ANN classifiers were practiced for five-class classification because of recording EEG signals in five different situations. The classifiers were trained by 80 data of each dataset from A–E. The rest 20 data of each dataset from A–E were used for testing. The classifiers were used to classify the data from datasets A–E.

14.3 Results and Discussion

The classification performance of the three cases is evaluated here. The experiment and simulation were operated with MATLAB R2017b on a 2.40 GHz Intel(R) Core(TM) i3-3110 M processor with 4 GB memory.

The test performance of a classifier can be determined by the following parameters.

$$\text{Accuracy} = \frac{\text{TP} + \text{TN}}{\text{TP} + \text{FN} + \text{FP} + \text{FN}} \tag{14.6}$$

$$\text{Sensitivity} = \frac{\text{TP}}{\text{TP} + \text{FN}} \tag{14.7}$$

$$\text{Specificity} = \frac{\text{TN}}{\text{TN} + \text{FP}} \tag{14.8}$$

True positive (TP)	the number of cases an ictal subject is predicted as ictal.
True negative (TN)	the number of cases a normal subject is predicted as normal.
False positive (FP)	the number of cases a normal subject is predicted as ictal.
False negative (FN)	the number of cases an ictal subject is predicted as normal.

14.3.1 Classification Results

In case-1, for epileptic seizures detection, the binary classification performance is shown in Table 14.1.

In the case of ANN, the classification performance fluctuated a little bit when it was trained multiple times by the same data without changing the hidden layer nodes number due to different initial conditions and sampling. To get a reliable result, ANN was trained five times for each particular wavelet and hidden layer nodes and the result was averaged. From Table 14.1, it is seen that the classification result varies slightly for different wavelet families. For db4 wavelet, the highest accuracy was 99.15% for ANN classifier and the lowest accuracy was 98.30% for fine k-NN and cubic SVM classifiers. The best accuracy was found for bior3.9 wavelet and for ANN composed of 25 hidden layer nodes, which was 99.54%.

In case-2, the EEG signals were separated into three groups. Group-1 contains ictal subjects, group-2 contains interictal subjects and group-3 contains normal subjects. The classification performance for three-class classification is shown in Table 14.2.

From Table 14.2, for the three-class classification, the highest accuracy was 98.22% for bior3.9 wavelet and for ANN composed of 25 hidden layer nodes. The accuracy varies for different wavelets and classifiers from 93.46% to 98.22% with a mean accuracy of 96.24%.

In case-3, five-class classification was executed. The EEG signals were classified from dataset A–E. The five-class classification performance is recorded in Table 14.3.

From Table 14.3, it is observed that for five-class classification, the accuracy was comparatively lower than binary classification and three-class classification. The highest accuracy, 87.00% was accomplished by bior3.9 wavelet and quadratic SVM classifier. The accuracy changed from 74.88% to 87.00% for different wavelets and classifiers. From Table 14.4, it is also seen that SVM and k-NN classifiers gave comparatively better accuracy than ANN. The accuracy increased slightly for ANN classifier as the number of hidden layer nodes increased.

14.3.2 Comparison with Other Works

In order to explore the significance of this work, our method is compared with other related works in the existing literature which used the same data for the binary classification in Table 14.4.

Table 14.1 Binary classification performance

Wavelet	Classifier	Hidden layer nodes	Accuracy (%)	Sensitivity (%)	Specificity (%)
Db4	Fine k-NN		98.30	95.00	99.06
	Quadratic SVM		99.50	98.75	99.69
	Cubic SVM		98.30	95.00	99.06
	ANN	5	98.38	94.04	99.44
		10	99.15	95.65	100.00
		15	98.88	96.25	99.52
		20	98.76	96.02	99.46
		25	98.83	95.80	99.59
Coif4	Fine k-NN		98.30	95.00	99.06
	Quadratic SVM		98.80	96.25	99.38
	Cubic SVM		99.30	96.25	100.00
	ANN	5	98.88	96.02	99.58
		10	97.88	94.80	98.64
		15	98.08	95.20	98.76
		20	98.58	97.42	98.82
		25	98.33	96.75	98.70
Bior3.9	Fine k-NN		98.30	95.00	99.06
	Quadratic SVM		99.00	96.25	99.69
	Cubic SVM		98.50	96.25	99.06
	ANN	5	98.38	95.54	99.06
		10	98.00	95.02	98.76
		15	97.74	94.52	98.50
		20	98.16	94.50	99.08
		25	**99.54**	**98.52**	**99.76**
Db9	Fine k-NN		97.50	92.50	98.75
	Quadratic SVM		99.00	97.5	99.38
	Cubic SVM		98.30	95.00	99.06
	ANN	5	98.88	96.78	99.38
		10	99.44	98.54	99.64
		15	99.24	98.02	99.52
		20	97.94	93.28	99.08
		25	99.04	96.78	99.58

(continued)

Table 14.1 (continued)

Wavelet	Classifier	Hidden layer nodes	Accuracy (%)	Sensitivity (%)	Specificity (%)
Sym6	Fine k-NN		98.30	95.00	99.06
	Quadratic SVM		99.30	97.50	99.69
	Cubic SVM		98.50	96.25	99.06
	ANN	5	98.18	91.78	99.52
		10	98.52	94.00	99.64
		15	99.16	96.78	99.76
		20	97.64	91.04	99.28
		25	99.18	96.02	99.94

Where, **bold** values represent best classification result

All authors in Table 14.4 used binary (A + B + C + D, E) classification. From Table 14.4, it is perceived that our proposed method is better for epileptic seizure detection than other methods.

The performance of the three-class classification of the EEG signals for epileptic seizure detection is compared with other works in Table 14.5.

The performance of the five-class classification is compared with other works in Table 14.6.

The aim of this work is to develop a method which can efficiently classify the EEG signals for epileptic seizures detection. As EEG signal is nonstationary in nature, DWT was performed for features extraction. For collecting information from the frequency domain, discrete Fourier transform was employed. To analyze the complexity of the EEG signals, multiscale entropy with sample entropy was exploited. A total of twenty-four features were extracted and selected for classification. For classification of the given EEG signal datasets, supervised learning classification methods such as k-NN, SVM, and ANN were used. The performance of this work for two-class classification is compared with other works in Table 14.4. From Table 14.4, it is seen that for two-class classification of the EEG signals to detect epileptic seizures, the highest accuracy was achieved for our method. Three-class and five-class classifications were also accomplished and shown in Table 14.5 and Table 14.6, respectively. From Table 14.4, it is shown that the proposed method is reliable for the detection of epileptic seizures using EEG signals.

14.4 Conclusions

This chapter proposes an effective classification method of the EEG signals based on multi-domain feature extraction as well as multiscale sample entropy analysis for automatic epileptic seizures detection. Two-class classification results of the presented method outstrip the existing reported results in the literature with an

Table 14.2 Performance of the three-class classification

Wavelet	Classifiers	Hidden layer nodes	Accuracy (%)
Db4	Fine k-NN		95.30
	Quadratic SVM		96.80
	Cubic SVM		97.30
	ANN	5	95.23
		10	95.12
		15	96.32
		20	96.14
		25	96.38
Coif4	Fine k-NN		95.50
	Quadratic SVM		96.80
	Cubic SVM		97.50
	ANN	5	93.46
		10	94.82
		15	96.82
		20	96.34
		25	96.15
Bior3.9	Fine k-NN		97.30
	Quadratic SVM		96.30
	Cubic SVM		97.50
	ANN	5	96.04
		10	94.64
		15	96.86
		20	96.22
		25	**98.22**
Sym6	Fine k-NN		95.30
	Quadratic SVM		95.30
	Cubic SVM		95.80
	ANN	5	96.42
		10	96.86
		15	95.96
		20	95.74
		25	94.24
Db9	Fine k-NN		96.30
	Quadratic SVM		96.80
	Cubic SVM		97.50
	ANN	5	96.62

(continued)

Table 14.2 (continued)

Wavelet	Classifiers	Hidden layer nodes	Accuracy (%)
		10	96.82
		15	96.48
		20	96.64
		25	97.58

Where, **bold** values indicate the highest accuracy

accuracy of 99.54%. Combination of features from several domains such as time, frequency, time-frequency, and multiscale sample entropy analysis ensures the better classification performance. For multiclass classifications, our method also outperforms other methods in the existing literature. Different mother wavelets were applied for discrete wavelet transform to observe differences in classification accuracy.

In this study, we used DWT to decompose EEG signal in five levels. It is very important in DWT to use an appropriate number of decomposition levels. Thus, an automatic best decomposition level can be developed in future. Besides, subbands which carry most discriminant information for epileptic seizures can be pinpointed. To achieve a more robust model, multiple EEG signals datasets can be used, specifically training the model with one dataset and testing with other datasets.

In future, researchers can address for higher recognition results with smart feature selections. Besides, recently some variants of multiscale entropy method like multiscale fuzzy entropy, multiscale permutation entropy, etc. have been introduced to the research community. Someone can compare our results with those recently introduced methods of feature extraction in future for rigor.

The better classification performance is obtained largely due to the feature fusion from several domains. Hence, one can explore different other features that may significantly enhance the recognition rates, especially for five-class case. A researcher can also explore various combinations of features. This work explored db4, db9, coif4, bior3.9, and sym6-based DWT, however, one can implement other wavelet bases.

In future, prediction of epilepsy can be unearthed instead of classification only. More datasets can be explored, e.g., the Bonn EEG database is a benchmark dataset in epileptic seizure detection, and a larger dataset like CHB-MIT Scalp EEG database [53] can be employed to verify the effectiveness of our method.

Table 14.3 Performance of the five-class classification

Wavelet	Classifiers	Hidden layer nodes	Accuracy (%)
Db4	Fine k-NN		80.80
	Quadratic SVM		83.50
	Cubic SVM		84.00
	ANN	5	74.88
		10	77.86
		15	81.04
		20	81.68
		25	80.78
Coif4	Fine k-NN		81.80
	Quadratic SVM		83.30
	Cubic SVM		84.80
	ANN	5	77.38
		10	81.64
		15	81.16
		20	80.36
		25	81.98
Bior3.9	Fine k-NN		84.80
	Quadratic SVM		**87.00**
	Cubic SVM		85.50
	ANN	5	77.38
		10	79.60
		15	81.88
		20	81.52
		25	82.28
Sym6	Fine k-NN		80.50
	Quadratic SVM		83.50
	Cubic SVM		86.00
	ANN	5	79.20
		10	79.42
		15	81.82
		20	82.18
		25	81.36
Db9	Fine k-NN		84.00
	Quadratic SVM		85.00
	Cubic SVM		86.30
	ANN	5	79.52

(continued)

Table 14.3 (continued)

Wavelet	Classifiers	Hidden layer nodes	Accuracy (%)
		10	81.18
		15	78.94
		20	81.46
		25	82.26

Where, **bold** values indicate the highest accuracy

Table 14.4 Comparison with other related works for the binary classification

Authors	Feature extraction	Classifiers	Accuracy (%)
Tzallas et al. [4]	Time-frequency analysis	ANN	97.73
Guo et al. [18]	Multiwavelet transform	MLPNN	98.27
Kaleem et al. [20]	Variation of empirical mode decomposition		98.20
Fu et al. [21]	HMS analysis	SVM	98.80
Lina et al. [22]	DWT, multi-domain feature extraction, and nonlinear analysis	SVM, k-NN, LDA, NB, NR	99.25
This work	**DWT, multi-domain feature extraction, and MSE analysis**	**k-NN, SVM, ANN**	**99.54**

Where, **bold** values indicate the best classification result

Table 14.5 Comparison with previous works for the three-class classification

Authors	Feature extraction	Classifiers	Subsets	Accuracy (%)
Mosabber [24]	MSE using SampEn, PermEn, LZEn	LOOC, NNC		90.00
Tzallas et al. [4]	Time-frequency analysis	ANN	(A + B), (C + D), E	97.72
This work	DWT, multi-domain feature extraction, and MSE analysis	k-NN, SVM, ANN		98.22
Yuanfa et al. [23]	LDWT, maximum, standard deviation	SELM	A, D, E	98.40

Table 14.6 Comparison with previous works for the five-class classification

Authors	Feature extraction	Classifiers	Accuracy (%)
Mosabber [24]	MSE using SampEn, PermEn, LZEn	LOOC, NNC	69.20
This work	**DWT, multi-domain feature extraction, and MSE analysis**	**k-NN, SVM, ANN**	**87.00**

Where, **bold** values indicate the best classification result

References

1. von Bartheld, C.S., Bahney, J., Herculano-Houzel, S.: The search for true numbers of neurons and glial cells in the human brain: a review of 150 years of cell counting. J. Comp. Neurol. **524**(18), 3865–3895 (2016)
2. Duncan, J., Shorvon, S., Fish, D.: Clinical epilepsy. Curr. Opin. Neurol. Neurosurg. **5**(2), 224–227 (1995)
3. Megiddo, I., Colson, A., Chisholm, D., Dua, T., Nandi, A., Laxminarayan, R.: Health and economic benefits of public financing of epilepsy treatment in India: an agent-based simulation model. Epilepsia **57**(3), 464–474 (2016)
4. Tzallas, A.T., Tsipouras, M.G., Fotiadis, D.I.: Automatic seizure detection based on time-frequency analysis and artificial neural networks. Comput. Intell. Neurosci. **2007** (2007)
5. Päivinen, N., Lammi, S., Pitkänen, A., Nissinen, J., Penttonen, M., Grönfors, T.: Epileptic seizure detection: a nonlinear viewpoint. Comput. Methods Programs Biomed. (2005)
6. Kobayashi, K., Jacobs, J., Gotman, J.: Detection of changes of high-frequency activity by statistical time-frequency analysis in epileptic spikes. Clin. Neurophysiol. (2009)
7. Guerrero-Mosquera, C., Trigueros, A.M., Franco, J.I., Navia-Vázquez, Á.: New feature extraction approach for epileptic EEG signal detection using time-frequency distributions. Med. Biol. Eng. Comput. (2010)
8. Samiee, K., Kovács, P., Gabbouj, M.: Epileptic seizure classification of EEG time-series using rational discrete short-time fourier transform. IEEE Trans. Biomed. Eng. (2015)
9. Ambulkar, N.K., Sharma, S.N.: Detection of epileptic seizure in EEG signals using window width optimized S-transform and artificial neural networks. In: 2015 IEEE Bombay Section Symposium: Frontiers of Technology: Fuelling Prosperity of Planet and People, IBSS 2015 (2016)
10. Sivasankari, K., Thanushkodi, K.: An improved EEG signal classification using neural network with the consequence of ICA and STFT. J. Electr. Eng. Technol. (2014)
11. Yuan, Y., Jia, K., Xun, G., Zhang, A.: A multi-view deep learning method for epileptic seizure detection using short-time Fourier transform. In: ACM-BCB 2017—Proceedings of the 8th ACM International Conference on Bioinformatics, Computational Biology, and Health Informatics (2017)
12. Xie, S., Krishnan, S.: Wavelet-based sparse functional linear model with applications to EEGs seizure detection and epilepsy diagnosis. Med. Biol. Eng. Comput. (2013)
13. Acharya, U.R., Sree, S.V., Ang, P.C.A., Yanti, R., Suri, J.S.: Application of non-linear and wavelet based features for the automated identification of epileptic EEG signals. Int. J. Neural Syst. (2012)
14. Rajendra Acharya, U., Vinitha Sree, S., Alvin, A.P.C., Suri, J.S.: Use of principal component analysis for automatic classification of epileptic EEG activities in wavelet framework. Expert Syst. Appl. **39**(10), 9072–9078 (2012)
15. Kumar, Y., Dewal, M.L., Anand, R.S.: Epileptic seizures detection in EEG using DWT-based ApEn and artificial neural network. Signal, Image Video Process. (2014)
16. Ahammad, N., Fathima, T., Joseph, P.: Detection of epileptic seizure event and onset using EEG. Biomed Res. Int. (2014)

17. Sharmila, A., Aman Raj, S., Shashank, P., Mahalakshmi, P.: Epileptic seizure detection using DWT-based approximate entropy, Shannon entropy and support vector machine: a case study. J. Med. Eng. Technol. (2018)
18. Guo, L., Rivero, D., Pazos, A.: Epileptic seizure detection using multiwavelet transform based approximate entropy and artificial neural networks. J. Neurosci. Methods **193**(1), 156–163 (2010)
19. Djemili, R., Bourouba, H., Amara Korba, M.C.: Application of empirical mode decomposition and artificial neural network for the classification of normal and epileptic EEG signals. Biocybern. Biomed. Eng. (2016)
20. Kaleem, M., Guergachi, A., Krishnan, S.: EEG seizure detection and epilepsy diagnosis using a novel variation of empirical mode decomposition. In: Proceedings of the Annual International Conference of the IEEE Engineering in Medicine and Biology Society, EMBS, pp. 4314–4317 (2013)
21. Fu, K., Qu, J., Chai, Y., Zou, T.: Hilbert marginal spectrum analysis for automatic seizure detection in EEG signals. Biomed. Signal Process. Control **18**, 179–185 (2015)
22. Wang, L., et al.: Automatic epileptic seizure detection in EEG signals using multi-domain feature extraction and nonlinear analysis. Entropy **19**(6), 1–17 (2017)
23. Wang, Y., Li, Z., Feng, L., Zheng, C., Zhang, W.: Automatic detection of epilepsy and seizure using multiclass sparse extreme learning machine classification. Comput. Math. Methods Med. **2017** (2017)
24. Ahmed, M.U.: Complexity analysis of brain electrical activity **2**(11), 146–152 (2013)
25. Kumar, T.S., Kanhangad, V., Pachori, R.B.: Classification of seizure and seizure-free EEG signals using local binary patterns. Biomed. Signal Process. Control **15**, 33–40 (2015)
26. Sharma, M., Pachori, R.B., Rajendra Acharya, U.: A new approach to characterize epileptic seizures using analytic time-frequency flexible wavelet transform and fractal dimension. Pattern Recognit. Lett. **94**, 172–179 (2017)
27. Tiwari, A.K., Pachori, R.B., Kanhangad, V., Panigrahi, B.K.: Automated diagnosis of epilepsy using key-point-based local binary pattern of EEG signals. IEEE J. Biomed. Heal. Informatics **21**(4), 888–896 (2017)
28. Bhattacharyya, A., Singh, L., Pachori, R.B.: Fourier–Bessel series expansion based empirical wavelet transform for analysis of non-stationary signals. Digit. Signal Process. A Rev. J. **78**(Vmd), 185–196 (2018)
29. Gupta, V., Pachori, R.B.: Epileptic seizure identification using entropy of FBSE based EEG rhythms. Biomed. Signal Process. Control **53**, 101569 (2019)
30. Bhattacharyya, A., Pachori, R.B.: A multivariate approach for patient-specific EEG seizure detection using empirical wavelet transform. IEEE Trans. Biomed. Eng. **64**(9), 2003–2015 (2017)
31. Ullah, I., Hussain, M., Qazi, E., Aboalsamh, H.: An automated system for epilepsy detection using EEG brain signals based on deep learning approach insight centre for data analytics, national university of Ireland, Galway, Ireland visual computing lab, department of computer science, college of Com. Expert Syst. Appl. **107**, 61–71 (2018)
32. Hussein, R., Palangi, H., Ward, R., Wang, Z.J.: Epileptic seizure detection: a deep learning approach 1–12 (2018)
33. Acharya, U.R., Oh, S.L., Hagiwara, Y., Tan, J.H., Adeli, H.: Deep convolutional neural network for the automated detection and diagnosis of seizure using EEG signals. Comput. Biol. Med. **100**, 270–278 (2018)
34. Zhou, M., et al.: Epileptic seizure detection based on EEG signals and CNN. Front. Neuroinform. **12** (2018)
35. Emami, A., Kunii, N., Matsuo, T., Shinozaki, T., Kawai, K., Takahashi, H.: Seizure detection by convolutional neural network-based analysis of scalp electroencephalography plot images. Neuro. Image Clin. **22**, 101684, May 2018 (2019)
36. Birjandtalab, J., Heydarzadeh, M., Nourani, M.: Automated EEG-based epileptic seizure detection using deep neural networks. In: Proceedings of 2017 IEEE International Conference on Healthcare Informatics (ICHI) **2017**(1), 552–555 (2017)

37. Wei, X., Zhou, L., Chen, Z., Zhang, L., Zhou, Y.: Automatic seizure detection using three-dimensional CNN based on multi-channel EEG. BMC Med. Inform. Decis. Mak. (2018)
38. Shamim Hossain, M., Amin, S.U., Alsulaiman, M., Muhammad, G.: Applying deep learning for epilepsy seizure detection and brain mapping visualization. ACM Trans. Multimed. Comput. Commun. Appl. (2019)
39. Lin, C., Hsin, Y.U.E.L.: The nonlinear and nonstationary properties in EEG signals : probing the complex fluctuations **1**(3), 461–482 (2009)
40. Richman, J.S., Moorman, J.R.: Physiological time-series analysis using approximate entropy and sample entropy. Am. J. Physiol. Heart Circ. Physiol. **278**(6), H2039–H2049 (2000)
41. Andrzejak, R.G., Lehnertz, K., Mormann, F., Rieke, C., David, P., Elger, C.E.: Indications of nonlinear deterministic and finite-dimensional structures in time series of brain electrical activity : dependence on recording region and brain state **64**, 1–8 (2001)
42. Teplan, M.: Fundamentals of EEG measurement. Meas. Sci. Rev. **2**(2), 1–11 (2002)
43. Acharya, U.R., Fujita, H., Sudarshan, V.K., Bhat, S., Koh, J.E.W.: Application of entropies for automated diagnosis of epilepsy using EEG signals: a review. Knowl. Based Syst. **88**, 85–96 (2015)
44. Kumar, N., Alam, K., Ḥasan Siddiqi, A.: Wavelet transform for classification of EEG signal using SVM and ANN. Biomed. Pharmacol. J. **10**(4), 2061–2069 (December, 2017)
45. Subasi, A.: EEG signal classification using wavelet feature extraction and a mixture of expert model. Expert Syst. Appl. **32**(4), 1084–1093 (2007)
46. Gonzalez, R.C., Woods, R.E.: Digital Image Processing (3rd edn.) (2007)
47. Orhan, U., Hekim, M., Ozer, M.: EEG signals classification using the K-means clustering and a multilayer perceptron neural network model. Expert Syst. Appl. **38**(10), 13475–13481 (2011)
48. Costa, M., Goldberger, A.L., Peng, C.K.: Multiscale entropy analysis of biological signals. Phys. Rev. E Stat. Nonlinear, Soft Matter Phys. **71**(2), 1–18 (2005)
49. Costa, M., Goldberger, A.L., Peng, C.-K.: Multiscale entropy to distinguish physiologic and synthetic RR time series. Comput. Cardiol. **1**, 137–140 (2002)
50. Bhatia, P.K., Sharma, A.: Epilepsy seizure detection using wavelet support vector machine classifier. Int. J. Bio-Science Bio-Technology **8**(2), 11–22 (2016)
51. AnarYegnayana, B.: Artificial Neural Networks. Prentice-Hall of India Pvt, Ltd (2004)
52. Nielsen, M.A.: Neural networks and deep learning, vol. 25. Determination press USA (2015)
53. Shoeb, A.: Application of machine learning to epileptic seizure onset detection and treatment. PhD Thesis, Massachusetts Institute of Technology (September, 2009)